MEDICINE IN THE VEDA

RELIGIOUS HEALING IN THE VEDA

Indian Medical Tradition

Edited by
DOMINIK WUJASTYK

VOL. I

Medicine in the Veda

RELIGIOUS HEALING IN THE VEDA

With translations and annotations of medical hymns from the Ṛgveda and the Atharvaveda and renderings from the corresponding ritual texts

KENNETH G. ZYSK

MOTILAL BANARSIDASS PUBLISHERS
PRIVATE LIMITED • DELHI

3rd Reprint : 2009
2nd Indian Ed. 1998
First Indian Edition: Delhi, 1996

First Published in U.S.A. in 1985

ISBN: 81-208-1400-2 (Cloth)
ISBN: 81-208-1401-0 (Paper)

Also available at:
MOTILAL BANARSIDASS
41 U.A. Bungalow Road, Jawahar Nagar, Delhi 110 007
8, Mahalaxmi Chamber, Warden Road, Mumbai 400 026
120 Royapettah High Road, Mylapore, Chennai 600 004
Sanas Plaza, Subhash Nagar, Pune 411 002
16 St. Mark's Road, Bangalore 560 001
8 Camac Street, Calcutta 700 017
Ashok Rajpath, Patna 800 004
Chowk, Varanasi 221 001

PRINTED IN INDIA
BY JAINENDRA PRAKASH JAIN AT SHRI JAINENDRA PRESS,
A-45 NARAINA, PHASE I, NEW DELHI 110 028
AND PUBLISHED BY NARENDRA PRAKASH JAIN FOR
MOTILAL BANARSIDASS PUBLISHERS PRIVATE LIMITED,
BUNGALOW ROAD, DELHI 110 007

To my mother and my father,
Madelein and Stanley Zysk

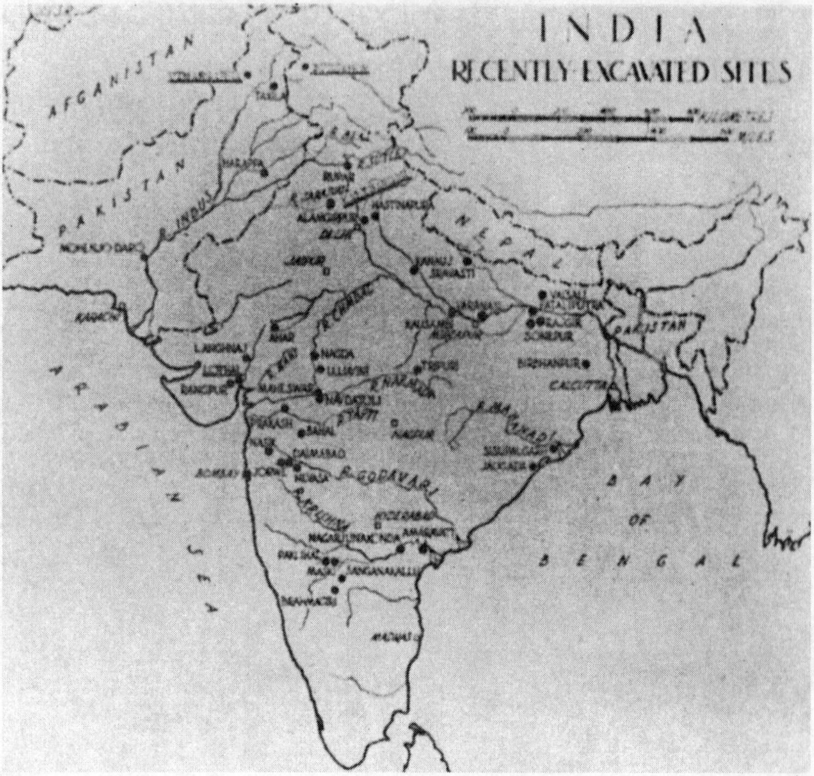
INDIA
RECENTLY EXCAVATED SITES
AFGANISTAN
PAKISTAN
R. INDUS
NEPAL
PAKISTAN
CALCUTTA
R. GODAVARI
BAY OF BENGAL

Map of India

CONTENTS

FOREWORD

Since its publication in 1985, Kenneth Zysk's study of medicine in the Vedic texts has established itself as a classic of the genre. It is an honour and a pleasure that this book should launch this new series. It is also particularly appropriate that this new publishing venture on the Indian medical heritage should be inaugurated by a work which examines the earliest textual evidence of medicine in India.

In its previous incarnation as a publication of the American Philosophical Association, Zysk's book did not reach a wide audience in India, and I sincerely hope that its appearance now will rectify this situation, enabling readers in India to take advantage of some of the best contemporary scholarship on the history of Indian medicine.

It will not escape notice that more than half this book consists of textual annotations. These notes are vital to the project that Zysk undertakes, of excavating all possible medical information from the *saṃhitās* and immediately related texts. The reader should not be tempted to skip this information: only by working through the full text and annotations does the rich, complex, and multi-valent nature of the Vedic medical situation emerge. History, one might paraphrase, is in the details.

Another important feature of this book is that it is the first work on medicine in the Vedic period to take account of the readings of the Orissan *Paippalāda Atharvaveda*.

There is something of a tradition in good books about *āyurveda* of placing valuable information in appendices: one thinks of Meulenbeld's *Mādhavanidāna*, and Kashikar's translation of Jolly's *Medizin*. Zysk's volume adheres to this tradition, and his excellent bibliography will be of enduring value to serious researchers. His bibliographical and historical essay is also a valuable survey of modern scholarship on the history of Indian medicine, both in India and abroad. In the decade since it was first published, of course the field has moved on a little. Some new faces have appeared on the scene, and some of the projects he mentions as being in progress have now been published, including all the articles by Zysk himself, listed in the bibliography as 'to appear.' (The reference to myself as a 'young scholar' of course requires no amendment!) Perhaps in another decade the essay should be updated, but today it still stands as a valuable and informative overview of the principal work done so far this century.

At the present time there is a popular interest in the earliest roots of Indian culture, and in particular in early Indian scientific traditions. It is all too easy to fall into the trap of talking about 'Vedic medicine' as though this were an integrated medical system. But there are, of course, no medical texts from the Vedic period, nor any evidence that such texts ever existed. The best we can do is comb meticulously through the surviving Vedic literature and try to reconstruct, from texts whose primary purpose was religious, a picture of medical thought and practice in those far-away times.

No one has done this more thoroughly than Zysk, whose book I warmly commend to all scholars of the history of Indian medicine.

DOMINIK WUJASTYK

INTRODUCTION TO THE INDIAN EDITION

Ten years have passed since this book appeared with the title *Religious Healing in the Veda*, as part of the Transactions of the American Philosophical Society, Vol. 75.7. The monograph received good, sometimes excellent reviews, and is now out of print. On the whole, I was very pleased with the work, and especially with the beautiful text produced by the American Philosophical Society, which is here reproduced. My only regret is that it did not reach a wider audience. It passed by many largely unnoticed. The subject-matter of the work, although specific, has relevance beyond the narrow focus of medicine and healing. Its content is useful to students of Indian religion and civilization, as well as of the history and science and medicine. Moreover, it almost never reached the Indian scholars with whose scientific and religious heritage the study is concerned. Fortunately, this reprint edition will now have the opportunity of coming to the notice of those who previously missed it and who might well find it useful and interesting.

Although my studies have moved me into later time-frames and literary genres in order to fill in the gap between Vedic and classical āyurvedic medicine, and more recently even into the related tradition of the India aesthetics of love, I have constantly returned to the Veda when new ideas and insights arose. Anyone who has embarked upon a study of the Veda can testify that it is a vast and fascinating subject that constantly beckons one to plunge ever deeper into its texts in an attempt to unlock the wonderful mysteries of the archaic mind. It is a life-long pursuit in which I shall always be engaged, reading and rereading the frequently enigmatic and clever hymns of the *Ṛgveda* and *Atharvaveda*.

Although the fundamental aspects of medicine in the Vedas are contained in the present monograph, there remain several points requiring further exploration. One important part of this healing tradition, only briefly mentioned in this work, is Vedic toxicology. Several hymns of the *Atharvaveda* and a few of the *Ṛgveda* concern themselves with poisoning usually caused by animals, and with the remedial measures to cure it. It is almost certain that India's long and renowned tradition of toxicology derives from a basic knowledge of poisons and poisonous animals found in the Veda. I have collected and examined the relevant hymns and passages from the early texts and hope to publish the results of my study in the near future.

My subsequent research and investigations have taken me to time periods not covered by the material in this book and have provided certain fresh ideas and a radically different interpretation of the origins of the āyurvedic system of healing. It might therefore be useful to outline here the development of the Indian healing arts from vedic medicine to classical *āyurveda*, based on my recent studies.

A distinctive part of Vedic medicine is its pharmacopoeia, especially its rich description of these substances and its knowledge of the local flora. This botanical wisdom occurs largely in the hymns of the *Atharvaveda* and is connected to a tradition of healing plant goddesses. The hymns of the *Ṛgveda* reveal less of a familiarity with indigenous plant life, and what is found there relates principally to a tradition of a male plant divinity. A homologization of these two botanical traditions is reflected in the mythological connections between the principal plant deities mentioned in each text, and occurs in mythical parts of the Atharvavedic medical hymns. Here are found myths of both the healing plant god Kuṣṭha, and the healing plant goddess Arundhatī. Kuṣṭha was the remedy *par excellence* for fever (*takmán*) and generally identified with the aromatic costus, native of Kashmīr and known to have been an important export from India in the spice trade. The healing plant goddess Arundhatī was used in the treatment of fractures and wounds, and is identified among others with *lākṣā*, the Sanskrit term for the resinous "lac". The mythology of Kuṣṭha links him closely both with the Ṛgvedic plant Soma, important to the sacrificial cults, and the Atharvavedic Arundhatī, significant to the medical cults. He is called Soma's brother, and, like Soma, is known to have grown high in the Himavant Mountains, the birthplace of eagles, the third heaven from earth and the seat of the gods. Likewise, several of the epithets associated with Kuṣṭha are identical to those given to Arundhatī. They are both perennial, life-giving, and harmless. Kuṣṭha's mythological link with Soma and his name-association with Arundhatī imply a conscious effort to homologize a Ṛgvedic botanical tradition dominated by a male plant divinity with a medical-botanical tradition of plant goddesses particular to the Atharvaveda.[1] This assimilation of useful (and thereby powerful) botanical knowledge concurs with the medical intellectuals' general tendency to appropriate wisdom which could render their healing rituals more efficacious. Further investigations of the mythological traditions of plant divinities in the *Ṛgveda* and *Atharvaveda* should reveal interesting aspects of the homologization of religious ideas and help identify elements of indigenous beliefs in ancient India.

Vedic medicine's dominant appeal to and reflection of popular beliefs have led to more profound comparisons between medicine in the Veda and Indo-European healing traditions. Using Georg Dumézil's tripartite division of ancient Indo-European society as a convenient framework, it is clear that Vedic medicine, along with most of the healing traditions of

---

1 See K.G. Zysk, *Asceticism and healing in ancient India* (New York and Oxford: Oxford University Press, 1991), pp. 17-19

Indo-European antiquity was most appropriately a function of the third social order. The ideology of this third estate was usually represented by members of peasant communities and reflected the society's popular folk culture. The Vedic healer's knowledge of the local flora tends to link him to an agrarian-oriented group of people; and his use of magical rituals, amulets, and incantations reflects fundamental folk beliefs. Literature of the third order has traditionally been in the form of folklore, often transmitted orally from generation to generation. In many Indo-European cultures, folk literature preserves the peoples' medical knowledge in the form of folk medicine and home remedies. Being produced by learned men closely associated with the third order, the healing hymns of the *Atharvaveda*, therefore, reveal one of the earliest forms of folk healing of Indo-European antiquity, and offer an excellent example of ancient folk literature.[2]

Although a highly specialized intellectual tradition of the third social level, medicine in the Veda reflects a homologization of knowledge from other levels of the society, most significantly the order of priests whose words and actions were thought to bring them into direct contact with the greater cosmic forces. The healers also required knowledge of the means to control the natural forces in order to set right again what had gone wrong in the first place. Combining their expertise in accessing and manipulating the spirit world with the knowledge they acquired from the sacrificial cults, the healers became the priests of the third estate, operating along with the sacrificial priests of the first estate. The roles of each type of priest were quite distinct, but outwardly they probably resembled each other in many respects. The medical priest probably enjoyed relative freedom in the social structure and was not confined to a particular social group, as he served the needs of all people regardless of their social standing. The sacrificial priest, on the other hand, fearing contamination from impure elements of the society, was restricted to the social milieu of the first order. It would not be unreasonable to assume that competition between priests for power and prestige may well have emerged. With time, the healers became recognized by their counterparts in the first estate as impure and contaminating, eventually being excluded from the higher, more sacred circles of the sacrificial cults. They were gradually forced to remain in their own communities of the third estate, located at the margins of society where contact with many sorts of people with different healing traditions might well have taken place. This removal of healers and their special craft from mainstream Vedic priestly culture led eventually to a radical shift in medical thinking. The result was the development

[2] See K.G. Zysk, "Reflections on an Indo-European system of medicine," in *Perspectives on Indo-European language, culture and religion. Studies in honor of Edgar Polomé*, Vol 2 (McLean, Virgina: Institute for the study of Man, 1992), pp. 321-36.

of a new approach to medicine which came to be known as classical *āyurveda*.

The chapters in the present book elucidate a healing tradition based on magico-religious beliefs and practices. The classical medical treatises of Caraka and Suśruta, which represent the earliest extant medical books of *āyurveda*, clearly indicate that this form of medicine never completely disappeared, but was probably superseded over time by a system of medicine based on empiricio-rational principles and practices, issuing from an active encounter with the world. It should not be assumed that empiricism or the process of observing and defining is evident only in the classical medical tradition. Vedic medicine relied on close observation of phenomena in order to develop its unique form of mythical and religious classifications and associations. The difference between these two epistemologies lies in their respective premises. The foundation of Vedic medicine was a belief in a multitude of benevolent and malevolent deities or spirits that populated the cosmos and caused good and bad effects in the human realm. Controlling and taming these entities were the ultimate goals of this healing system. In *āyurveda*, a basic understanding of the interrelationship between humans and their environment prefaced every observation. Ideally humans and nature should be in perfect harmony. Disease occurred when the equilibrium between these two was disrupted. Restoration of a fundamental balance was the goal of this medical system. Reasons for this shift in modes of medical thought have puzzled scholars of ancient Indian medicine for many years. My recent socio-historical study of medicine during the intervening period between the medical tradition of the early Vedic texts and the occurrence of the classical medical treatises, roughly from the ninth century B.C.E. to the beginning of the common era, offers a plausible explanation for this paradigm shift.[3]

We noticed that a social event occurring in Vedic antiquity was probably a key factor in initiating change. A forthright denigration of medicine by the priestly order and the brāhmaṇic hierarchy resulted in the healers' exclusion from the orthodox ritual cults because of the defilement they incurred from contact with impure people with whom they found fellowship. This type of "excommunication" transformed the medical priests into members of a fringe-group. Other important marginalized people included the heterodox wandering ascetics who renounced the trappings of orthodox ideologies and practices, and abandoned society for the wilderness in search of higher spiritual goals. Unencumbered by the strictures of brāhmaṇical orthodoxy, these ascetics, who included among others the Buddhists, acquired a radically different view of the world and humankind's place in it, fostered by their intense meditative discipline. In fact, early Buddhist literature reveals that their understanding of the relationship between humans and nature was not very different from that

3 See K.G. Zysk, *Asceticism and healing in ancient India*, pp. 1-70.

which contributed to āyurvedic medical thought. An intellectual sympathy seemingly was shared by both the wandering ascetics on a spiritual quest and the roving physicians whose professional curiosity led them to encounters with different sorts of people from whom they could obtain useful medical knowledge.

Finding rapport with the communities of heterodox ascetics and renunciants who were not inclined to censure their philosophies, practices and associations, the healers, like the knowledge-seeking ascetics, wandered the countryside performing cures and acquiring ever new remedies, treatments and medical information. They eventually became practically indistinguishable from the mendicants with whom they were in close contact. A vast storehouse of medical knowledge soon developed among these wandering physicians who, like the ascetics, were unhindered by brāhmaṇic strictures and taboos. With the help of ideas from the intellectual ascetics, the doctors began to conceive a radically new epistemology with which to codify and systematize this body of efficacious medical data.

Fitting into the Buddha's key teaching of the middle way between world indulgence and self-denial, medicine became part of Buddhism by providing the means to maintain a healthy bodily state characterized by an equilibrium—both within the body and between the body and its surroundings. Portions of the repository of medical lore were codified in the early monastic rules, thereby giving rise to a Buddhist monastic medical tradition. The early Buddhist community of monks or *saṅgha* was where wandering intellectuals would gather and exchange information which often included medical knowledge. As the *saṅgha* established more permanent dwellings and fixed abodes for ascetics, the intellectual life turned more scholarly, and a formal systematization of information and instruction ensued. The symbiotic relationship between Buddhism and medicine facilitated the spread of Buddhism in India, led to the teaching of medicine in the large conglomerate monasteries *(vihāras)*, and expedited the acceptance of Buddhism in other parts of Asia. Probably during the early centuries of the common era, Brāhmaṇism assimilated the storehouse of medical knowledge into its socio-religious and intellectual tradition and by the application of an orthodox veneer rendered it a brāhmaṇic science. Over the nine centuries of this transitional phase of Indian medicine, the medical system represented in the early Vedic literature gradually diminished in significance until medicine became part of Brāhmaṇism, whose intellectuals consciously revived the ancient medical wisdom in order to legitimize a largely heterodox body of knowledge and make it orthodox. The technique by which this was accomplished is revealed in the opening portions of the two classical medical treatises, which are characteristic of an ubiquitous and ingenious Brāhmaṇization process by which seemingly contradictory and disruptive ideas are reconciled and assimilated. Returning to Dumézil's paradigm, a social evolution of Indian medicine may be explained as follows: medicine originated in the third order, maintained its position or fell out of the social system in the intervening or transitional period, and vaulted to the first order in the classical phase, a position it appears to hold at the present time. With this brief outline of Indian medical history, we are perhaps better able to understand and appreciate the content and significance of Vedic medicine as it is presented in the following chapters.

PREFACE

The medicine of the Vedic Indians is inextricably connected with their religion and must not be considered in isolation from it. Just as there is a pantheon of gods, there also occurs a pantheon of demons in the Vedic religious tradition. Our aim is to understand the particular group of demonic beings and forces which were considered to have brought about disease and the religious rites by which these malady-causing demons were evicted and kept away. The hymns employed in the rites are the principal sources of information and have been translated in their entirety. An examination and a translation of later ritual prescriptions provide continuity in the tradition and offer a basis for comparison with the practices found in the earlier hymns. The selection of hymns is based on the data which they contain rather than exclusively on the traditional classification of the charms offered in the *bhaiṣajya* (medical) section of the *Kauśika Sūtra* (25–36). The translations have been undertaken according to the strict principles of Vedic philology in order to assure their accuracy. Historians of religion, historians of medicine and Indologists are given an analysis of the fundamental doctrines and practices of India's earliest medical tradition and provided with a good basis from which to undertake further research.

The work is divided into two major sections: the first examines the various diseases which afflicted the Vedic people and the treatments used to cure them. Translations of the particular hymns devoted to the eradication of specific maladies and symptoms and to the consecration of the medicines are offered in their appropriate places. The classification of internal and external diseases and medicines has been suggested by the hymns themselves. The second section encompasses the textual annotations to the individual hymns. Within the notes I have included the text and translation of corresponding and relevant passages from the *Paippalāda* recension of the *Atharvaveda.* I have used the texts of both the Kashmir and Orissa recensions of the *Paippalāda.* The editions of Barret and Raghu Vira were the principal sources for the Kashmir readings.

For the Orissa readings, the first four published books edited by D. M. Bhattacharyya were consulted. Recently, Professor Michael Witzel of the Kern Institute in Leiden has kindly given me the readings from most of the remaining books. They are based on photocopies and films made in Orissa. Readings from Orissa books 5–15, 17–18, and part of book 20, are indicated by 'O,' signifying the Orissa manuscripts and those from books 16, 19 and part of book 20, by manuscript 'P,' referring to Witzel's photographs of a seventeenth-century palm-leaf manuscript written in Oriya script by a certain Raghunātha Śarma. This manuscript comes from Parikula in Northern Orissa. Verses 16.12.5–14.7 and 16.74.8 were blurred and 19.3–19.7 were unavailable. Every effort has been made to incorporate the most recent textual information pertaining to the *Atharvaveda*.

Although some modern scholars discount the explanations of the Sanskrit commentaries as merely fanciful, contrived in an age too far removed from the time of the original to be of any real value, I have included them so that we may better comprehend how the later tradition understood the earliest notions of religious medicine. Likewise, their comments provide data for the history of traditional Indian medicine in more recent times. I regret that I have had to omit a section on "toxicology." It is hoped that it will be published at a later date. I have included an appendix which traces the bibliographical history of studies in Indian medical history. Historians of medicine should find this particularly useful.

Finally, I should like to express my sincere gratitude to all those individuals who have helped me in the preparation of this work which, in an earlier form, was submitted as a Ph.D. thesis in the Department of Asian Civilisations, Faculty of Asian Studies, The Australian National University. In particular I wish to thank Professor Arthur L. Basham, my principal supervisor for the thesis, from whose insights and expertise, I have greatly benefitted, and Professor Michael Witzel, who unselfishly provided important material from his personal collection in order to enhance my work. Professor J. W. de Jong, Professor R. E. Emmerick, Professor W. Rau, Dr. G. J. Meulenbeld, Professor H. P. Schmidt, Professor S. Insler, Professor G. B. Risse and Dr. P. M. H. Mazumdar, all of whom took the time to read all or parts of the manuscript, also deserve my humble appreciation. I have considered all of their comments while preparing the final version of the work. Likewise to all those individuals who have offered advice and words of encouragement since I began the project in 1977, I am deeply grateful. Lastly, I wish to thank the Associated Medical Services, Inc. and the Hannah Institute for the History of Medicine for giving me the necessary financial support to see the final version of this work into the press.

Toronto, 1985 K. G. Zysk

ABBREVIATIONS

(Full citations found in bibliography)

AĀ	*Aitareya Āraṇyaka*
AB	*Aitareya Brāhmaṇa*
AH	*Aṣṭāṅgahṛdaya Saṃhitā* of Vāgbhaṭa
AJPh	*American Journal of Philology*
Anu	*Sarvānukramaṇī (Ṛgveda)*
AOS	*American Oriental Series*
ĀpGS	*Āpastamba Gṛhya Sūtra*
ĀpMB	*Āpastamba Mantra Brāhmaṇa (Mantrapāṭha)*
ĀpŚS	*Āpastamba Śrauta Sūtra*
ĀśvŚS	*Āśvalāyana Śrauta Sūtra*
AthPariś	*Pariśiṣṭas of the Atharvaveda*
AV	*Atharvaveda*
AVŚ, Śau.	*Atharvaveda Saṃhitā* (Śaunakīya recension)
Bar., Barret	Leroy Carr Barret, editor of *The Kashmirian Atharva Veda*
BB	*Beiträge zur Kunde der indogermanische Sprachen*
BD	*Bṛhad Devatā*
Bergaigne-Henry, *Manuel*	A. Bergaigne and V. Henry, *Manuel pour étudier le sanscrit védique*
Bh, Bh.	Durgamoham Bhattacharyya, editor of *Paippalāda Saṃhitā of the Atharvaveda,* Books 1–4 (Orissa recension)
Bloomfield, *Hymns*	Maurice Bloomfield, *Hymns of the Atharva-Veda* (SBE, vol. 42)
BŚS	*Baudhāyana Śrauta Sūtra*
Ca	*Caraka Saṃhitā*
Caland, AZ	W. Caland, *Altindisches Zauberritual*
Chowdhury, JBORS	T. Chowdhury, "On the Interpretation of Some Doubtful Words in the Atharva-Veda"
CiSth	*Cikitsāsthāna*
CU, CUp	*Chāndogya Upániṣad*
Dutt and King, *Materia Medica*	U. C. Dutt and George King, *Materia Medica of The Hindus*
ERE	*Encyclopaedia of Religion and Ethics,* ed. James Hastings
EVP	Louis Renou, *Études védiques et pāṇinéennes,* 17 vols.

Filliozat, *La doctrine*	J. Filliozat, *La doctrine classique de la médecine indienne; ses origines et ses parallèles grecs*
Geldner, *Der Rigveda*	K. F. Geldner, *Der Rig-Veda,* 3 pts., (HOS vols. 33–35)
Grassmann, Wb	H. Grassmann, *Wörterbuch zum Rig-Veda*
Griffith	Ralph T. H. Griffith, trans. *The Hymns of the Atharvaveda,* 2 vols.
Henry, *Les livres*	Victor Henry, trans., *Les livres . . . de l'Atharva-Véda,* Livres VII–XIII
Henry, *La magie*	Victor Henry, *La magie dans l'Inde antique*
Hoffmann, *Aufsätze*	Karl Hoffmann, *Aufsätze zur Indoiranistik,* 2 vols.
HOS, H.O.S.	*Harvard Oriental Series*
IAL	R. L. Turner, *A comparative dictionary of the Indo-Aryan languages*
IIJ	*Indo-Iranian Journal*
IS	*Indische Studien*
JA	*Journal asiatique*
JAOS	*Journal of the American Oriental Society*
JASB	*Journal of the Asiatic Society of Bengal*
JB	*Jaiminīya Brāhmaṇa*
JBORS	*Journal of the Bihar and Orissa Research Society*
JOIB	*Journal of the Oriental Institute,* Baroda
JRAS	*Journal of the Royal Asiatic Society of Great Britain and Ireland*
K	Kāśmīri text of the Paippalāda recension from editions of Barret and Raghu Vira. Books 1–20
KaiNi	*Kaiyadevanighaṇṭuḥ*
KaSth	*Kalpasthāna*
KapS	*Kapiṣṭhala Kaṭha Saṃhitā*
KaṭhUp	*Kaṭha Upaniṣad*
KauśS	*Kauśika Sūtra*
Keith, VBYS	A. B. Keith, *The Veda of the Black Yajus School entitled Taittirīya Sanhitā* (HOS vols. 18–19)
KS	*Kāṭhaka Saṃhitā*
KŚS	*Kātyāyana Śrauta Sūtra*
KZ	*Zeitschrift für vergleichende Sprachforschung auf dem Gebiete der indogermanischen Sprachen*
Macdonell-Keith, *Vedic Index*	A. A. Macdonell and A. B. Keith, *Vedic Index of Names and Subjects,* 2 vols.
MahānārUp	*Mahānārayaṇa Upaniṣad*
Mahīdh.	Mahīdhara
manuscript 'P'	Orissa manuscript of Paippalāda Atharvaveda (photograph) belonging to Professor Michael Witzel of the Harvard University, Books 16, 19 and part of 20

Mayrhofer, Wb	Manfred Mayrhofer, *Kurzgefasstes etymologisches Wörterbuch des Altindischen,* 3 vols.
Mbh	*Mahābhārata*
Meulenbeld, *The Mādhavanidāna*	G. J. Meulenbeld, trans., *The Mādhavanidāna and its chief commentary, chapters 1–10*
MS	*Maitrāyaṇī Saṃhitā*
MSL	*Mémoires de la société de linguistique de Paris*
MŚS	*Mānava Śrauta Sūtra*
MV	*Mahāvagga*
MWSED	Monier Monier-Williams, *A Sanskrit-English Dictionary*
Nadk.	Nadkarni's *Indian Materia Medica,* 2 vols.
Nir	*Niruka*
NiSth	*Nidānasthāna*
O	Orissa Manuscripts of the Paippalāda (*Atharvaveda*) (Books 5–15, 17–18, part of 20)
Oldenberg, *Vedic Hymns* 2	H. Oldenberg, trans., *Vedic Hymns, II. Hymns to Agni* (SBE, vol. 46)
Oldenberg, *Noten*	H. Oldenberg, *Ṛgveda, Textkritische und exegetische Noten,* 2 vols.
P	*Atharvaveda Saṃhitā* (Paippalāda recension): combined readings from Kāśmīri and Orissa texts and manuscripts. Books 1-20
Pāṇ., Pāṇ	*The Aṣṭādhyāyī of Pāṇini*
PraUp	*Praśna Upaniṣad*
PW	Böhtlingk and Roth, *Sanskrit-Wörterbuch,* 7 vols., i.e. *Petersburger Wörterbuch*
ṚV	*Ṛgveda*
ṚVKh, RVKh	*Ṛgveda Khila*
ŚāSth	*Śārīrasthāna*
ŚB	*Śatapatha Brāhmaṇa*
SBE	*Sacred Books of the East*
ŚGS	*Śāṅkhāyana Gṛhya Sūtra*
Sharma, *Beit. z. Ved. Lex.*	Aryendra Sharma, *Beiträge zur vedischen Lexikographie*
ŚŚS	*Śāṅkhāyana Śrauta Sūtra*
St.II.	*Studien zur Indologie und Iranistik*
Su	*Suśruta Saṃhitā*
SūSth	*Sūtrasthāna*
SVB	*Sāmavidhāna Brāhmaṇa*
TĀ	*Taittirīya Āraṇyaka*
TAS	Toḍarānanda's *Āyurveda Saukhyaṃ or Materia Medica of Āyurveda*
TB	*Taittirīya Brāhmaṇa*
TS	*Taittirīya Saṃhitā*
TU, TUp	*Taittirīya Upaniṣad*
Utt	*Uttaratantra, Uttarasthāna*

VaitS	*Vaitāna Sūtra*
VIJ	*Vishveshvaranand Indological Journal*
ViSth	*Vimānasthāna*
VS	*Vājasaneyi Saṃhitā*
Whitney-Lanman	W. D. Whitney and C. R. Lanman, *Atharva-veda-saṃhitā*. 2 pts. (HOS, vols. 7–8)
Wise	T. A. Wise, *Commentary on the Hindu System of Medicine*
ZDMG	*Zeitschrift der deutschen morgenländischen Gesellschaft*
Zimmer, *Leben*	H. Zimmer, *Altindisches Leben*

LIST OF TRANSLATED AND ANNOTATED HYMNS

LIST OF RITUAL VERSES RENDERED

Kauśika Sūtra (*continued*)	Translation (Page No.)
27.29–31	22
28.5–6, 14	74
28.15–16	45
28.17–20	27
29.18–19	39
29.20–26	66
29.30	33
30.8–10	88
30.13	92
30.14–16	84–85
31.6	77
31.7	39
31.11–15	94
31.16–17	85
31.20–21	85
31.27	45
31.28	88
32.8–10	85
32.17	38
32.18–19	47

LIST OF ILLUSTRATIONS

INTRODUCTION

Tracing the history and evolution of Indian medicine is a difficult enterprise. Continuities of doctrine and practice occur rarely, preventing us from positing an unbroken succession of development from earliest times. We must look at Indian medicine rather in terms of distinct phases. Although not well defined, the first may be called prehistoric or pre-Vedic medicine, dating from about 2700 B.C. to 1500 B.C. The second is that of Vedic medicine which looks back to a time around the second millennium B.C. It is the earliest period in which a clearly discernible medical lore can be ascertained. Vedic medicine is the focus of the present work. The next distinguishable stage is characterized by the presence of separate Sanskrit treatises on Indian medical science or *āyurveda*, 'the science of longevity.' The earliest of these medical books are the *saṃhitās* of Bhela, Caraka and Suśruta, which date from around the Christian era. The subject matter of these works is quite unlike that of Vedic medicine. Most diseases are defined in terms of a humoral theory. The Indian physicians understood there to be three 'humors' (*doṣas*): wind (*vāta, vāyu*), bile (*pitta*) and phlegm (*kapha, śleṣman*), which, on analogy with the humors of the Hippocratic and Galenic systems, were vitiating forces in the body. In a normal state, the humors are in a state of equilibrium in the body. When something called a *nidāna*, 'primary cause,' which could be of climatic, organic, or less commonly, demonic origin, acted upon the humors, an imbalance occurred, bringing about the manifestation of disease. The principal aim of the physician was to recognize which humor or humors were out of balance and to reestablish the equilibrium through allopathic treatments, which usually included drugs with opposite qualities, diet, and daily regimen, although surgery was also sometimes recommended.

This thumbnail sketch of early āyurvedic medicine serves to illustrate that at its basis lies a theoretical and a rational understanding of disease and cure. The origin of this new approach to medicine is a point of controversy. It is quite certain that little of it can be traced to Vedic medicine. Although the theoretical framework of *āyurveda* may not be Vedic, the basis of its materia medica could indeed have evolved from Vedic medicine or even from prehistoric, pre-Vedic medicine.

Prehistoric medicine

A clear and detailed picture of medicine prior to the Vedic phase is difficult to ascertain. Evidence of this prehistoric period in South Asia derives primarily from archaeological remains excavated from the sites of the Harappan Culture, sometimes referred to as the Indus Valley Civilization. Its dates are from about 2700 B.C. to 1500 B.C., making it roughly contemporaneous with the Old, Middle, and New Kingdoms of Egypt and the period of Sumer and Akkad in Mesopotamia. The mosaic of Harappan settlements illustrates a highly developed, urbanized culture, established principally along the Indus River (in modern Pakistan), stretching from the Arabian Sea to as far north as the Panjab (sites have also been found further south in present-day Gujarat). The area covered was nearly twice as large as the Egyptian civilization and almost four times as great as that of Sumer and Akkad.[1] This vast civilization had two main centers or capitals: one in the south, Mohenjo-Dāro (near modern Sukkur) and one in the north, Harappā (near Lahore).

The architecture of the Harappan sites was unique for its time. Streets were planned on a north–south and east–west grid. Houses were usually two-story and made of baked brick. Many homes contained a bathroom, built near the wall facing the street so that water could be drained through a pipe into a covered sewer running under the street. The bathrooms were either square or rectangular, with a sloping floor with an opening in the corner through which the water could drain. Several of the houses even had latrines with a drainage system similar to that of the bathrooms.[2] These architectural designs point to a conscious concern for public health and sanitation and suggest an implicit belief in ritual purity and pollution, which is so prevalent in later Indian thought. The Great Bath found in the citadel area of Mohenjo-Dāro perhaps epitomizes the Harappan penchant for purification through bathing. The man-made pool measured 108 by 180 feet with a center basin 23 by 39 feet and a sloping floor which reached a depth of 8 feet. This giant structure was filled with water from a large well.[3] The central purifying agent was water which, as we shall see, was an important medicine of the Vedic people. It is quite possible, therefore, that hydrotherapy was a therapeutic measure used by the Harappans to restore and to preserve health, which brings to mind the purpose of the Roman baths of a later period.

The material remains excavated from the Indus cities point to a socially and technically advanced urban culture supported by an agrarian subculture. Highly sophisticated sculptures in stone and bronze, and jewelry fashioned by skillful artisans from precious and semiprecious stones and metals, indicate an affluent class, and evidence of land and sea trade suggests a significant merchant class.[4] Less artfully sculptured terra-cotta fi-

---

[1] Henry E. Sigerist, *A History of Medicine* (New York: Oxford University Press, 1961) 2: 137.

[2] Ibid., 143. See fig. 4, 91, below.

[3] Ibid. See fig. 3, 91, below.

[4] See A. L. Basham, *The Wonder that was India* (New York: Grove Press, 1954, 1959), 18–19. At the Indus site of Lothal (in Gujarat), there is a large structure which appears to be a shipping dock (see S. R. Rao, *Lothal and the Indus Civilization*, New York: Asia Publishing House, 1973). See also Gregory L. Possehl, ed., *Ancient cities of the Indus* (Durham, North Carolina: Carolina Academic Press, 1979), 203–22, on Lothal and 96–97 and 113–75 on contacts with Mesopotamia.

gurines of an Earth Mother Goddess point to the worship of the soil by farmers, and by lower orders in general (see fig. 5, 114, below).

The most interesting artifacts discovered at the various Indus sites are the small square or rectangular seals and sealings, on many of which are found short inscriptions written in a pictographic script which has yet to be deciphered. The precise purpose of these seals and sealings is uncertain. They may have been used as a type of identification tag, with the inscription providing the pertinent information, or perhaps as amulets, worn to ward off various kinds of evil and to bring good luck, the inscriptions being magico-religious utterances (*mantras*). Many of the seals are perforated in the back, suggesting that a string or cord was used to bind them to some part of the body. Until the code to the script is broken—unfortunately, there is no counterpart of the Rosetta stone to aid scholars—the seals will remain an enigma, and many important facts about this magnificent civilization will be kept shrouded in mystery.

Images of a species of bull, elephant and rhinoceros found on many seals suggest the particular importance of these animals. Several seals and sealings appear to portray mythological episodes.[5] The representation of a goddess standing between the branches of a pīpal tree and being worshipped by seven devotees is significant. It depicts the worship of a female plant divinity or a Tree Goddess and points to a reverence for plants and their products.[6] Similarly, an oblong sealing from Harappā illustrates a mythological story in which a woman, presumably the Earth Mother Goddess, standing on her head, gives birth to what appears to be a plant or tree. On the reverse, a man, bearing a sickle, stands waiting in front of the woman (see fig. 6, 115, below). These scenes point to a deep sentiment felt towards the earth and its offspring, the plants, and suggest that certain rituals were performed at the time of harvesting. A reverence for the medicinal plant or simple is also quite evident in Vedic medicine; and in the later tradition of āyurvedic medicine, pharmacopoeias, detailing the medicinal virtues of numerous plants, became fundamental components of the medical tradition. We may, therefore, look to the Harappan Culture for the seeds of traditional Indian pharmaceutical knowledge.

Another seal portrays a multi-faced figure, adorned with a horned headdress and ritual clothing, seated in a yogic posture, and surrounded by different kinds of animals. It is generally assumed that this horned deity represents a forerunner of the later Hindu god, Śiva, Lord of Beasts (*paśupati*), and it has been styled, "proto-Śiva."[7] The elaborate headdress, the costume with bangles and the implication of trance states achieved through the intense concentration or meditation of yoga suggest that this figure depicts a type of medicine-man, shamanistic in character.

Evidence is available that the magically based surgical technique of trepanation may also have been practiced during the period of the Indus

---

[5] See Basham, *The Wonder*, pl. IX, a, e, f.

[6] Cf. ibid., 23–24. See fig. 9, 220, below.

[7] Basham, *The Wonder*, 23.

Valley Civilization. Two skulls said to exhibit signs of trepanation have been discovered at two Harappan sites. Skull H. 796B from cemetery R 37 of Harappā appears to have one man-made hole in the temporo-parietal region. The hole is thought to have been made by a small circular gouge with an alabaster handle, which was discovered in the same strata from which the skull came.[8] Since no mention of this hole is made in the original report of this skull, strong doubt is cast on its authenticity as an example of trepanation.[9] It remains a mystery how the hole was made. The second skull, KLB-8/69, from Kalibangan (a Harappan settlement on the dried bed of the Ghaggar-Hakra River in the deserts of Rajasthan, India) is that of a child who may have suffered from hydrocephaly. Three small holes occur on the right side of the skull. They are on the squamous temporal bone, above the right acoustic meatus. A black streak joining the upper holes appears to have been made by a glowing hot, pointed instrument. It is possible that the operation was performed with a hot iron in order to relieve the pain caused by the swelling of the skull. As the wounds show signs of healing, it is likely that the child survived the operation.[10] If indeed this skull was trepanned, it demonstrates a unique method of performing it. Trepanation is not mentioned in ancient Indian medical literature. A reference to such a surgical procedure does, however, occur in a Pāli Buddhist text from about the fourth century B.C.[11]

The decline and eventual collapse of the Harappan Culture is an enigma. We know that the process took place gradually over a period of about two hundred years. The cities were completely abandoned, but post-urban settlements in the area indicate that part of the population survived. Theories of the cause of the decline of the Indus Civilization range from the invasions of the charioteering Āryan tribes from the north to the persistent flooding of the Indus River, leading to its economic decline and eventual fall.[12] No one is quite sure why or how the end came, but we know that this great culture had ceased by around 1500 B.C.

In the absence of written sources, the general picture of Harappan medicine derived from the available data illustrates a definite concern for public health and suggests a tradition of medicine which involved the use of plants in a religious ceremony. This spiritually based method of healing was characteristic of the medical traditions of ancient Egypt and Mesopotamia and, as we shall shortly discover, typifies Vedic medicine.

Sources of Vedic medicine

Unlike the ancient Egyptian and Mesopotamian medical traditions which have specific treatises outlining their medical systems, the earliest Indian

---

[8] Amiya K. Roy Chowdhury, "Trepanation in Ancient India," *Asiatic Society of Calcutta, Communications*, 25 (1972): 203–206. See fig. 7, 209, below.

[9] P. Gupta, et al., *Human Skeletal Remains from Harappa* (Calcutta: Anthropological Survey of India, 1963), 19, 21, 30–31, 184; fig. 18, pls. VII, VIII.

[10] A. K. Sharma, "Kalibangan Human Skeletal Remains—An Osteo-archaeological Approach," *Journal of the Oriental Institute*, Baroda 19 (1969): 109–14. See fig. 8, 209, below.

[11] See 67, below.

[12] See Gregory L. Possehl, ed., *Ancient cities of the Indus*, 287–326.

textual evidence of medicine is randomly inserted in the corpora of its principal religious literature, primarily in the *Atharvaveda* and to a much lesser extent in the *Ṛgveda.*

The medical material contained in these two ancient texts is not wholly free from problems. Because we have well edited texts with which to work, we stand on fairly firm ground when laboring with these bodies of literature, which have been preserved by an extraordinarily accurate oral tradition from very early times until comparatively recently when they were recorded in written form. Doubts concerning the meaning of specific words and phrases are present; but these uncertainties are not unexpected in such ancient documents. Of all the religious literature of ancient India, these Vedic texts have received the most extensive philological investigation. With this background of scholarship at our disposal we have a solid basis upon which to test new hypotheses and to construct new theories. Although we may not be able to eliminate all the doubts which the literature still contains, we can, nevertheless, contribute significantly to the elucidation of India's antique medical lore.

The actual medical doctrines we shall study are found mostly in the *Atharvaveda,* a religious text which contains much material of a secular nature. The *Ṛgveda* is almost entirely religious in character and therefore provides for the most part mythological stories illustrating the healings performed by various gods of the Vedic pantheon.[13] These episodes along with other scattered medical references will be utilized in order to explain more fully the medical philosophy and practice of the Vedic people; but they cannot in themselves be viewed as representing a separate medical tradition.[14] It is only when the two texts are examined together that the fundamental doctrines of the Vedic medical tradition can be fully appreciated. The three hymns we have rendered from the *Ṛgveda* are close in style to those of the *Atharvaveda* and for this reason may be considered as representing the same textual tradition.

We have included translations of the corresponding ritual practices which are found in the *Kauśika Sūtra* (to the *Atharvaveda*) and in the *Ṛgvidhāna* (to the *Ṛgveda*). Although these texts are much later (perhaps from the second or third century B.C.), they preserve the ritual prescriptions which often reflect an older attitude, not unlike those implied in the original hymns which they accompany. At other times, the ritual actions are merely interpretations, conjured up in an attempt to fit a particular hymn or group of hymns. We shall draw on materials from later religious and medical traditions in order to elucidate more completely this phase of Indian med-

[13] See in particular the healing feats of the twin horsemen, Aśvins at ṚV 1.112.8, 15; 116.10, 15, 16; 117.9, 13, 17–18, 24; 118.6–8; 5.74.5; 75.5; 7.68.6; 71.5; 10.39.3, 4, 8; and 10.40.5; the connection of Rudra with healing at ṚV 1.43.4; 114.5; 2.33.2, 4, 7, 12; 5.42.11; 7.35.6; 46.3; and 8.29.5; of the Maruts at ṚV 2.33.13; and 8.20.23–26; of Soma and Rudra at ṚV 6.74.3; of Indra at ṚV 2.21.6; 4.19.9; 8.1.12 and especially 8.91(80), where Indra cures Apālā of the loss of hair and of ugly skin. Cf. also Filliozat, *La doctrine,* 72–81.

[14] An examination of R. Müller's research into the medicine of the *Ṛgveda* illustrates this point well ("Die Medizin im Ṛg-Veda," *Asia Major,* 6 [1930]: 315–76; 386–87).

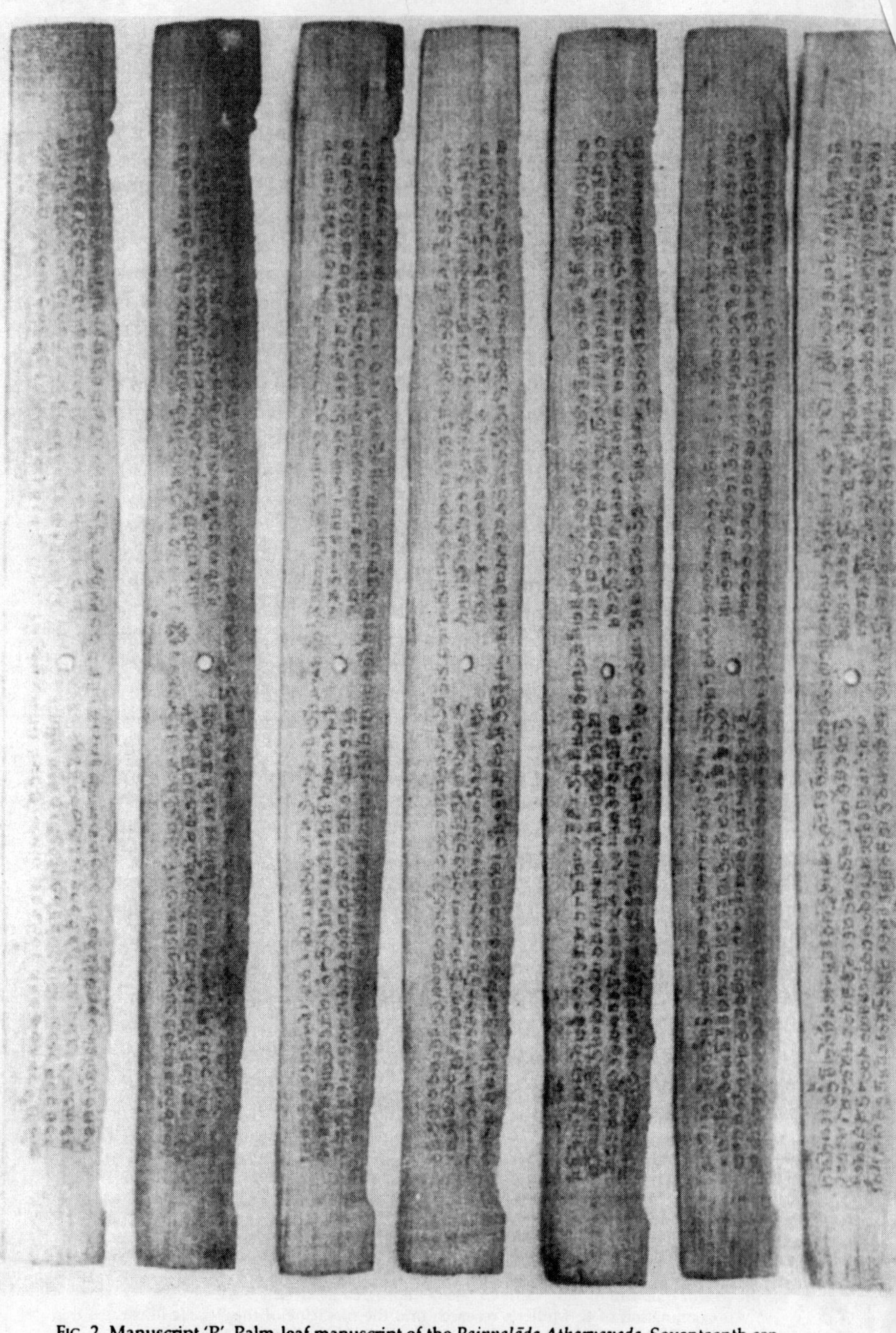

FIG. 2. Manuscript 'P'. Palm-leaf manuscript of the *Paippalāda Atharvaveda*. Seventeenth century. Oriya script. Written by Raghanātha Śarma. Courtesy of M. Witzel.

icine and to trace any possible continuities and changes. Similarities in other Indo-European traditions will also be mentioned in order to point to ancient beliefs which may well have derived from a common source.

Anatomical knowledge in ancient India

A work of this type should include a discussion of anatomy. We refrain, however, from an examination of individual anatomical terms, as this has already been undertaken by A. F. R. Hoernle, F. S. Hammett and especially J. Filliozat, to whose works the reader should refer for the best discussion of the subject.[15] For all their painstaking work on anatomy, Filliozat and the others have neglected to explain adequately the basis of ancient Indian anatomical knowledge.

Anatomical knowledge in ancient India was derived principally from the sacrifice of the horse and of man; chance observations of improperly buried bodies and examinations of the corporal members made by medical men during treatment contributed comparatively little to the body of anatomical knowledge. As a result of the precise ritual procedures of the sacrifice, which called for the recitation of the name of each part of the body as it was cut (for the horse this is documented at *Ṛgveda* 1.162.18; for man no early references are found, but later tradition specifies that the action should follow that of the immolation of the horse), fairly accurate lists of anatomical parts of the horse and of man have been preserved and transmitted, primarily through the exegetical *Brāhmaṇa*-texts. Filliozat's efforts at defining many of these parts have greatly advanced our understanding of the individual terms. Difficulties, however, still remain in the proper identification of many of the internal parts, which tend to be described by the native authorities in terms of a locality or as attached to a known organ. These enumerations provided the principal sources of anatomical knowledge until the time of the classical treatises (*saṃhitās*) of āyurvedic medicine, when the visual inspection of the body by a type of dissection was introduced, perhaps from the West, into the traditional system of medical education, thus contributing a wholly new dimension to the understanding of the human body.[16]

Characteristics of Vedic medicine

Vedic medicine may be characterized essentially as a magico-religious system. Such a hackneyed definition implies more that it expresses. Space does not permit a complete discussion of magico-religious medicine and

---

[15] A. F. Rudolf Hoernle, *Studies in the Medicine of Ancient India*, Part I: Osteology or the Bones of the Body (Oxford: Clarendon Press, 1907); Frederick S. Hammett, "The Anatomical Knowledge of the Ancient Hindus," *Annals of Medical History* (New Series) 1 (1929): 325–33; and Jean Filliozat, *La doctrine*, 117–37.

[16] See my "The Evolution of Anatomical Knowledge in Ancient India, with special reference to cross-cultural influences," JAOS, 106.4 (1986): 687-705.

its apparent opposite, empirical medicine.[17] In this work however the concept of magico-religious medicine is understood to be as follows: Causes of diseases are not attributed to physiological functions, but rather to external beings or forces of a demonic nature who enter the body of their victim and produce sickness. The removal of such malevolent entities usually involved an elaborate ritual, often drawing on aspects of the dominant local religion and nearly always necessitating spiritually potent and efficacious words, actions and devices. The empirical medicine evident during this period, on the other hand, involved both observation and experience in order to determine the cause of disease and to effect an appropriate treatment.

The Vedic Indian's attitude toward disease, therefore, was dominated by the belief that evil spirits, demons and other malevolent forces invaded the body and caused their victims to exhibit a state of dis-ease. These demons were often personified and deified, giving rise to an entire pantheon of gods of disease. The impetus for the attack may have come from a breach of a certain taboo, from a sin committed against the gods or from witchcraft and sorcery. Injuries such as broken bones or wounds, however, were considered to be accidentally caused or the result of warfare. Other external diseases and afflictions were noticed to have been caused by noxious insects and vermin, often thought to be demonic in character.

The idea of health in a positive sense is wanting in Vedic medicine. Any notion of the concept is to be found in the negative or opposite of what was understood to be disease, or more specifically in the absence of particular disease-causing demons, of injuries and damages and of toxins.

As among most cultures of the world, an individual was considered to be healthy if his life-time was long, i.e. if he could repeatedly witness the rising sun, and if he showed complete recovery from illness. There are also indications that a wholesome body was associated with the intake of nutritious food.[18]

An elaborate healing ritual was performed to restore a patient, attacked by a disease-demon or suffering an injury, to a sound state of mind and body. The principal figure in the rite was the healer (*bhiṣáj*) who, like the medicine-man of the North and South American Indians among other peoples, is known for his dancing and his recitation of incantations, being called a shaker (*vípra*) and a chanter (*kaví*). The contents of the hymns suggest that he possessed a special knowledge of the preparation and use of medicines, including medicinal herbs or simples, and often water. The consecration of these remedies formed a significant part of his sacred utterances. In certain instances the healer waved or stroked plants over the

---

[17] In a lengthy review Rahul Peter Das has broached the topic of magic, religion and science in the medical context (*Indo-Iranian Journal,* 23.3 [1984]: 232–44). His comments could serve as a point of departure for a complete examination and reappraisal of these terms in the light of modern scholarship in the history of medicine, the history of religions, and anthropology.

[18] See my article, "Towards the notion of health in the Vedic phase of Indian medicine," ZDMG, 135.2 (1985): 312–18.

patient in the course of his ritual performance. The healer, like the professional carpenter who fixed something broken, was also known to be one who repaired the fracture, suggesting that one of his professional activities was the setting of bones.[19]

The healing ritual always required the recitation of religious incantations or charms. An analysis of these verses illustrates certain apotropaic devices which included the use of sympathetic magic, of the rhetorical question, of onomatopoeic sounds, of the identifying name, of the esoteric word or phrase which, when properly uttered focused the demon's attention on the healer, leading to its loss of grip and power. Disease-demons were often transferred from the patient to enemies or less desirable people, dispelled into the ground or carried away by birds to places where they could no longer be a menace to the community. Amulets or talismans (*maṇí*, literally 'jewel'), usually of vegetal origin, were ritually bound to drive out demons and to act as prophylactic measures in preventing further attacks. Fragrant plant substances were burnt to help expel the patient's demon, to protect him, and to make his environment pure and generally favorable for healing. Early morning (dawn), noon, and early evening (twilight) seem to have been the most auspicious times of the day to carry out healing rituals. Some rites were performed when certain stars were in a particular part of the heavens, suggesting that astrology may have played an important role in Vedic medicine.

Mythology also formed a significant part of the charms and hymns recited by the healer. Major disease-demons, in addition to being deified, were often mythologized, pointing to the important and long-lasting impact they had on the people. Likewise, certain curative herbs were given mythical beginnings, often personified, and worshipped as gods and more commonly as goddesses. The uttering of mythological stories about plant divinities imbued the herbs and plants used in the rite with supernatural powers, and therefore made them extremely potent. Reverence for plant-life was an integral part of the Vedic Indian's medical tradition and gave rise to an elaborate pharmacopoeia which is evident in all phases of Indian medical history.

As far as we can gather from the texts, the ancient practice of divination by means other than astrology, often encountered in antique medicine, was not employed by the Vedic healers. Diagnosis and prognosis were rather undertaken by the isolation and identification of dominant and recurring symptoms, many of which were considered to be separate demonic entities. This technique illustrates the importance which the recording of observable facts played in Vedic medicine. Various characteristics of a patient were noticed, given names and recorded. Plants and herbs were also put under the same rigorous scrutiny and their important features and qualities noted. The technique was a method for recording valuable facts and is an example of the very beginnings of the Indians' "empirical" mode

[19] ṚV 9.112.1.

of thought, exemplified in their penchant for enumeration, so prevalent in later Indian philosophical, religious and scientific literature.

In addition to the evidence of a systematic, classificatory way of thinking, the Vedic healers showed that they were familiar with more empirical procedures of healing. These therapeutic actions, however, are found in the context of the magico-religious rite, implying that their efficacy was inextricably connected with the magical or spiritual operation. The treatments worked because the proper words were recited, the correct actions performed, and the right devices used.

Quite naturally these procedures are encountered most frequently in the treatment of external diseases and afflictions. For example, a form of surgery, utilizing a reed as a catheter, was performed to cure urine-retention; lancing and salt were used in the treatment of certain pustules; cauterization with caustic medicines and perhaps with fire was practiced; sand and perhaps also reeds were applied to stop the flow of blood issuing from a wound and perhaps from the uterus; a resin was applied to wounds to prevent them from bleeding and to aid in the healing process; ointments and dyes were applied to the skin; a special plant was used which evidently promoted the growth of hair; and certain plants may also have been used in salves or poultices. Perhaps the most important empirical method of healing was the use of water as a type of hydrotherapy. It was employed for numerous ailments, both internal and external, suggesting that it was looked on as a significant therapeutic agent. The medicinal uses of water may well have evolved from the medical tradition of the Harappans.

Before examining and presenting in translations the most significant hymns which constitute the principal doctrinal remains of the Vedic phase of Indian medicine, we should have some idea of the Vedic medical lore in later centuries.

Vedic medicine in the later medical tradition

In the earliest āyurvedic treatises of Bhela, Caraka and Suśruta a reverence for Vedic medicine, as exemplified in the *Atharvaveda,* is advocated.[20] In actual practice, however, few of these early techniques seem to have survived. As an example, magico-religious utterances or *mantras,* which form the cornerstone of Vedic medicine, are found to have been used principally in five ways: 1. the treatment of swellings or tumors and wounds or sores (*śotha, vraṇa*); 2. the treatment of poison (*viṣa*); 3. the treatment of mental disorders (*unmatta, apasmāra*); 4. the treatment of fever (*jvara*); and 5. the collection and preparation of certain medicines. Parallels in Vedic medicine occur for each category. Often the similarities between the archaic and the āyurvedic uses of *mantras* are remarkable. Vestiges of Vedic medicine are clearly represented by these five groups. The infrequent use of magico-religious medicine, however, implies that *āyurveda* had su-

[20] CaSūSth 30.21.

perseded Vedic medicine and, more importantly, that it was seriously considered to be an alternative to the more antique, yet firmly established, Vedic medical tradition. The theoretical foundation of early āyurvedic medicine seemed to provide rather more rational than magical and religious explanations of disease and cure. Although magical medicine did not completely vanish from traditional Indian medical lore, it was never to acquire the status in the āyurvedic treatises which it had enjoyed in the *Atharvaveda*. Further research into the different phases of Indian medical history will shed considerable light on the causes and motivations behind changes and developments in traditional Indian medicine.[21]

---

[21] See my "Mantra in *āyurveda*: a study of the use of magico-religious speech in ancient India," in Harvey Alper, ed., *Understanding Mantra* (Albany, New York: SUNY Press, 1989), 123-43.

I. INTERNAL DISEASES

The ancient Indians' concept of internal disease was based on the fundamental notion that illnesses were caused by demonic entities which entered the body. Each demon had a specific name and caused particular morbid bodily conditions.

We have divided the analysis of the medical lore surrounding the internal diseases into two sections: A. those related to *yákṣma* and/or *takmán;* B. those unrelated to *yákṣma* and/or *takmán.* The first section examines the disease-entities which demonstrate a definite connection with one or the other of the major internal disease-demons, *yákṣma* and *takmán.* Since many of the symptoms are shared by both, some overlapping can be expected. The second section investigates the demonic diseases which exhibit the general characteristic of being in the body, but which do not bear a close relationship either to *yákṣma* or to *takmán.*

A. Internal Diseases related to yákṣma *and/or* takmán

1: *YÁKṢMA* (CONSUMPTION; TUBERCULOSIS)

Charms AVŚ 2.33, 6.85, 19.36, 19.38 are devoted specifically to the removal of *yákṣma.* AVŚ 2.33, called Kaśyapa's spell (verse 7), appears to have been very popular and very effective, having been preserved in three closely related forms both in the AVŚ (2.33; 20.96.17–22) and ṚV (10.163). AVŚ 6.85, 19.36, 19.38 seem to be more prophylactic in nature, being concerned with protecting one from the harmful effects of the disease-demon.

yákṣma, the general, internal disease-demon,[1] found both in humans and cattle,[2] is characterized as entering and possessing each and every part of the body.[3] It causes disintegration of the limbs, fever in the limbs, heartache and pain in all parts of the body.[4] Such a description of the disease led H. Zimmer to the conclusion that *yákṣma* referred to a class of diseases whose principal characteristics were those of consumption.[5] R. Müller, on the

---

[1] See R. E. Emmerick, "Indo-Iranian Concepts of Disease and Cure," unpublished paper delivered at The International Conference on Traditional Asian Medicine, Canberra, September 1979, 11–12.

[2] AVŚ 8.7.15, 12.2.1.

[3] ṚV 1.122.9, 10.97.12, 10.161.5, 10.163; AVŚ 2.33, 6.85.1, 9.8.7, 9, 12; cf. AVŚ 14.2.69.

[4] AVŚ 5.30.8, 9; 9.8.5, 13–19, 21, 22; 19 19.44.1–2.

[5] *Leben,* 375 f.; cf. also Macdonell-Keith, *Vedic Index,* 2: 182–83. More recently Filliozat has come to the same conclusion (*La doctrine,* 88).

other hand, discounts this view of Zimmer and considers that, in the eyes of the Vedic people, *yákṣma* was simply a demon or external force who, when entering the body, caused malady.[6] It appears from the point of view of the ancient Indian that Müller is quite correct; but one cannot overlook the similarities between the description of *yákṣma* and those of consumption, or more generally, those of any disease which brings about a general condition of bodily decay.

The hymns or charms speak of many *yákṣmas*[7] who are classified as speaking like a child and like an adult, suggesting that their victims were both children and adults.[8] Specifically, there is the *ajñātayakṣmá* (unknown-*yákṣma*)[9] and the *rājayakṣmá* (royal-*yákṣma* or *yákṣma* of kings).[10] They are often associated with other internal disease-entities, many of whom have separate charms devoted to their removal,[11] and with various demons.[12] In one important verse, the *yákṣmas* are said to have their origin in the relatives of the bride and to follow the wedding procession.[13] More particularly, *yákṣma* is said to be divinely sent[14] and caused by sin (*énas*).[15] At ṚV 1.122.9 we read that it is the dishonest man himself who, in a sly way, presses the Soma and causes the *yákṣma* to enter his heart.[16] This, then, illustrates a type of sin which must be committed before the gods send the affliction.[17]

The principal cures for one afflicted by *yákṣma* included the recitation of spells, of which the most efficacious was AVŚ 2.33, along with the use of herbs[18] which, from ṚV 10.97.11–13, appear to have been held in the

[6] "Medizin im Ṛg-Veda," *Asia Major*, 6: 357; see also "Yakṣma. Medizingeschichtliche Untersuchungen zur Entwicklungswertung der indischen Krankheitslehre," *Mitteilungen des Instituts für Orientforschung*, 4: 278.

[7] AVŚ 9.8.10–12; at 19.36.4 and VS 12.97 there is mention of a hundred *yákṣmas*.

[8] AVŚ 19.36.3.

[9] AVŚ 6.127.3; 3.11.1; 20.96.6; ṚV 10.161.1; see Filliozat, *La doctrine*, 87–88, 89.

[10] AVŚ 3.11.1; 11.3.39; 12.5.22 where he appears to attack a cow during the vulnerable time of urination, and ṚV 10.161.1. See myth of its origin below.

[11] Among the afflictions with which he has a connection, there is yellowness, *jāyā́nya*, disintegration of the limb and *visálpaka*, at AVŚ 19.44.2; *takmán* at 5.4.9; 5.30.16; head diseases at 9.8.1, 13, *balā́sa* at 9.8.10; *visalpá, vidradhá, vātīkārá* and *alají*, at 9.8.20 (cf. also 9.8.5) and *kṣetriyá* at 2.10.5, 6.

[12] Among the other demonic entities, there is death and *nírṛti* ('destruction') at AVŚ 8.1.21 and *grā́hi* ('seizure') at ṚV 10.161.1, AVŚ 3.11.1, 20.96.6.

[13] ṚV 10.85.31 (=AVŚ 14.2.10) *yé vadhvàś candrám̐ vahatúm̐ yákṣmā yánti jánād ánu, púnas tā́n yajñíyā devā́ náyantu yáta ā́gatāḥ.* On the interpretation of *jánād*, see L. Alsdorf, "Bemerkungen zu Sūryasūkta," ZDMG, 111: 493 (*Kleine Schriften*, 30). Note: In *cd*, worshipful gods are requested to lead the *yákṣmas* back from where they came.

[14] AVŚ 8.7.2.

[15] AVŚ 8.7.3.

[16] *jáno yó mitrāvaruṇāv abhidhrúg apó ná vām̐ sunóty akṣṇayā́dhrúk, svayám̐ sá yákṣmam̐ hṛ́daye ní dhatta ā́pa yád īm̐ hótrābhir ṛtā́vā*; cf. also R. Müller, "Medizin im Ṛg-Veda," 354.

[17] See also AVŚ 12.4.8 where the master's children die and a mild form of *yákṣma* (?) attacks him because he allowed his cow's hair to become injured (*yád asyā gópatau satyā́ lóma dhvā́ṅkṣo ájīhiḍat, tátaḥ kumārā́ mriyante yákṣmo vindaty anāmanā́t*; on the difficult word *anāmanā́t*; see Mayrhofer, Wb 1: 33).

[18] Among the most beneficial herbs, there is *kúṣṭha* at AVŚ 5.4.9 and *cīpúdru* at 6.127.1, 3, with whose help the *yákṣma* is dispelled downward; *arundhatī́*, also makes man free from *yákṣma* at AVŚ 6.59.2.

hand of the healer and stroked or waved over the patient, causing the demon to leave the body and to fly away with birds. Elsewhere we learn that a lead amulet dispels the *yákṣma* downward[19] and that ointment (*ā̆ñjana*) has the power to remove it from the limbs.[20] Likewise, since it is divinely sent, gods also have the power to destroy it. The divinities most helpful for the eradication of *yákṣma* included Agni,[21] Savitṛ, Vāyu[22] and Āditya.[23] Water was also used in the therapy.[24] Charms, gods and other plant materials were utilized to prevent attacks from the *yákṣmas*. At AVŚ 6.85, an amulet fashioned from the *varaṇá*-tree is able to restrain *yákṣma;* at AVŚ 19.36, the *śatávāra*-amulet protects one from the *yákṣmas*; and at AVŚ 19.38, the scent of the burning *gulgulú*-plant is said to disperse them.

The *varaṇá*-plant is called thousand-eyed and is described as being yellow and gold in color. In the later medical tradition, it was employed for a wide variety of ailments.[25] The *śatávāra*-amulet, whose name suggests that it was used to 'ward off a hundred [demons],' appears to have been fashioned from a small bifurcated plant, whose fork at the apex was, like the *varaṇá*-tree, gold in color, resembling the auspicious 'golden-horned bull.' The *gulgulú* (*gúggulu*)-plant or bdellium was brought from afar by means of maritime trade.[26] This tended to make it a valuable and expensive commodity which is listed along with gold, *aukṣá* (perhaps an ointment) and fortune at AVŚ 2.36.7*ab.*[27] Such an early mention of the auspicious uses of this scent is significant especially in light of the later uses of incense and fumigation in India.

The ritual prescribed in the later *Kauśika Sūtra* and *Ṛgvidhāna* points to a healing-practice different from that implied in the hymns: With AVŚ 2.33, the healer tears off bandages which have been wrapped around the patient and sprinkles him from head to foot with water mixed with the dregs of ghee. Likewise, while constantly whispering ṚV 10.163, the priest touches the patient's head, two ears, two eyes, chin and two nostrils, with his hand which has been anointed with ritually prepared ghee; or he should remove *yakṣma* with the ritual mentioned perhaps at *Ṛgvidhāna* 4.16.1–5 (to ṚV 10.161) which entails the sprinkling of the patient (with water) by means of *darbha*-grass, the sacrificing of ghee in the fire and the giving to the patient of a concoction of ghee and milk and a spirituous decoction made from water, pieces of *khadira*-wood, and flour mixed with honey and

---

[19] AVŚ 12.2.1, 2, 14.

[20] AVŚ 19.44.1–2.

[21] AVŚ 5.29.13.

[22] AVŚ 4.25.5.

[23] AVŚ 9.8.22; here Āditya is said to appease the limb-disintegrating *yákṣma*.

[24] AVŚ 3.12.9 (=9.3.23); 19.2.5; cf. also ṚV 9.49.1.

[25] See AVŚ 6.85.1n below. Cf. also H. C. Patyal, "Significance of Varaṇa-(*Crateava Roxburghii*) in the Veda," *Oriens,* 21–22: 300–306, for a good discussion of the plant in Vedic literature.

[26] AVŚ 19.38.2.

[27] *idáṃ híraṇyaṃ gúlgulv (gúggulv) ayáṃ aukṣó átho bhágah.* Sāyaṇa understands *gúlgulu* (*gúggulu*) as a 'well known type of substance for fumigation' (*dhūpanadravyaviśeṣaḥ prasiddhaḥ*). Note: accent of *gulgulu* is irregular. It occurs either on first or last syllable.

ghee, to drink. With AVŚ 6.85, the healer binds that mentioned in the hymn (i.e. an amulet made from the wood of the *varaṇá*-tree) to the patient.[28]

Ghee or clarified butter is not mentioned in the hymns; nor are *gulgulú* and *sátávāra* prescribed in the later healing rites. They are, however, used in later non-medical rites at *Śāntikalpa* 17.4, 19.6 and AthPariś 4.4, suggesting their employment as a prophylactic.

Because of the obvious effect this disease had on the people and the great respect the ancient Indians had for it, a mythological story concerning its origin developed and is recorded at TS 2.3.5.1–2 (MS 2.2.7 and KS 11.3). In this myth, King Soma was given thirty-three wives, the daughters of Prajāpati. Soma, however, took a fancy only to Rohiṇī. This angered the other thirty-two; so they returned to their father. Soma followed and requested them back; but Prajāpati would not return them unless Soma swore an oath to consort with all of them equally. He did this and his wives were returned to him; but again he associated only with Rohiṇī. Because he broke the oath to Prajāpati, Soma was seized by *yákṣma;* since it had attacked a king, that was the origin of *rājayakṣmá;* since Soma had become corrupted, that was the origin of *pāpayakṣmá* (vile-*yákṣma*); and since he contracted it from his wives, that was the origin of *jāyénya.* In order to be freed of this affliction, one must make an offering to the Ādityas, who, as we have seen, have the power to appease a *yákṣma.*[29] It is interesting to note also that this later tradition has preserved the older notion that the *yákṣmas* are sent by the gods because of a sin committed against them.

In the *Suśruta Saṃhitā,* the word *yakṣman* occurs in the compound *rājayakṣman* and tends to denote a state of general decay and specific atrophy or paralysis of a particular limb or organ, characterized by the symptoms of food-aversion (*bhakta-dveṣa*), fever (*jvara*), asthma (*śvāsa*), cough (*kāsa*), appearance of blood (*śoṇitadarśana*) and laryngitis (*svarabheda*).[30]

2.33

From your eyes, from [your] nostrils, from [your] ears, from [your]
chin, from [your] brain, from [your] tongue, I tear away for you
the *yákṣma* who is in the head. 1.

---

[28] KauśS 27.27–28; *Ṛgvidhāna* 4.19.3–5 and KauśS 26.37: 27.27. *akṣībhyāṃ ta iti vībarham;* 28. *udapātreṇa saṃpātavatāvasiñcati;* 4.19.3. . . . *ājyaṃ saṃskṛtya juhuyād akṣībhyāṃ ta iti dvijaḥ;* 4. *pāṇinā tu ghṛtāktena mūrddhānaṃ saṃspṛśet tataḥ, karṇau netre ca cubukaṃ nāsike caiva saṃspṛśet;* 5. *etad eva japen nityaṃ yakṣmaṇo vipramucyate, pūrvoktenaiva kalpena yakṣmanāśanam ācaret;* 26.37. *tṛtīyena mantroktaṃ bandhnāti.* See Bloomfield, *Hymns,* 327, 505; Caland, AZ, 80, 85 and Gonda, *The Ṛgvidhāna,* 112-13 and 114-15.

[29] See Keith, VBYS, Pt. 1: 168; cf. also TS. 2.5.6.4–5, where King Soma again is stricken with these *yákṣmas* because, of his wives who were the nights of the half-month, he only consorted with the new and full moon night (Keith, ibid., 195); cf. also Filliozat's analysis of the myth, *La doctrine,* 84–86. A version of this legend is also found at *Caraka Saṃhitā,* CiSth, 8.1–11; see Filliozat, ibid., 86–87; cf. also *Suśruta Saṃhitā,* Utt. 41.5.

[30] Utt. 41.1–11; see also Filliozat, *La doctrine,* 83–84, 87.

From your neck, from the nape of [your] neck, from [your] vertebrae, from [your] spine, from [your] shoulders, from [your] forearms, I tear away for you the *yákṣma* who is in the arm. 2.

From your heart, from [your] lungs, from [your] *hálīkṣṇa*, from [your] two sides, from [your] two *mátasnas*, from [your] spleen, from [your] liver, we tear away for you the *yákṣma*. 3.

From your bowels, from [your] intestines, from [your] rectum, from [your] stomach, from the lateral parts of [your] abdomen, from [your] *plāśí*, from [your] navel, I tear away for you the *yákṣma*. 4.

From your thighs, from [your] kneecaps, from [your] heels, from the front of [your] feet, from [your] haunches, from [your] *bháṃsas*, I tear away for you the *yákṣma* who is in the backside. 5.

From your bones, from [your] marrows, from [your] tendons, from [your] (blood) vessels, from [your] hands, from [your] fingers, from [your] nails, I tear away for you the *yákṣma*. 6.

By means of Kaśyapa's exorcising spell, we tear completely away the *yákṣma* who is of your skin, who is in your every limb, every hair [and] every joint. 7.

6.85

May this *varaṇá*-tree, god [and] lord of the forest, check [him]; [for] the gods also have checked that *yákṣma* who has entered this [man]. 1.

We check your *yákṣma* with the spell of Indra, of Mitra and of Varuṇa, [in fact] with the speech of all the gods. 2.

As Vṛtra restrained these ever-flowing waters; just so I, with Agni Vaiśvānara, check your *yákṣma*. 3.

19.36

Ascending with brilliance, the *śatávāra*-amulet, which is the dispeller of the evil-named ones, has destroyed, by [its] efficacy, the *yákṣmas* [and] the *rákṣas*-demons. 1.

[It] nudges away the *rákṣas*-demons with [its] two horns [and] the sorceresses with [its] root; [and it] repels *yákṣma* with [its] middle. [Indeed,] evil does not overcome it. 2.

The *śatávāra*-amulet, the killer of the evil-named ones, has destroyed all the childish *yákṣmas* and those who speak as adults. 3.

[It] has produced a hundred heroes [and] has dispersed a hundred *yákṣmas*; having killed all the evil-named ones, it shakes off the *rákṣas*-demons. 4.

Having crushed all the evil-named ones, this *śatávāra*-amulet, [as it were] the golden-horned bull, has trampled down the *rákṣas*-demons. 5.

With *śatávāra,* I ward off a hundred evil-named females, a hundred Gandharvas and Apsarases [and] a hundred dog-accompanied (females) (Apsarases). 6.

19.38

Neither the *yákṣma*s, O Arundhatī, nor a curse reaches him whom the pleasant scent of the medicinal *gulgulú* (bdellium) reaches. 1.
From him [who is permeated with its scent], the *yákṣma*s disperse in all directions, like deer [or] horses. Whether, O *gulgulú,* you are from the Sindhu or whether [you are] from the ocean, I have taken the name of both [kinds], so that this man may be unharmed. 2(-3).

2: *JĀYĀNYA*

AVŚ 7.76 (80).3–5 is a charm concerned with the disease-entity known as *jāyā́nya* which, in the form *jāyénya* at TS 2.3.5.1–2, is closely associated with the demonic disease, *yákṣma*. Much controversy surrounds the exact nature of this disease Filliozat and some, because of its inclusion in a hymn which begins with the removal of the skin disorder, *apacít*, consider it to be a term designating various types of suppurating skin-ulcers.[1] In addition to its inclusion in a charm involving the *apacíts*, the *jāyā́nya* mentioned at AVŚ 7.76 (80).2(4), possesses the characteristic of flight, which is also shared by the *apacíts*.[2] At ṚV 10.97.13, however, there is a suggestion that *yákṣma* may also be a disease-demon who can fly. Others, based on Sāyaṇa, who equates it with *jāyénya* in the TS, understand him to be a form of *yákṣma*, etymologically signifying perhaps a type of venereal or congenital disease.[3] This latter explanation is supported by verse 3(5) which mentions the demon's mythological origin which is fully detailed in the TS. Likewise at verses 1, 2, he, like the *yákṣma*, invades every part of the body from the head to the feet, including the spinal column. In fact, at 19.44.2, he is considered to be a *yákṣma* and at P 19.40.9 he appears to be a *yákṣma* which enters the abdomen and causes it to swell. This demonstrates that, according to the tradition, he was a type of *yákṣma* which invaded the body and produced the symptomatic condition of a swollen belly. At verse 2, he is also called *ákṣita* (*ákṣata*) and *súkṣata* (*súkṣita*) whose meanings are in this context uncertain.

The cure for *jāyā́nya* included the performance of an offering in the house of the patient by a healer who, through his knowledge of its origin, establishes his power over the demon (verse 3). At verse 2, there is also mentioned a medicine which is effective against him. This medicine may be ointment (*ā́ñjana*) which, at AVŚ 19.44.1–2, is able to expel, among other *yákṣmas*, *jāyā́nya*.

---

[1] *La doctrine*, 89. See also Henry, who, because of its connection with *apacít* in the first two verses, defines it as "la diathèse générale dont les apacít sont la manifestation extérieure" (*Le livre*: VII, 30, 98; see also *La magie*, 194). This view is followed by Griffith (1: 365 and n.).

[2] See AVŚ 6.83.1, 3; P 1.59.4.

[3] Sāyaṇa explains *jāyā́nya* to be 'the disease of decay, produced by sexual union with a lawful wife' (*nirantarajāyāsaṃbhogena jāyamāna kṣayarogam*). He cites TS 2.3.5.2 as support and equates the *jāyénya* mentioned there with the *jāyā́nya* found in the AVŚ (*tatra jāyenya iti paṭhyate atra tu jāyānya iti ākāravattvena iti viśeṣaḥ*). Zimmer accepted this equation (*Leben*, 377) and Bloomfield, on this basis and on etymological grounds, considers him to be either congenital disease (root *jan*, 'to be born') or venereal disease (*jāyā*, 'woman') (*Hymns*, 561). Whitney-Lanman also suggests the possibility of venereal disease (Pt. 1: 442; cf. however Caland's remarks, AZ, 105 n. 6).

7.76 (80) 3–5

I have driven away every *jāyā̃nya* who crushes the vertebrae, who reaches down to the sole of the foot [and] who is attached to the apex [of the head]. 1(3).

The winged *jāyā̃nya* flies [and] he enters the man. This is the medicine of both the *ákṣita* and the *súkṣata.* 2(4).

O *jāyā̃nya,* [since] we know your origin [and] whence, O *jāyā̃nya,* you were born, how then could you harm [him] there, in whose house, we made the oblation? 3(5).

3: *KṢETRIYÁ*

AVŚ 2.8 and 3.7 are charms used to heal one afflicted with the internal disease-demon *kṣetriyá*. The former, however, is concerned principally with the consecration of the *kṣetriyá*-destroying plant.

Because of the paucity of symptoms present in the charms, an exact determination of the disease is problematic. Etymologically, the word is derived from *kṣétra*, 'field,' 'land,' 'soil,' and, in addition to the Atharvavedic references, occurs at KS 15.1 and TB 2.5.6.1–3, where a repetition of the Atharvavedic material is to be found. Based on *Aṣṭādhyāyī* 5.2.92:*kṣetriyac parakṣetre cikitsyaḥ*, "*kṣetriya* is curable in another womb," [1] Sāyaṇa and the native tradition consider it to be an anomalous word signifying a 'disease beginning with consumption, skin-disease and epilepsy, derived from the limbs of the father or mother, etc., contaminated by the defilements [causing] consumption, skin-disease, etc. [and] curable in the body of a grandson or son, etc.' [2] A type of hereditary disease was clearly understood by the word. Western interpreters, however, are in disagreement about its meaning: Weber considered it to be either crop-damage or a type of disease which afflicted new-born children.[3] Bloomfield originally followed the native tradition,[4] but later suggested that it may be of the "scrofulous or syphilitic order." [5] Filliozat, after having examined the passage of Pāṇini, its commentaries, in particular the *Kāśikāvṛtti* which associates the disease with *kuṣṭha*, a class of skin-diseases which includes leprosy, and Suśruta's description of *kuṣṭha* at NiSth 5.23–27, concluded that it most probably designated "les maladies imprégnant intimement l'organisme comme les lèpres incurables." [6] Karambelkar has also undertaken an extensive investigation of the word in the Vedic and post-Vedic texts as well as the treatment of it as prescribed in the KauśS and has suggested that it is "the name for a disease or diseases caused by grass-poisoning." [7] Although it is clear that there are widely differing opinions about the disease, it may be possible to offer a more plausible hypothesis.

---

[1] Here *kṣetra* has the medical meaning 'healthy womb' (see SuŚāSth 2.33 and P. Kutumbiah, *Ancient Indian Medicine* [1964; rpt. Bombay Orient Longman, Ltd., 1974], 184; cf. Bloomfield, *Hymns*, 287–88).

[2] Sāyaṇa to AVŚ 2.8.1: . . . *putrapautrādiśarīre cikitsyaḥ kṣayakuṣṭhādidoṣadūṣitapitṛmātrādiśarīrāvayavebhya āgataḥ kṣayakuṣṭhāpasmārādirogaḥ kṣetriya ity ucyate. 'kṣetriyac parakṣetre cikitsyaḥ' iti kṣetriyaśabdo nipātyate.*

[3] IS 13: 149, 156, 17: 208, see also notes to AVŚ 3.7, 121 below.

[4] *Hymns*, 13, 14, 15.

[5] *The Atharvaveda* (Strassburg: Karl J. Tübner, 1899), 60; see also Macdonell-Keith, *Vedic Index* 1: 211.

[6] *La doctrine*, 96.

[7] *The Atharva-Veda and The Āyur-Veda* (Nagpur, 1961), 240.

Some of his characteristics allow us to place him among the general class of internal disease-demons associated with *yákṣma*. He was definitely looked upon as a demon or evil by the Vedic people, as is indicated at AVŚ 2.10 1–6 by the following refrain: "I release you from *kṣetriyá*, from destruction, from the curse of a relative, from the foe [and] from the bond of Varuṇa. I make you sinless with the spell. May both heaven and earth be favorable to you." [8] Likewise, he is associated with seizure (*grā́hi*), at AVŚ 2.10.6, with the curse (*śapátha*), sorceresses (*yātudhānī́*) and evil spirits (*arā́yī*), female demons (*abhikṛ́tvarī*) and demons belonging to the magical realm (*saṃdeśyà*) at 2.8.2,5; and at 2.14.5 the Sadānvā-demons are said to be part of the *kṣetriyás* (plural). He is specifically mentioned in relation to *yákṣma* at AVŚ 2.10.5–6 and, like him, is said to dwell internally (3.7.2). At P 5.17.1, he is mentioned as a cause of insanity (see 187, below). The only clue to a direct cause for the malady is found at 3.7.6, where it is said that he enters and takes possession of his victim because of a prepared mixture. Although we cannot be completely certain, it is likely that this mixture was a type of food derived from various cultivated plants which, when magically concocted and then consumed, was believed to cause the disease.

In the Buddhist literature written in Pāli, we learn of a monk who suffered from a disease caused by drinking a liquid made poisonous by witchcraft. The remedy for this condition is said to be a concoction of clay, turned up by a ploughshare, mixed with water.[9] It is significant that the cause of the malady mentioned in the Pāli text is the same as that which we assume for *kṣetriyá;* likewise, its cure incorporated ingredients which included cultivated soil. A connection with the field or soil (*kṣétra*) is fundamental to its meaning, as is seen by its symbolic association with agricultural elements (2.8.3–5). Further support is therefore given to the notion that *kṣetriyá* originally denoted a disease whose cause was considered to be the consumption of a substance made harmful by sorcery. The citation of the word early in the grammatical text of Pāṇini points to a disease which is transmitted from generation to generation. The major symptoms included sunken eyes (2.8.5), pain in the chest (3.7.2), and perhaps a severe rash.

The cure for one afflicted by this demonic disease necessitated the use of a *kṣetriyá*-destroying plant, which may have been called *apāmārgá*,[10] consecrated by 2.8, for at 4.18.7 it is said to wipe away the *kṣetriyá*.[11] Barley and sesame were also used in the treatment and, together with the plant,

---

[8] *kṣetriyā́t tvā nírṛtyā jāmisaṃsā́d druhó muñcāmi váruṇasya pā́śāt, anāgásaṃ bráhmaṇā tvā kṛṇomi śivé te dyā́vāpṛthivī́ ubhé stām.*

[9] MV 6.14.7: *tena kho pana samayena aññatarassa bhikkhuno gharadinnakābādho hoti. [bhagavato etamattham ārocesum.] anujānāmi, bhikkhave, sītāloḷiṃ pāyetuṃ ti.* Cf. Buddhaghosa at *Samantapāsādikā* (5: 1092): *gharadinnakābādho ti- vasikaraṇapānakasamuṭṭhitarogo; sītāloḷin ti- naṅgalena kasantassa phāle laggamattikaṃ udakena āloḷevtā pāvetum anujānāmī' ti attho.*

[10] Later *apāmārga* is prescribed against warts on the penis and other parts of the body, as a laxative and a promoter of secretions and against ascites and anasarca. *apāmārga taila* or oil is poured into the ear as a treatment against ringing in the ear and deafness (Dutt and King, *Materia Medica*, 222).

[11] *apāmārgó 'pa mārṣṭu kṣetriyáṃ. . . .*

may have been originally fashioned into an amulet (2.8.2–5). From the passage in the Pāli text, we may assume that clay was also used; this is confirmed by the later ritual (see below). The horn of a buck deer (3.7.1–3) and water (3.7.5) were employed in the rite which commenced at dawn, when the two "unbinding" stars were visible in the sky and may have lasted for several days (2.8.1, 2; 3.7.4, 7). In the rite, the healer employed the often encountered technique of stating that he possesses the proper knowledge for the eradication of the demon (3.7.6.).

The ritual prescribed in the later texts may not be too different from that originally performed:

> With AVŚ 2.8.1 [the healer] washes [the patient] outside [of the house]; with verse 2, [he performs this action] at dawn; with verse 3, after having pulverized [together the plants] mentioned in the verse [and ordinary] clay and clay from an anthill; and after having sewn [this] up in the skin of a [recently killed] healthy animal, he binds [it as an amulet] around [the patient]; with verse 4, [he places] the plow yoked [with oxen] over [his] head [and] sprinkles [water over it]; with verse 5, in an empty house, he pours [some] dregs of ghee in [a cup of] water; [he pours] the remainder [of the dregs] in an old pit into which grass-thatch from the same house has been placed; [and he puts the patient in it], gives [him the water] to sip and washes [him with it]. With AVŚ 3.7 (the following action is performed): the binding [of an amulet made from antelope-horns], the giving [of water] to drink [to the patient], the spitting out [of the water]; when the stars begin to fade, [the healer] sprinkles [the patient with water heated] by the burning of a peg-holed piece of [antelope] skin; from an indeterminate quantity of barley, he takes exactly one handful [and] scatters it; he offers [the patient food].[12]

The mention of deer's horns or antlers is significant.[13] From archaeological evidence we notice that horns constitute one of the dominant motifs on many of the seals and sealings recovered from the various Indus Valley sites. Perhaps one of the most famous examples is found on a seal excavated from Mohenjo-dāro. It depicts a horned deity seated in what appears to be a "yogic" posture. The exact interpretation of this seal, however, is a very hotly debated topic. E. Mackay has pointed out that the horn of the rhinoceros may have had medical importance: "The horns of the rhinoceros are greatly esteemed in Eastern Asia, at the present day for their medicinal qualities and it may well be that they were valued for the same reason at Mohenjo-dāro";[14] and in a note, he adds that the cups made from the

---

[12] KauśS 26.41–27.4; 27.29–31: 26.41. *udagātām ity āplāvayati bahiḥ;* 42. *apeyam iti vyucchantyām;* 43. *babhror iti mantroktam ākṛtiloṣṭavalmīkau parilikhya jīvakoṣaṇyām utsīvya badhnāti;* 27.1. *namas te lāṅgalebhya iti sīrayogam abhiśiro 'vasiñcati;* 2. *namaḥ sanisrasākṣebhya iti śūnyaśālāyām apsu saṃpātān ānayati;* 3. *uttaraṃ jaratkhāte saśālātṛṇe;* 27.29. *hariṇasyeti bandanapāyanācamanaśaṅkudhānajvālenāvanakṣatre 'vasiñcati;* 30. *amitamātrāyāḥ sakṛdgṛhītān yavān āvapati;* 31. *bhaktaṃ prayacchati.* Cf. in particular Bloomfield, *Hymns,* 287, 336 and Caland, AZ, 81–82, 85; see also Henry, *La magie,* 204, 205.

[13] Bloomfield has pointed out that the parts of the deer are often used in magical rites. In addition to the use of its skin and horns at KauśS 27.29–31, he mentions that its skin is employed as an amulet at KauśS 16.13 and that its horn is used at ŚB 3.2.2.20, ĀpŚS 10.9.17 and *Śāntikalpa* 17 and 19 (*Hymns,* 337).

[14] *Further Excavations at Mohenjo-Daro,* 1 (Delhi: Manager of Publication, Government of India Press, 1938), 291.

rhinoceros horn are revered for their ability to reveal the presence of poison.[15] At Mohenjo-dāro, Sir John Marshall discovered pieces of the antlers of four different species of deer: the Kashmīr stag (*Cervus cashmerianus*), and Sambar deer (*Cervus unicolor*), the Hog deer (*Cervus porcinus*), and the Spotted deer (*Cervus axis*).[16] In describing these antlers Marshall explains that many of the fragments, "in addition to the flat end, have cuts and notches on the sides of the horns, where small fragments have been removed. The flat end may have been produced either by sawing when it was removed from the original antler, or may subsequently have been ground down during the process of making powder, in which form the horn is utilized as medicine." [17] The antlers of the Sambar deer were also found at Rangpur (Period III), at Rupar[18] and at Chanhu-dāro.[19]

It is difficult to know exactly what function the horns of the deer played in the healing rites of the early Indians. From the description of the fragments presented by Marshall it appears that the Indus people may have used small pieces removed from the horns as amulets;[20] or, as Marshall has suggested, powdered horn could have been used as a medicine.[21] From the representation of the horned images on the various seals from the Indus sites, one is drawn to the interpretation that horns or antlers may have been utilized as part of a headdress. Similar antler-adorned headpieces are worn by shamans and witch-doctors in various parts of the world.[22] We can notice, therefore, that the horns constituted a part of healing ritual against the internal disease-demon *kṣetriyá* and were also excavated from archaeological sites of the early Indians, suggesting that they were used prior to the Āryan invasions.

2.8

The two illustrious stars, "unbinders," by name, have ascended. Let them release the lowest [and] the highest bond of *kṣetriyá*. 1.
Let this night disappear; let the female demons disappear; let the *kṣetriyá*-destroying plant [cause] the *kṣetriyá* to disappear. 2.
For your sake, let the *kṣetriyá*-destroying plant with the stalk of the white-sectioned, dark-brown barley, with the sesame-blossom of the sesame plant [cause] the *kṣetriyá* to disappear. 3.

---

[15] Ibid., note 1.

[16] *Mohenjo-Daro and the Indus Civilization*, 2: 671–72.

[17] Ibid.

[18] S. R. Rao, "Excavations at Rangpur and Other Exploration in Gujarat," *Ancient India*, 18, 19 (1962–63): 158.

[19] Ernest J. H. Mackay, *Chanhu-Daro Excavations, 1935–36* (New Haven, Connecticut: American Oriental Society, 1943), 52–53.

[20] Cf. KauśS 27.29 where such a use of an antler fragment is suggested (22 above).

[21] Such a usage is prescribed in *The Bower Manuscript*, Pt. 2, vs. 21: *śikhināḍaṃ ruroḥ śṛṅgam ṛṣyaskandhaṃ ghṛtāplutam, dagdham antaḥ puṭe śvāsī lihyāt tan madhusarpiṣā.* See also A. F. Rudolf Hoernle, *The Bower Manuscript*, Pt. 2 (Calcutta: Office of the Superintendent of Government Printing, 1895): 79 and note.

[22] See Willard R. Trask, trans. Mircea Eliade, *Shamanism: Archaic Techniques of Ecstasy* (Princeton: Bollingen Foundation, 1964), 155, 462.

Obeisance to your ploughs; obeisance to [your] poles and yokes. Let
the *kṣetriyá*-destroying plant [cause] the *kṣetriyá* to disappear. 4.
Obeisance to those with very sunken eyes; obeisance to those demons
belonging to the magical realm; obeisance to the lord of the field.
Let the *kṣetriyá*-destroying plant [cause] the *kṣetriyá* to disap-
pear. 5.

3.7

Medicine is on the head of the speedy deer. By means of [his] horn,
he has destroyed the *kṣetriyá,* everywhere. 1.
The buck-deer has chased you with [its] four feet. You, O horn, untie
the *kṣetriyá* who is knotted in this man's heart. 2.
With that which glistens in the distance like a four-pinioned (sided)
canopy, we cause every *kṣetriyá* to vanish from your limbs. 3.
Let those two auspicious stars, "unbinders," by name, which [are]
in the sky, release the lowest [and] the highest bond of *kṣetriyá.* 4.
The waters [are] indeed medicinal; the waters [are] *ámīvā;*-dispellers;
[and] the waters [are] medicines for every [disease]. [Therefore,]
let them release you from *kṣetriyá.* 5.
I know the medicine for that *kṣetriyá* who, because of a prepared
mixture, has taken possession of you. [Therefore,] I [now] destroy
your *kṣetriyá.* 6.
With the departure of the stars and with the departure of the dawns,
let every evil [and] the *kṣetriyá* disappear from us. 7.

4: *RÁPAS*

AVŚ 4.13, 6.91 and ṚV 7.50 are charms devoted to the removal of *rápas* (neuter), a word which is difficult from the point of view both of etymology and of medical history.[1] As early as the *Nirukta* (4.2), Yāska equated *rápas* with *pāpa*, 'evil.' [2] This then served as the basis for the traditional interpretation of the term.[3] More recently, R. Müller has suggested that it is a general expression for fragility and sickness;[4] while R. Emmerick understood it to be a "local morbid symptom," corresponding to the classical Indian medical use of *roga*.[5]

The association of *rápas* with *yákṣma*[6] and with *harimán* ('yellowness'),[7] its cause being stated as a transgression[8] and its connection with the ground, like *kṣetriyá* and *takmán*, all point to a generalized internal disease-demon, occasionally equated with *viṣá* (neuter), 'poison.' [9] Likewise, it is said to have a divine origin[10] and is allied with various evils and demonically caused problems which may, on occasion, suggest the symptoms of the infirmity or the physical and mental states of the individual suffering from the attacks of such a disease-demon.[11]

It was a bodily affliction[12] which often attacked the foot.[13] At ṚV 8.20.26, it is used to describe a sick person who seems to have been suffering from a crooked or deformed limb.[14] In addition to its being divinely sent because of a transgression, its form as a foot-*rápas* appears to have been caused by an evil-looking, crawling animal called *ajakāvá* which was known to have

---

[1] See Mayrhofer, Wb. 3: 41.

[2] *rapo ripram iti pāpanāmanī bhavataḥ.*

[3] See in particular Sāyaṇa to AVŚ 1.22.2, ṚV 10.137.2, etc.

[4] "Medizin im Ṛg-Veda," *Asia Major,* 6 (1930): 345.

[5] "Indo-Iranian concepts of disease and cure," 15; cf. also AVŚ 4.13.4n (127, below), where the equation may be rather with *gada,* which in the tradition of *āyurveda* means 'poison,' and G. J. Meulenbeld, *The Mādhavanidāna,* 505.

[6] AVŚ 4.13.5.

[7] AVŚ 1.22.2.

[8] AVŚ 4.13.1.

[9] AVŚ 6.57.3; 6.91.1, 2 and note; ṚV 8.20.26; 10.59.8–10; 10.60.11.

[10] ṚV 2.33.7; cf. AVŚ 6.57.1.

[11] At ṚV 1.34.11 and 1.57.4 it is connected with *sédhata* ('hostility'); at ṚV 2.33.3, with *áṅhas* ('misery'); at ṚV 8.67.21, *aṅhatí* ('misery'), *dvéṣas* ('enmity') and *sáṃhita* which is obscure. Sāyaṇa glosses it as 'net' (*jālam*) and Geldner follows this interpretation (*Der Rigveda,* 2: 391). Renou suggests: "*sáṃhita* ep. de *rápas* ou plutôt mot indépendant. En ce dernier cas, 'compacité (de liens ou de forces adverses)'; . . ." (EVP 7: 98). At ṚV 8.18.8, it is associated with *srídh* ('failure'); and at ṚV 10.59 there is a possibility that it is connected with *nírṛti* ('destruction').

[12] ṚV 7.34.13; 10.97.10; AVŚ 5.4.10; 6.91.1; cf. also ṚV 8.18.16, where Geldner renders *rápas* as "Leibesschaden" (*Der Rigveda,* 2: 318).

[13] ṚV 7.50.1–3.

[14] *kṣamā́ rápo maruta ā́turasya na (n)íṣkartā víhrutaṃ púnaḥ.*

lived under the skin and to have formed a swelling or eruption which occurred on the *vijā́man* (twin?)-joint and covered the two knees and two ankles.[15] Likewise, it seems to have developed after contact with polluted water.[16] Such a description of the bodily affliction of foot-*rápas* implies an external malady; but its close association with the internal disease-demons makes it rather difficult to isolate as one or the other.[17]

The remedies for *rápas* included water[18] or watery medicines,[19] wind for resuscitation[20] and the plants, barley[21] and *kúṣṭha;* the latter at AVŚ 5.4.10, is requested to eradicate, among other afflictions, bodily *rápas* (*tanvò rápaḥ*). We learn that in the healing rite the healer held the medicinal herbs in one hand, probably his left, while, with his other (right) hand, he stroked the patient;[22] the end result being that the *rápas* was forced downward and into the ground. *takmán*[23] and the unknown-*yákṣma*[24] were also dispelled down into the ground; and a remedy for the *kṣetriyá*-disease required amulets composed of barley.[25] There is also the suggestion that cauterization with fire was used to eradicate the disease.[26] In the *Ṛgveda,* various deities are said to effect the removal of *rápas.*[27]

---

[15] ṚV 7.50.1–2.

[16] ṚV 7.50.3.

[17] There are two other possible occurrences of the word *rápas* in the Ṛgveda; yet there is a debate over the correct reading for each. At ṚV 1.69.8, we read: *tát tú te dáṅso yád áhan samānáir nṛ́bhir yád yuktó vivé rápāṅsi.* Geldner renders: "Das aber ist dein [Agni] Meisterstück, dass was du zerstörtest, du diesen Schaden wieder gutmachst im Bunde mit den gleichgearteten Herren" (*Der Rigveda,* 1: 90). Aufrecht, on the strength of other occurrences of *ápas* with the root *viṣ,* has suggested the reading: *tát tú . . . yuktó vivér ápāṅsi,* and translates: "Das aber ist eine ausserordentliche that von dir, dass du an einem und demselben Tage mit Helden verbündet Werke vollführtest" (KZ 25: 601; cf. Oldenberg, *Vedic Hymns* 2:67). Likewise, at ṚV 6.31.3, the traditional reading is: *dáśa prapitvé ádha sū́ryasya muṣāyáś cakrám ávive rápāṅsi.* Geldner renders: " 'Stachle (deine Rosse) an und raube im Vorlauf das Rad der Sonne!' (So) hast du [Indra] die Scharten ausgewetzt" (*Der Rigveda,* 2: 130 and note). Aufrecht would suggest *áviver ápāṅsi,* i.e. "You have carried out the works" (KZ 25: 601; cf. Oldenberg, *Vedic Hymns* 2: 69).

It is difficult to know if Aufrecht's emendations are correct. Since the occurrence of *ápas* with the root *viṣ* is not uncommon (see, in particular, ṚV 4.19.10; 7.21.4 and 10.147.1 which has the phrase *vivér apáḥ;* but, the emended reading for *apáḥ* is *ápaḥ,* Aufrecht, KZ, 25: 601–602 and Oldenberg, *Vedic Hymns,* 2: 68–69), the suggested changes to the text at first seem reasonable. It should be noted, however, that, according to the traditional reading, Agni, a known healer, at ṚV 1.69.8, was said to have repaired the *rápas;* while Indra, who is not noted as a healer, at ṚV 6.31.3, was said to have performed the same task. Moreover, only in this one instance do we find Indra in association with *rápas;* whereas Agni is connected with it at ṚV 7.50.2. A complete resolution to the problem is, therefore, not to be found.

[18] ṚV 7.50.4; AVŚ 6.91.3.

[19] ṚV 8.20.23–25; cf. also AVŚ 6.57.1–3.

[20] AVŚ 4.13.2–3; ṚV 8.18.9 and 10.137.2–3.

[21] AVŚ 6.91.1.

[22] AVŚ 4.13.6–7; cf. also ṚV 10.97.11–12.

[23] AVŚ 5.22.2, 4.

[24] AVŚ 6.127.3.

[25] AVŚ 2.8.3.

[26] ṚV 7.50.2.

[27] The Aśvins at 1.34.11, 157.4 and 8.18.3; the Viśvedevas at 7.34.13; 10.137.5; Heaven and Earth at 8.18.16; 10.59.8–10; Rudra at 2.33.3 and The Ādityas at 8.67.21.

The later ritual tradition, to which AVŚ 6.91 (and 5.9) is attached, points to a possible use of barley in the original rite:

With AVŚ 5.9 and 6.91, [the healer] pours four [portions] of the dregs of ghee into a water-jar; two [portions are poured] on the earth; having recovered those two, he washes [the patient with them]; and [putting the dregs] in [a cup] with barley, he binds [to the patient] a barley [-amulet], while [reciting] the latter [hymn, i.e. 6.91].[28]

The characteristics mentioned above suggest that in at least one aspect *rápas* was conceived to be a demonically caused infirmity which, in the form of an ugly, worm-like creature, attacked its victim from the water and poisoned him. It was found to inhabit an area of the body, under an eruption of the skin, around the joints of both extremities. This description, along with the general internal symptoms of jaundice, consumption and mental unrest, strongly suggest dracunculiasis or guinea-worm disease.[29] It is significant that a part of its ritual cure seemed to have required that the creature be extracted with barley which may have been used in a type of poultice or as an amulet,[30] for barley is employed in the later ritual as an amulet and barley-meal which, along with buttermilk, is made into ball-poultices, is mentioned in the *Bhāvaprakāśa* (midsixteenth century A.D.) as an effective means for drawing out the thread-like string of the guinea worm.[31]

4.13

O gods, you gods bring [him] up again who was put down; and then, O gods, you gods revive him again who has committed a sin. 1.

These two winds blow here from the Sindhu, from afar. Let the one blow dexterity to you; let the other blow away *rápas*. 2.

O wind, blow medicine here; O wind, blow away *rápas*. For you, who are medicine for all [diseases], go [about as] messenger of the gods. 3.

Let the gods rescue this [man]; let the troops of the Maruts rescue [him] and let all beings rescue [him], so that he may be devoid of *rápas*. 4.

---

[28] KauśS 28.17–20: 17. *dive svāhemaṃ yavam iti catura udapātre saṃpātān ānayati;* 18. *dvau pṛthivyām;* 19. *tau pratyāhṛtyāplāvayati;* 20. *sayave cottareṇa yavaṃ badhnāti.* Cf. Bloomfield, *Hymns,* 507, and Caland, AZ, 90–91. On ritual using 4.13 (variant at ṚV 10.137), see notes to 4.13, 124–28 below.

[29] See Thomas T. Mackie, et al., *A Manual of Tropical Medicine* (Philadelphia: W. B. Saunders Company, 1945), 362–66.

[30] See notes to 6.91.1, 128–30 below.

[31] Claus Vogel, "On the Guinea-Worm Disease in Indian Medicine," *Adyar Library Bulletin* 25 (1961): 62. Vogel contends that dracunculiasis did not occur in India until the eighth century A.D., when it was introduced by the Muslims and was given the name *snāyuka* ('sinew-worm') (58). This assertion will have to be reexamined in light of the foregoing analysis.

I have come to you with beneficial and healthy means; I have brought to you powerful dexterity [and] I [now] dispel your *yákṣma.* 5.

This [is] my propitious hand; that [is] my more propitious one. This [is] my [hand] with medicines for all [diseases]; and that [is] the one with a beneficial stroke. 6.

[It is said that] the tongue precedes words; [thus,] I stroke you by means of those two curative hands—hands which are ten-branched. 7.

6.91

I draw out backward (unwrap) your bodily *rápas* with this barley [grown on land which] they repeatedly ploughed with yokes of eight [and] with yokes of six [oxen]. 1.

[As] the wind blows downward, the sun shines downward [and] the cow gives milk downward, [just so] let your *rápas* go. 2.

The waters [are] indeed medicinal; the waters [are] the *ámīvā*-dispellers [and] the waters [are] medicines for every [disease]. [Therefore,] let them make (be) medicine for you. 3.

ṚV 7.50

Protect me, O Mitra and Varuṇa, in this world and do not let that which nests and forms a swelling come to us. I remove that evil-looking *ajakāvá.* Do not let the crawling creature befall me with the foot-*rápas.* 1.

Let the flaming Agni expel from here that *vándana* which may occur in the *vijā́man*-joint [and] which may cover over the two knees, the two ankles. Do not let the crawling creature befall me with foot-*rápas.* 2.

Let all the gods drive away from here that poison which is in the *śalmalí*-tree, which is in the stream [and] which is produced from herbs. Do not let the crawling creature befall me with foot-*rápas.* 3.

Let all those divine rivers, swelling with water [and] auspicious to us, which [flow] from the slopes, from the depths (springs?) and from the heights (rain?), which are rich in water and waterless, be devoid of *śípada,* devoid of *śímidā.* 4.

5: *HṚDDYOTÁ (HṚDROGÁ)* (CHEST-PAIN; ANGINA PECTORIS?), *HARIMÁN* (JAUNDICE)

AVŚ 1.22 is a charm directed against the removal of two internal disease-entities or better, disease-symptoms, *hṛddyotá* and *harimán*. *hṛddyotá* or *hṛdrogá* (ṚV 1.50.11) is a controversial term which Filliozat has fairly convincingly shown to mean "éclat qui est dans le coeur" or simply heart-affliction, probably referring to a burning pain in the chest (angina pectoris?), and synonymous with *hṛdayāmayá*[1] which at AVŚ 6.14.1 is an affliction associated with *balā́sa* and, at 5.30.9 and 6.127.3, is connected with the *yákṣma*s and *balā́sa*. *hṛddyotá* is said to be an ailment sent to foes[2] and a disease or symptom characteristic of internal diseases.[3] *harimán* means 'yellowness' and quite naturally suggests jaundice, which is rather a symptom than an actual malady.[4] It is equally associated with a wide range of demons, in particular internal disease-demons, including *rápas* (1.22.2), and its residence is stated as being in the limbs.[5] Since both are so closely connected with a vast majority of the internal disease-entities, it would seem likely that *hṛddyotá*, 'heart-affliction' or 'chest-pain,' and *harimán*, 'yellowness,' 'jaundice,' represented the most obvious symptoms which these demons manifested. R. Müller has also come to this conclusion.[6] He has, however, gone too far by asserting that both *hṛdrogá* (*hṛddyotá*) and *harimán* exemplify the essential fiery nature or association with the god Agni which lies at the root of all Vedic diseases.[7] Both Filliozat[8] and Karambelkar[9] suggest a causal relationship between these two entities, i.e. the heart-affliction or chest-pain is the cause of, or a complication of, the yellowness or jaundice. Since they often occur separately, however, the theory faces certain difficulties.[10] The evidence suggests rather that they represent major disease-symptoms which, because of their frequency and intensity of occurrence, were looked upon as demons.

The principal remedy for *hṛddyotá* was water,[11] while that for *harimán* was ointment (*ā́ñjana*).[12] The present charm (1.22) demonstrates the use

---

[1] *La doctrine*, 89–90 and n.
[2] AVŚ 5.20.12.
[3] AVŚ 6.24.1.
[4] Filliozat, *La doctrine*, 89. Karambelkar, however, asserts that it is a proper disease (*The Atharva-Veda and the Āyurveda*, 205).
[5] AVŚ 9.8.9.
[6] "Die Gelbsucht der Alt-Inder," *Janus*, 34 (1930): 188–89.
[7] "Medizin im Ṛg-Veda," *Asia Major*, 9 (1930): 359–61, and "Die Gelbsucht . . . ," 186.
[8] *La doctrine*, 89.
[9] *The Atharva-Veda and the Āyurveda*, 207–209.
[10] See also R. Müller, "Medizin im Ṛg-Veda," 360–61.
[11] AVŚ 6.24.1.
[12] AVŚ 4.9.3; 19.44.2.

of associative magic for the removal of these two symptoms. The purpose of the healing rite as illustrated by this charm was to eliminate the undesired bodily condition and to replace it with the desired one. The sun, which is the source of heat and is yellow in color, is a suitable place to send the patient's burning chest-pain and jaundice. The redness of the bull, approximating the normal hue of a healthy individual, is the desired color. In every way, the healer endeavors to surround the victim with redness (verses 1–3). His aim was to overwhelm and to drive away the undesired color with the desired one. In the final verse, the healer exorcises the demon, i.e. jaundice, with the use of birds which are naturally yellow and thus suitable hosts for jaundice.[13] He requests them to remove the yellowness and to carry it completely away to a place, perhaps near the sun, where it could no longer affect anyone. This charm represents one of the best examples of associative or sympathetic magic among the healing hymns of the *Ṛg-* and *Atharva-Veda*s.

The often quoted ritual practice prescribed in the *Kauśika Sūtra* is an excellent example of this principle found among many archaic and primitive peoples, as is well illustrated by Sir James Frazer.[14] The actions may, therefore, be not too different from those originally performed:

> With AVŚ 1.22, [the healer] makes [the patient] sip [water] mixed with the hair of that mentioned in the hymn (i.e. a red bull); and, after having poured [water] over the back [of the bull], [he makes the patient sip it]; having seated [the patient] on the [red] hide, he binds a [piece of] peg-holed [hide steeped] in cow's milk and smeared with the dregs of ghee [as an amulet around his neck]; he gives [him the milk] to drink; [he gives him] food of rice-pap mixed with turmeric (*haridrā*); having smeared [him from the head,] ending with the tip of the toe, with both the remnants [of the pap] and [the pap] not yet eaten, and then having bound [the birds] mentioned in the hymn [i.e. the parrot, the *ropaṇākā* (thrush) and *hāridrava* (yellow wagtail)—all yellow in color] by the left legs at the foot of a couch [on which the patient is placed], he washes [the birds and the patient] with water; [after having given him a stirred food or pap,] he makes [the patient] step forth; [he] allows [the patient] to address the noisy [birds with the hymn, in order to quieten them]; [finally], having smeared the breast-hairs [of the red-bull's hide] with gum [in order to make them stick together] and having covered them with gold (?), [he binds it as an amulet around the patient].[15]

---

[13] Henry, *La magie*, 182.

[14] *The Golden Bough* (New York: The Macmillan Company, 1963, abridged edition), 12–55.

[15] KauśS 26.14–21: 14. *anu sūryam iti mantroktasya lomamiśram ācamayati*; 15. *pṛṣṭhe cānīya*; 16. *śaṅkudhānaṃ carmaṇy āsīnāya dugdhe saṃpātavantaṃ badhnāti*; 17. *pāyayati*; 18. *haridraudanabhuktam ucchiṣṭānucchiṣṭenā prapadāt pralipya mantroktān adhas talpe haritasūtreṇa savyajaṅghāsu baddhvāvasnāpayati*; 19. *prapādayati*; 20. *vadata upasthāpayati*; 21. *kroḍalomāni jatunā saṃdihya jātarūpeṇāpidhāpya*. See also Bloomfield, *Hymns*, 263–64 and Caland, AZ, 75–76, who has a slightly different rendering for the last *sūtra*. Cf. also Henry, who explains that the charm and the later rite are examples both of homeopathic and of allopathic magic, *La magie*, 182 and n.

1.22

Let your *hṛddyotá* (chest-pain) and yellowness go up to the sun. [For] we surround you with the color of the red bull. 1.

We surround you with the red colors so that you may live for a long time. In order that he be without *rápas,* likewise, let him be yellowless. 2.

In [their] every shape [and] in [their] every nourishment, we surround you with those cows whose divinity is red (Rohiṇī) and who are [themselves] red. 3.

We put your yellowness on to the parrots [and] on to the *ropaṇā̄kā̄s*. Also we deposit your yellowness on to the *hā̄ridravas*. 4.

6: *BALĀ́SA* (SWELLING)

AVŚ 6.14 and 6.127 are charms devoted principally to the eradication of the disease-demon *balā́sa* who appears to have been a type of symptomatic swelling commonly associated with internal diseases. The native commentators Sāyaṇa and Mahīdhara (to VS 12.97) have understood the word to mean consumption or tuberculosis; and this was followed by H. Zimmer. Grohmann considered it to be a type of aqueous sore or swelling commonly found on a fever-patient. Ludwig has rendered it as 'dropsy'; Bloomfield, however, has explained that its exact meaning is uncertain.[1] Filliozat, after examining the occurrence in the Vedic literature and the texts of classical Indian medicine, concluded that it probably referred to "affections oedémateuses";[2] and Karambelkar, considering that *balā́sa* is related to *kilā́sa*(leukoderma) in form, posited that it was a skin-disease.[3]

The Atharvavedic hymns imply that *balā́sa* was a type of internal disease, *yákṣma,*[4] being called specifically, the brother of *takmán.*[5] He is said to be seated in the limbs, in the joints, to loosen the bones and the joints and to afflict the heart.[6] He is described as testicle-like lumps situated in the armpit[7] and perhaps as having a red color similar to *vidradhá* (abscess) and *visálpaka* (*visalpá*),[8] a type of cutaneous swelling.[9] One of his causes appears to have been excessive emotion, for he is said to arise out of desire, abhorrence, and from the heart.[10]

The healer removed him by cutting him out (surgically), requesting him to dry up, become like ash, and fly away.[11] The principal remedy for him was the *cīpúdru*-plant,[12] which may have been called specifically the

---

[1] Macdonell-Keith, *Vedic Index,* 2: 61–62.

[2] *La doctrine,* 98.

[3] *The Atharva-Veda and the Āyurveda,* 219.

[4] AVŚ 9.8.10; cf. also AVŚ 6.127.3.

[5] AVŚ 5.22.11–12.

[6] AVŚ 6.14.1; cf. also AVŚ 5.30.9; 6.127.3 and 9.8.8.

[7] AVŚ 6.127.2.

[8] AVŚ 6.127.1, 3; cf. 9.8.2, 20 and VS 12.97 at ṚV 10.97.23n, where *upacít* (cf. *apacít*), and *pākārú* (hemorrhoids?) are mentioned along with *bā́lasa* (248–49, below).

[9] *visálpaka* (*visalpá*) appears also to be a type of *yákṣma* affecting all limbs (AVŚ 6.127.3; 9.8.3, 5; 19.44.2; cf. also VS 12.97 at ṚV 10.97.23n) which is specified as a type of head affliction, located in the two ears, the two eyes and the *káṅkūṣas* (?) (AVŚ 6.127.3; 9.8.1–2). He is said to contain poison and is associated with *vidradhá* (abscess), *vātīkārá* (a symptom of injury caused by a wound) and *alají* (a type of abscess) (AVŚ 9.8.20). Like *balā́sa* and jaundice, etc., one of its remedies included *ā́ñjana* (ointment) (AVŚ 19.44.2). It is, therefore, likely that *visálpaka* was also a demonically caused cutaneous swelling, symptomatic of internal diseases.

[10] AVŚ 9.8.8.

[11] AVŚ 6.14.2, 3; 9.8.10; see also Karambelkar, *The Atharva-Veda and the Āyurveda,* 220.

[12] AVŚ 6.127.2.

balāsa-destroying plant.[13] Ointment (*āñjana*) was also said to be effective against him and against yellowness or jaundice, both of whom were symptoms of *takmán*,[14] and the *jaṅgiḍá*-amulet was employed to protect the patient from further attacks from *balāsa* and *takmán* by making them powerless.[15]

Being derivative and secondary, the ritual mentioned in the later text has very little to offer to our understanding of the original practice:

> With AVŚ 6.14, [the healer] sprinkles [the patient] with water by means of a woodchip which is smeared with the dregs of ghee on a reed-mat [situated] in water. With AVŚ 6.127, [the healer] anoints [the patient] with a [pulverized piece] of *palāśa*-wood, four fingers wide (or long) and pours the dregs of ghee over the head of one seized by Varuṇa (i.e. suffering from ascites).[16]

There is the faint possibility that the plant *cīpúdru* mentioned at AVŚ 6.127.2 is the same as the *palāśa*-tree referred to in the ritual text.

The implication, therefore, is that *balāsa* was considered to be a swelling or an eruption on the skin, symptomatic, like jaundice, of internal disorders. This then could have given rise to its inclusion as one of the internal demons of disease.

6.14

Destroy every *balāsa*, who is seated in the limbs and in the joints, the indwelling one who loosens the bones and the joints [and] afflicts the heart. 1.

I eradicate the *balāsa* of the *balāsa*-victim, like a *muṣkará* (or *puṣkará*, 'lotus') [and] I cut through his link [to the body] as the root of the *urvārú*-plant (gourd). 2.

O *balāsa*, fly forth out of here, as the very young *āśuṃgá* (-bird?), and like the annual grass, pass away without destroying [our] men. 3.

6.127

O tree, O herb, do not let even a small bit of the red *balāsa*, the *vidradhá* (abscess), the *visálpaka* (swelling) remain. 1.

O *balāsa*, your two withdrawn testicles which are hidden in the armpit, I know the splendid medicine for that—*cīpúdru*. 2.

We tear away the *visálpaka* (swelling) who is in the limbs, in the two ears [and] in the two eyes, the *vidradhá* (abscess) [and] the heart-affliction; [likewise] we dispel down [and] away that unknown *yákṣma*. 3.

---

[13] AVŚ 8.7.10; cf. VS 12.97 at ṚV 10.97.23n (248–49 below).

[14] AVŚ 4.9.3, 5.

[15] AVŚ 19.34.10.

[16] KauśS 29.30; 26.34; 26.39: 29.30. *asthisraṃsam iti śakalenāpsv iṭe saṃpātavatāvasiñcati*; 26.34. *upottamena palāśasya caturaṅgenālimpati*; 26.39. *pañcamena varuṇagṛhītasya mūrdhni saṃpātān ānayati*. Cf. Bloomfield, *Hymns*, 463, 530, and Caland, *AZ*, 79, 80, 95. See also chapter on Ascites, below, 62.

7: *TAKMÁN* (FEVERS; MALARIA, ETC.)[1]

AVŚ 1.25; 5.22; 6.20 and 7.116(121) are charms against the internal disease-demon, *par excellence, takmán,* and AVŚ 5.4; 6.95 and 19.39 are charms used in the consecration of its principal cure, the *kúṣṭha*-plant.

Since V. Grohmann made the astute observation that *takmán* bore a very close resemblance to malarial fever, nothing new has been advanced on the subject.[2] As many of the symptoms and characteristics, which we are about to outline, demonstrate, the disease *takmán* in many of its qualities resembles malaria as it was first described in the Hippocratic works and in the writings of Celsus.[3] Likewise, the references to its most severely felt occurrence during the rainy season allude to the *anopheles* mosquitoes which breed abundantly during this time of the year and act as vectors of the disease. Not all of the symptoms, however, correspond precisely to what we know to be the tropical disease malaria, suggesting that all similar types of disease characterized by high fever and chills must be meant. The dominant febrile malady indicated by *takmán* is, nevertheless, malaria; in which case, this would be the earliest recorded testimony of the occurrence of the disease.

We hope to show that to the Vedic Indians, its cause—indeed, the demon itself—was conceived to be something quite different: they considered, above all, *takmán* to be a divinity,[4] who, in the form of the thunder and lightning which accompanied the monsoon rains, attacked his victim, bringing about the morbid bodily condition characterized by intermittent and recurring fevers, chills along with other symptoms.

---

[1] A shorter version of this chapter has appeared; see my "Fever in Vedic India," JAOS, 103.3 (1983): 617–21.

[2] "Medizinisches aus dem Atharva-Veda, mit besonderem Bezug auf den Takman," IS, 9: 381–423; Weber was perhaps the first western scholar to make the connection between *takmán* and fever, IS 4: 419. For other references see in particular Macdonell-Keith, *Vedic Index,* 1: 294–96; R. Müller, "Der *Takman* des *Atharvaveda* . . . ," *Artibus Asiae* (Leipzig) 6(1937): 230–42; Filliozat, *La doctrine,* 96–7; Karambelkar, who tried to find three separate febrile diseases in the word: malarial fever, influenza and typhoid fever, *The Atharva-veda and The Āyur-veda,* 289, and K. Hoffmann, *Aufsätze,* 1: 153–54.

[3] See A. Castiglioni, *A History of Medicine,* trans. from Italian by E. B. Krumbhaar, second rev. ed. (New York: Alfred A. Knopf, 1947), 163, 207–208.

[4] It became deified by its association with other gods: Homage is paid to it along with Rudra and King Varuṇa (AVŚ 6.20.2); it is called the son of Varuṇa (AVŚ 1.25.3); it is given the epithet the thousand-eyed immortal (P 5.21.7 = 13.1.14) which at AVŚ 11.2.3 is Rudra. It is associated with Yama (P 19.12.11); it accompanies the gods (P 1.45.1) and it is extolled and called breath at AVŚ 11.4.11.

Symptoms and associations

The chief symptom which the *takmán*-victim exhibits is a hot-cold fever-syndrome.[5] He also suffers from severe headaches, pounding in the eyes, bodily *rápas,*[6] thirst,[7] and redness and soreness of the joints.[8] He is often jaundiced,[9] coughs, and is afflicted by the disease-entities of *balā́sa* (swelling), *udyugá* (uncontrollable shaking?), *pāmán* (rash), *anvṛja* (*anvṛju*) (?) and *yákṣma.*[10] In fact, *takmán* is put in a familiar relationship with *balā́sa* (swelling), his brother, cough, his sister and *pāmán* (rash), his evil cousin.[11]

Types

The ancient Indians understood the types of *takmán* to be that which recurs daily (quotidian), in two days, every third day (tertian), and that which has the third day free (quartan?), that which is continual, that which lasts the entire year, and that which attacks in the autumn, in the summer and in the rainy season.[12]

Various epithets

As we have noticed, *takmán* has a special connection with the yellow color of jaundice; in fact, he is called the god of the yellow one.[13] He is also known to be of a red, a brown and a grey color.[14] He is called the fist-striker of the *śakambhará* (?),[15] malicious,[16] powerful,[17] unruly,[18] wild,[19] shaking, driving and violent,[20] evil, awesome, indestructible and inciting.[21] He is said to enter men[22] and to make them tremble.[23] He also has an esoteric name, *hrū́ḍu,* which is important for his removal.[24]

---

[5] See AVŚ 1.25.4; 5.22.2, 10, 13; 7.116(121).1; P 1.45.1–3; 16.74.6.
[6] AVŚ 5.4.10; 19.39.10.
[7] P 1.45.1.
[8] AVŚ 5.22.3.
[9] See AVŚ 1.25.2, 3; 5.22.2; 6.20.3; cf. also AVŚ 4.9.3, 8; 19.44.1, 2.
[10] See AVŚ 4.9.8; 5.4.9; 5.22.10–12; P 1.45.4; 5.21.6; see also AVŚ 5.30.16 where the hundred pains (*śátaṃ rópīś*) of *takmán* are said to have been exorcised along with *yákṣma*.
[11] See AVŚ 5.22.12.
[12] See AVŚ 1.25.4; 5.22.13; 9.8.6; 19.34.10; 19.39.10; P 1.32.5; 1.45 1.
[13] AVŚ 1.25.2, 3.
[14] See AVŚ 5.22.3; 6.20.3; P 1.45.2; 19.12.10.
[15] AVŚ 5.22.4.
[16] AVŚ 5.22.6.
[17] AVŚ 5.22.9.
[18] AVŚ 6.20.1; 7.116(121).2.
[19] AVŚ 6.20.3.
[20] AVŚ 7.116(121).1.
[21] P 1.45.1–3.
[22] P 1.45.2.
[23] AVŚ 9.8.6.
[24] AVŚ 1.25.2, 3.

Cause and identification with lightning and thunder

At AVŚ 11.2.22 and 26, fever and cough are called Rudra's missiles or arrows which were conceived to be lightning streaks accompanied with thunder, i.e. the noise of a stallion horse.[25] Likewise, *takmán* is said to strike with a thunderbolt,[26] to possess dreaded missiles,[27] to be flashing and possessing fiery weapons,[28] to be a flame-thrower[29] and to be a flash of lightning.[30] He is characterized as resounding thunder[31] whose fading noise may resemble that of a chattering drunkard.[32] In his aspect as lightning, the poet-healer relates a mythological story which recounts how, as Agni, he was born from the waters (the rain-clouds).[33]

In another charm (AVŚ 1.12) whose use, according to the tradition, is both in a medical rite[34] and in a rite against bad weather,[35] there are similarities between the afflictions caused by *takmán* and those brought about by lightning and thunder. In verse 2, the healer makes obeisance and worships that demon who takes possession of every limb by heat and is known as the seizer who seized the joints.[36] Likewise, in verse 3, the demonic lightning and thunder is said to have entered the victim's every joint and made his head ache and caused him to cough.[37] The charm's first verse

---

[25] Vs.22. *yásya takmā́ kā́sikā hetír ékam áśvasyeva vŕ̥ṣaṇaḥ kránda éti, abhipūrvám̐ nirṇáyate námo astv asmai.* Vs.26: *mā́ no rudra takmánā mā́ viṣéṇa mā́ naḥ sáṃ srā divyénāgnínā, anyátrāsmád vidyútaṃ pātayaitā́m.*

[26] AVŚ 5.22.6.

[27] AVŚ 5.22.7.

[28] AVŚ 6.20.1.

[29] AVŚ 6.20.3.

[30] P 19.12.10.

[31] P 13.1.9.

[32] AVŚ 6.20.1; P 19.12.10.

[33] See AVŚ 1.25.1; P 1.45.1.2; cf. also AVŚ 5.22.3 where it is called the son of the grey one (i.e. rain-cloud).

[34] Sāyaṇa prescribes its use in a rite against disease "born of the derangement of the *vāta, pitta* and *śleṣman*" at KauśS 26.1–9 (*vātapittaśleṣmavikārajeṣu*); see also Keśava: *atha vātapittaśleṣmāṇi bhaiṣajyāny ucyante.* At AthPariś 34.7 it is counted as among "the group of hymns for the destruction of *takmán*" (*takmanāśanagaṇa*); and the *AV-Anukramaṇī* describes it as a hymn for the "destruction of *yákṣma*" (*yákṣmanāśanaṃ sūktam*). Verse 3 is found among the *mr̥gāra*-hymns at KauśS 27.34 against all diseases (cf. Bloomfield, *Hymns,* 247–48 and Whitney-Lanman, Pt. 1, 12–13).

[35] Sāyaṇa mentions that it is also to be used in a rite for the warding off of bad (cloudy) weather and heavy rain at KauśS 38.1–7 (*tathā durdinanivāraṇe ativr̥ṣṭer nivāraṇe ca*). Cf. Keśava: *atha naimittikāny ucyante,* i.e., *durdinavināśakarmaṇāṃ vidhiṃ vakṣyāmaḥ* (cf. Whitney-Lanman, Pt. 1, 13).

[36] *áṅge-aṅge śocíṣā śiśriyāṇáṃ namasyántas tvā havíṣā vidhema, aṅkā́nt samaṅkā́n haviṣā vidhema yó ágrabhīt párvāsyā grábhītā.* P 1.17.2 has in *ab:* . . . *śiśriyāṇo yo agrabhīt parurasya grabhītā* and in *cd:* . . . *yajāmi hr̥di śrito manaso yo jajāna,* "I sacrifice . . . [of him] who, contained in the heart, was born of the mind(?)" (cf. Renou, JA, 252: 427).

[37] *muñcá śīrṣaktyā́ utá kāsá enaṃ páruṣ-parur āvivéśā yó asya, yó abhrajā́ vātajā yáś ca śúṣmo vánaspatīnt sacatāṃ párvatāṃś ca.* In *cd,* the notions of the flash (*śúṣma,* cf. Bloomfield, ZDMG, 48: 565–74 and *Hymns,* 7 and Filliozat, *La doctrine,* 140 n) and being born of the wind and of the thundercloud, which is requested to direct itself to the trees and the mountains, brings to mind the technique employed by the healer who sends the *takmán* back to the mountains where it originated (AVŚ 5.22.5, 8, 9, 12; P 13.1.9, 15) to attack others (AVŚ 5.22.6, 7; 6.20.1; cf. P 1.45.3; 13.1.9).

presents an interesting mythological episode in which the thunder and lightning are called the first bright bull, born of the *jarāyujá* (cloud conceived as after-birth?),[38] of the wind and of the thundercloud, which proceeds with the rain making a roaring noise.[39] This mythological story suggests the origin of *takmán* who, like Agni, was born of the rain-clouds. Although this charm does not specifically mention *takmán*, it does present elements which point to a connection between the demonic power of lightning and thunder and the disease-demon *takmán*.[40]

It is not difficult, therefore, to see why these ancient people sympathetically associated their morbid bodily condition with a demonic deity who struck with a thunderstorm. To be sure, there was the connection between the rains and the outbreak of fever. The people, however, were quite unaware of any further association. The jaundice and the cough were to them caused by the yellow streak of lightning, and the thunder which accompanied it—a deep cough could quite easily resemble the sound of thunder. Similarly, the severe heat of the fever and the delirium were aspects of the fiery, unruly, wild and violent nature of the demon. Likewise, the throbbing and heat in the head and the pounding in the eyes were his flashing and thundering qualities manifesting themselves in the victim's body. In almost every instance, this connection seems to hold true. The most dreaded disease-demon of ancient India, *takmán*, therefore, was conceived to be the lightning and thunder which entered an unsuspecting victim.

Cure

The cure for one possessed by such a demonic force required a rather elaborate ritual. First, the healer had to appease the demon. He did this by paying homage to him.[41] He then had to gain access to his world. This was accomplished by knowing the secret key, the demon's esoteric name, *hrū́ḍu*.[42] Once he had appeased him and had entered his realm, he could then dispel him. He sent him, like other internal demons of disease, back to where he originated,[43] and also downward, deep into the ground, where he would be harmless to living things.[44] Because of his awesome destructive

---

[38] Cf. Filliozat, *La doctrine*, 124.

[39] *jarāyujáḥ prathamá usríyā vŕ̥ṣā vātābhrajā́ stanáyann eti vr̥ṣṭyā́, sá no mr̥ḍāti tanvà r̥jugó ruján yá ékam ójas tredhā́ vicakramé*. P 1.17.1 has in *b*: *vātabhrajā́* (so also, Roth-Whitney for Śau) *etu*; and in *c*: *mr̥ḍā́t* (cf. Renou, JA, 252: 427 and Hoffmann, IIJ, 11: 2–3.). The request of the lightning and thunder to spare the body in *cd*, brings to mind the refrain of AVŚ 1.25.1–3 in which the healer beseeches the *takmán* to pass over its intended victims.

[40] Weber went as far as to entitle the charm: "Gegen hitzige Fieber (Against Burning Fever)," IS, 4: 405; similarly, Bloomfield: "Prayer to lightning, conceived as the cause of fever, headache, and cough," *Hymns*, 7.

[41] See AVŚ 1.25.1–4; 6.20.1–3; 7.116(121).1; P 1.45.1, 2, 4.

[42] AVŚ 1.25.2–3.

[43] See AVŚ 5.22.5, 8, 9, 12, 14(?); P 13.1.9, 15.

[44] See AVŚ 5.22.2–4; cf. AVŚ 19.39.10.

force, he often sent him to attack enemies and other undesirables.[45] Perhaps the most interesting substitute victims to which the healer dispatched *takmán* were frogs[46] which, as we know from the famous Frog-hymn of ṚV 7.103, were most active during the rains, filling the air with the melodious notes of their chorus.[47] The use of a frog is also found in later ritualistic literature from which we may gain insight into its purpose. At KauśS 32.17 the prescription is as follows:

While reciting AVŚ 7.116(121) the healer does as in the case of birds (see KauśS 26.18), i.e. he binds with a red thread and a blue thread a frog, stripped like reeds, by the feet (or armpits) [to the bed on which the patient is made to lie down and sprinkles him with water].[48]

From this, we notice that the frog, whose nature is cool and wet, served as the receptacle for the hot fever. Bloomfield[49] and Henry[50] consider that such a practice is an example of allopathic, as opposed to homeopathic, medicine which is exemplified at KauśS 26.14–21 (AVŚ 1.22), where yellow birds are used to carry away the yellowness (jaundice) of a patient. This is, indeed, one explanation. Filliozat, however, has proposed a different, equally valid, interpretation:

La présence de la grenouille pourrait contrebalancer la fièvre proprement dite mais non pas le froid du frisson. D'autre part, dans la prescription, les mots "comme les oiseaux" se rapportent à ce qui est dit dans une prescription antérieure (26.18) d'après laquelle on doit attacher au bas de la couche du malade "ceux qui sont mentionnés dans le vers védique à réciter à cette occasion" (AV 1.22.4), c'est-à-dire des oiseaux jaunes auxquels on renvoie le jaune d'un malade atteint de jaunisse. Dans ce cas les oiseaux jaunes, loin d'être utilisés pour combattre le symptôme morbide le sont pour attirer le jaune anormal chez le malade vers le jaune qui est normal chez eux. La grenouille a donc chance de représenter plutôt un habitat d'élection pour le froid du frisson qu'un élément ennemi de la fièvre.[51]

In this way, Filliozat understands both the yellow birds and the frog to be used homeopathically or, to use Frazer's term, sympathetically, in the healing rite. Both explanations seem valid in their own way. Bloomfield and Henry have taken into account the hot aspect of the fever, but have neglected the cold (*śītá*). Filliozat, on the other hand, has focused upon an explanation of the fever's chilly nature, but has not given due consideration to its hot (*rūrá*) aspect. It seems that, by its very nature, the frog, both in the original ritual and in that prescribed in the later *sūtra*, may have been

---

[45] See AVŚ 5.22.6, 7, 12(?); 6.20.1; cf. P 1.45.3; 13.1.9.

[46] AVŚ 17.116(121).2.

[47] See Geldner, *Der Rigveda*, 2: 271–73 and L. Renou, *Hymnes spéculatifs du Véda* (Paris: Gallimard, 1956), 45, 235 and EVP, 16: 112–13.

[48] *namo rūrāyeti śakunīn iveṣīkāñjimaṇḍūkaṃ nīlalohitābhyāṃ sūtrābhyāṃ sakakṣaṃ baddhvā.* See also Caland, AZ, 106, and Bloomfield, *Hymns*, 565–66.

[49] Ibid., 566–67.

[50] *La magie*, 181.

[51] *Magie et médecine* (Paris: Presses Universitaires de France, 1943), 101.

purposely and symbolically used, so that both qualities of the demonic *takmán* could find a suitable host. In this way, both interpretations, though different are in basic agreement.

On the use of frogs in healing rites in Europe, Grohmann has noted an interesting Bohemian practice in which a frog is used to cure the chills of fever. Accordingly, a green frog, which is caught on a dewy morning preceding St. George's day, is sewn into a bag which is hung around the neck of a patient unaware of its contents. It is to remain there for nine days, during which time the patient is to recite nine Lord's Prayers, one each day before sunrise. On the ninth day, he must go, praying, to a river, throw the bag into it, return home praying, and never look back.[52]

The remainder of the *sūtra*s connected with *takmán* also indicate a fundamentally symbolic ritual, reflecting a definite archaism:

> With AVŚ 1.25, [the healer] heats an axe, while muttering [the hymn]; [then,] plunging [the axe] into water in order to bring the liquid to a boil, he sprinkles [it over the patient]. With AVŚ 5.22 (also 6.20), [the healer] gives [the patient] a gruel made from fried rice to drink; by means of a copper vessel, he pours the dregs [of the gruel] over the head [of the patient and] into [a fire stemming from] a conflagration.[53]

The two basic remedies or medicines which the healer employed were *ā̃ñjana,* ointment, probably used to remove the jaundice and *balā̃sa* (cutaneous swelling) symptoms of the fever,[54] and the plant *kúṣṭha.* As a prophylactic measure the *jaṅgiḍá*-amulet was worn to render the fever powerless.[55]

kúṣṭha was considered to be the principal medicine for one suffering from fever.[56] He was known to be a divine, aromatic plant[57] with all-pervading strength,[58] the medicine for all diseases,[59] and the choicest among herbs.[60] He was said to be thrice-born from various divinities[61] and known by ancient venerable men.[62] Most importantly, he was closely connected with Soma,[63] even being called his brother.[64] For his consecration, the

---

[52] IS, 9: 414. Cf. also Bloomfield, *Hymns,* 567–68. See also Bloomfield's excellent discussion of the use of frogs and the water-plant *ávakā* for the quenching of fire, AJPh, 11: 342–50.

[53] KauśS 26.25; 29.18–19(31.7): 26.25. *yad agnir iti parasúṃ japaṃs tāpayati kvāthayaty avasiñcati;* 29.18–19(31.7).18. *agnis takmānam iti lājān pāyayati;* 19. *dāve lohitapātreṇa mūrdhni saṃpātān ānayati.* Cf. Bloomfield, *Hymns,* 270, 443; 468 and Caland, AZ, 77, 93, 96. See also Henry, *La magie,* 181, 183, 186–87.

[54] See in particular AVŚ 4.9.3, 8; cf. AVŚ 19.44.1, 2.

[55] AVŚ 19.34.10.

[56] See in particular AVŚ 5.4.1, 2.

[57] AVŚ 19.39.1; P 1.45.4.

[58] AVŚ 5.22.3; 19.39.10.

[59] AVŚ 19.39.5–9.

[60] AVŚ 5.4.9; 19.39.4.

[61] These included the *Śāmbus* (?), the descendants of the Aṅgiras, Ādityas and Viśvedevas (AVŚ 19.39.5). At P 1.93.1 he is said to have been born three times from Vṛtra, three times from the sky, three times from Soma and three times from the Ādityas.

[62] I.e. Ikṣvāka, Kāmya, Vasa and Mātsya (AVŚ 19.39.9).

[63] See AVŚ 19.39.5–8; P 1.93.1; cf. also A. Hillebrandt, *Vedische Mythologie* (1927; rpt. Hildesheim: Georg Olms, 1965), 1: 244–47 and notes to AVŚ 5.4.2–3, 151, below.

[64] P 2.32.3.

healer quite insistently relied on mythological events concerning his origin. He is said to have been born and acquired by the gods from the divine place where there is the appearance of immortality. This place was said to be in the third heaven from here, where there is the seat of the gods, the *aśvatthá*-tree. It is where golden boats with golden rigging sail about and where there are the highest peaks of the Himavant,[65] the birthplace of eagles.[66] We are told that the golden boats with golden oars, traveling on golden courses, transported the plant to the mountain.[67] His mother's name is *jīvalā́* ('perennial') and his father's name is *jīvantá* ('life-giving')[68] or *uttamá* ('choicest').[69] He is given three names, *naghamārá* ('non-destroying'), *naghā́riṣa* ('harmless') and *kúṣṭha*[70] or *uttamá* ('choicest')[71] which the healer was to recite individually at evening, in the morning, and during the day (i.e. continually).[72] He is also referred to as rescuing.[73] It is interesting to note that the healing plant-goddess Arundhatī is also said to be *naghāriṣā́* ('harmless') and a rescuer as well as *jīvalā́* ('perennial') and *jīvantī́* ('life-giving').[74] Apparently, the poet-healer was intentionally associating the male plant *kúṣṭha* with the already recognized female healing plant-divinity Arundhatī in an effort, perhaps, further to increase his efficacy.[75] He is given the epithet of the embryo of the herbs, of the Himavant and of every being.[76] We are also informed that he was a valuable item of trade brought from the mountains in the north to the people in the east where the choicest types were bartered.[77] He was also used, among other things, with ointment (*ā́ñjana*), as a means of winning a woman's love,[78] and in a treatment against poison.[79]

The hymns themselves do not tell us how or in which form the *kúṣṭha*-plant was employed. At KauśS 28.13, however, the plant is to be crushed, mixed with fresh butter and rubbed on the patient from his head to his feet.[80] In the tradition of later Indian medicine, its aromatic root is used, among other things, for cough and fever and also as a pastille for fumigation.[81] Because *kúṣṭha* is termed an aromatic plant with all-pervasive

---

[65] AVŚ 5.4.1, 3–4; 6.95.1–2; 19.39.1, 6–8; cf. also P 1.93.3–4; 5.21–3; 13.1.9.

[66] AVŚ 5.4.2.

[67] AVŚ 5.4.3; cf. P 5.21.3.

[68] AVŚ 19.39.3; cf. P 1.93.2.

[69] AVŚ 5.4.9.

[70] AVŚ 19.39.2.

[71] See AVŚ 5.4.9.

[72] AVŚ 19.39.2–4.

[73] AVŚ 19.39.1.

[74] See AVŚ 8.7.6; cf. AVŚ 8.2.6 *abd*.

[75] See chapter 21 below, 96.

[76] AVŚ 6.95.3.

[77] See AVŚ 5.4.2, 8: cf. P 1.93.4, where he is said to have been dug up from the Himavant with sharp spades.

[78] AVŚ 6.102.3.

[79] P 1.93.

[80] *kuṣṭhaliṅgābhir navanītamiśreṇāpratihāraṃ pralimpati;* see also Caland, AZ, 89 and cf. Bloomfield, *Hymns*, 415.

[81] See Dutt and King, *Materia Medica*, 181.

strength, one might speculate that the healer originally utilized the plant as a type of fumigant to help ward off and dispel the demon.

1.25

Because Agni burned the waters by entering [them], the place where those, who uphold the law, perform obeisance, they say, is [*takmán*'s] highest birthplace. You, O *takmán,* who are all-knowing, pass over us. 1.

Whether you are a flame, or whether [you are] a hot glow, or whether your birthplace is desirous of the wood chips, you, O god of the yellow one, are, by name, *hrū̆ḍu.* You, O *takmán,* who are all-knowing, pass over us. 2.

Whether [you are] burning, or whether [you are] consuming, or whether you are the son of King Varuṇa, you, O god of the yellow one, are, by name, *hrū̆ḍu.* You, O *takmán,* who are all-knowing, pass over us. 3.

I perform obeisance to the chilly *takmán;* [I perform] obeisance to the deliriously hot [and] to the radiant [*takmán*]. Let there be obeisance [to the *takmán*] who approaches daily (quotidian) and in two days [and] to the [*takmán*] who recurs every third day (tertian). 4.

5.22

Let Agni expel the *takmán* from here; [let] Soma, the pressing stone [and] Varuṇa of refined dexterity [expel him]; [let] the sacrificial altar, the *barhís* (sacrificial grass) and the blazing sacrificial fuel [expel him]. Let the enemies be gone! 1.

May you now, O *takmán,* who turns everybody yellow [and] who heats [them] like a scorching fire, become completely powerless; and then, go downward ever so deep. 2.

You, [O herb,] who have all pervading strength, dispel down [and] away the *takmán* who [is] grey, son of the grey one [and] red like (saw-) dust. 3.

After having made obeisance to *takmán,* I drive [him] downward. Let the fist-strik̄er of *śakambhará* return to the Mahāvṛṣas. 4.

His home is [both among] the Mūjavants [and among] the Mahāvṛṣas. Whenever you come into being, O *takmán,* among the Balhikas is the place where you should reside. 5.

O malicious *takmán,* keep silent; O deformed one, keep amply away [from us]; seek out the escaping slave-girl; strike her with a thunderbolt. 6.

O *takmán,* go to the Mūjavants or to the Balhikas further on; seek out the lustful-young Śūdra-girl [and], O *takmán,* shake her up a bit. 7.

When you have departed, [go and] consume your kinsmen: the Mahāvṛṣas and the Mūjavants. We [shall] point out to *takmán* these [and] those others' fields. 8.

If you aren't satisfied with the others' field [and must return; then,] may you, being powerful, look favorably upon us. [Since] *takmán* has now become anxious, [we hope] he will travel to the Balhikas. 9.

Since you, being chilly and then deliriously hot, make [this man] shiver [and] cough, indeed, O *takmán*, pass over us with those your dreaded missiles. 10.

I conjure you, O *takmán*, that you surely do not make these [your] companions: *balā̃sa* (swelling), cough [and] *udyugá* (uncontrollable shaking?); and to be sure, do not return here again from there. 11.

You, O *takmán*, accompanied with [your] brother *balā̃sa* (swelling), [your] sister cough [and your] evil cousin *pāmán* (rash), depart to that distant tribe. 12.

Destroy [, O plant,] the *takmán* who recurs every third day (tertian), who has the third day free (quartan?), who is continual, who is autumnal, who is hot and cold, who arises in the summer and in the rainy season. 13.

With the Gandhāris, with the Mūjavants, with the Aṅgas [and] with the Magadhas, we entrust the *takmán*, as [we entrust with riches] the man about to be despatched to the treasury. 14.

6.20

As if from Agni, he arises from this burning and flashing; and so like a chattering drunkard may [he] go away [again]. Let the unruly one seek out someone other than ourselves. Obeisance to *takmán* who possesses a fiery weapon. 1.

Let there be obeisance to Rudra, to *takmán*, to the splendid King Varuṇa, to heaven, to earth [and] to the herbs. 2.

I make obeisance to that wild *takmán*—he, the flame-thrower, who turns all forms yellow—[and] to your red [and] brown [color]. 3.

7.116(121)

Obeisance to the deliriously hot, shaking, driving [and] violent [*takmán*]. Obeisance to the chilly [*takmán* and to the *takmán*] who brings about the previous desire [for rain]. 1.

Let that unruly [*takmán*], who approaches daily [and] in two days, go unto the frog. 2.

5.4

You, O destroyer of *takmán*, O *kúṣṭha*, who were born on the mountains [and who are] the mightiest of plants, come here, destroying the *takmán*. 1.

Indeed, they know [you as] the destroyer of *takmán*, born from the Himavant, on the mountain where eagles are born; [and], having heard about [you], they approach [you] with riches. 2.

The seat of the gods, the *aśvatthá*-tree [is] in the third heaven from here. There, the gods acquired the *kúṣṭha*, the appearance of immortality. 3.

The golden boat with golden rigging sailed about in heaven. There, the gods acquired the *kúṣṭha*, the flower of immortality. 4.

Golden were the courses, golden the oars [and] golden were the boats by which they transported the *kúṣṭha* [from heaven to the mountain]. 5.

For me, O *kúṣṭha*, retrieve this man, heal him and further make him healthy for me. 6.

[Since] you are born from the gods [and] you are Soma's established companion, [therefore] be propitious to this my *prāṇá*-breath, *vyāná*-breath [and] faculty of sight. 7.

Born in the north from the Himavant, you are brought to the people in the east. There, they distributed the choicest types of *kúṣṭha*. 8.

You are, by name, choicest, O *kúṣṭha*, [and] your father [is], by name, choicest; [therefore] destroy every *yákṣma* and make *takmán* powerless. 9.

The throbbing in the head, the pounding in the eyes [and] the bodily *rápas*, all that may the *kúṣṭha* eradicate; [for he is] indeed divinely potent. 10.

6.95

The seat of the gods, the *aśvatthá*-tree [is] in the third heaven from here. There, the gods acquired the *kúṣṭha*, the appearance of immortality. 1.

The golden boat with golden rigging sailed about in heaven. There, the gods acquired the *kúṣṭha*, the flower of immortality. 2.

[Since] you are the embryo of the herbs, the embryo of the Himavant and the embryo of every being, [therefore] make this man healthy for me. 3.

19.39

Let the divine, rescuing *kúṣṭha* come here from the Himavant. [O plant,] destroy every *takmán* and all the sorceresses. 1.

Three [are] your names, O *kúṣṭha*: non-destroying (*naghamārá*), harmless (*naghāriṣa*) [and *kúṣṭha* or *uttamá* (choicest)]. Indeed, may this man, for whom I pronounce you at evening, in the morning, and during the day, not be injured. 2.

Your mother, by name, is perennial (*jīvalā́*); your father, by name, is life-giving (*jīvantá*). Indeed, may this man, for whom I pronounce you at evening, in the morning, and during the day, not be injured. 3.

You are the choicest among the herbs as the draft-ox among the domestic animals [and] as the tiger among the wild beasts. Indeed, may this man, for whom I pronounce you at evening, in the morning, and during the day, not be injured. 4.

Thrice born from the Śāmbus, the descendants of the Aṅgirases, from the Ādityas [and] from the Viśvedevas, this *kúṣṭha,* the medicine for all [diseases] stands with Soma. [Thus, O plant,] destroy every *takmán* and all the sorceresses. 5.

The seat of the gods, the *aśvatthá*-tree, [is] in the third heaven from here. There, the appearance of immortality [is found; and] from that place *kúṣṭha* was born. This *kúṣṭha,* the medicine for all [diseases], stands with Soma. [Thus, O plant,] destroy every *takmán* and all the sorceresses. 6.

A golden boat with golden rigging sailed about in heaven. There, the appearance of immortality [is found; and] from that place, *kúṣṭha* was born. This *kúṣṭha,* the medicine for all [diseases], stands with Soma. [Thus, O plant,] destroy every *takmán* and all the sorceresses. 7.

Where the boat descended [and] where [there is] the summit of the Himavant, there, the appearance of immortality [is found and] from that place, *kúṣṭha* was born. This *kúṣṭha,* the medicine for all [diseases], stands with Soma. [Thus, O plant,] destroy every *takmán* and all the sorceresses. 8.

[Since, we know] you whom the ancient Ikṣvāka knew, or you, O *kúṣṭha,* whom Kāmya, or whom Vasa or [even] whom Mātsya [knew], therefore, you are the medicine for all [diseases]. 9.

You, [O *kúṣṭha,*] who have all pervading strength, dispel down [and] away the *takmán* who racks the head with heat, who recurs every third day (tertian), who is continual and who lasts the entire year. 10.

8: *KĀ́SĀ* (*KĀ́S*) (COUGH)

AVŚ 6.105 is a charm against the morbid symptom *kā́sā* (*kā́s*) (feminine), a word which is onomatopoeic for 'cough.' It is closely associated with *takmán*, even being given the epithet, 'the sister of *takmán*.' [1] Likewise, along with *takmán*, she is considered to be one of Rudra's weapons;[2] and with headache, she is looked on as one of the harmful effects of thunder and lightning.[3] Her connection with *takmán* and thunder and lightning suggests the obvious sympathetic or symbolic association with the noise of thunder which may resemble the deep hacking-sound of a cough. Although cough does not normally accompany malaria, it does occur in the most severe kinds, in particular, "estivoautumnal malaria," and tends to indicate a very advanced stage of the disease.[4] It is also common among other types of febrile diseases.

The cure for this symptom involved an incantation with which the healer implored the demon to speed quickly away from the victim. The ritual practice found in the *Kauśika Sūtra* has very little to do with the eradication of cough; rather it prescribes the performance of a rite used in the case of one suffering from *ariṣṭa*, 'epilepsy.' [5] Such a treatment is mentioned at KauśS 28.15–16, which is connected with AVŚ 5.6(4.1): The healer first makes a woman, who has recently borne a child, and the patient, possessed of the evil, take one step forward (to the east, from the house); he then gives them a medicinal concoction to drink, lets them sip water and makes them worship the sun.[6]

6.105

As the mind flies quickly away with its perceptions, so also, you, O
cough, fly forth in conformity with the mind's stream. 1.
As a keenly honed arrow flies quickly away, so also, you, O cough,
fly forth in conformity with the land's contour. 2.
As the sun's rays fly quickly away, so also, you, O cough, fly forth
in conformity with the ocean's ebb. 3.

---

[1] AVŚ 5.22.10–12.

[2] AVŚ 11.2.22.

[3] AVŚ 1.12.3.

[4] T. R. Harrison, et al., *Principles of Internal Medicine*, fifth edition (New York: McGraw-Hill, 1966), 1766.

[5] KauśS 31.27: *yathā mano 'va diva ity ariṣṭena*. Cf. Bloomfield, *Hymns*, 513–14; M. Bloomfield, ed., *The Kauśika Sūtra of the Atharva Veda with extracts from the commentaries of Dārila and Keśvu* (1889; rpt. Delhi: Motilal Banarsidass, 1972) XIV; and Caland, AZ, 103 and especially 90 n.13. In later Indian medicine *ariṣṭa* is a name of the nīm-tree which is used to cure malaria and the name of the soap-nut tree, used against epilepsy, see Nadk, 1: 776f. and 1102–103.

[6] 15. *brahma jajñānam iti sūtikāriṣṭakau prapādayati;* 16. *manthācamanopasthānam ādityasya*. Cf. Bloomfield, *Hymns*, 513–14 and Caland, AZ, 99.

9: THE GENERAL REMOVAL OF INTERNAL DISEASES RELATED TO *YÁKṢMA* AND *TAKMÁN*

AVŚ 9.8 is a charm devoted to the exorcism of various types of internal-disease demons characterized as either *yákṣma-* or *takmán-*types. One disease-entity not previously mentioned, which occurs in verse 9, is the female *apvā́*. In addition to being located in the stomach, she is said, at ṚV 10.103.12, to confuse her victim's mind, to seize his limbs and then to depart, to burn him in the heart and to cause the unfriendly ones to suffer from blind darkness.[1] Yāska at *Nirukta* 6.12 (cf. 9.33) considered her to be either a disease or fear (*vyādhir vā. bhayaṃ vā*). Later scholars, using these pieces of information as a guide, have suggested that she represents a type of stomach disease, perhaps dysentery, or diarrhea, induced by fear.[2] Geldner has suggested that she was probably the personification of fright or panic, conceived to be an internal disease[3]; and Karl Hoffmann, along similar lines, has posited that, strictly speaking, *apvā́* is not a disease, defining the term as "lähmender Schrecken, Panik, Todesangst." [4] Whereas, she may not be a proper disease, she does appear to have been looked upon as a disease-demon, who may have been called upon in battle to bring about in the enemy certain internal bodily sensations associated with fear or panic. These sensations, like jaundice (*harimán*, verse 9), then, may have been considered as manifestations or symptoms of a morbid internal bodily state. The internal residence of the demon is quite clearly evidenced both at ṚV 10.103.12 and at AVŚ 9.8.9. Her inclusion at AVŚ 9.8 suggests that she was considered as one of the most dreaded demons causing abnormal bodily conditions.

In general, the healer desires, through AVŚ 9.8, to exorcise the most dangerous types of internal disease-demons out of the body. In verse 10, he implores the venom of all *yákṣma*s to be discharged with urine and in verse 11, he requests, moving down the body, both the *yákṣma*s and various other types of agents of pain to be excreted from the anus with the on-

[1] *amī́ṣāṃ cittáṃ pratilobháyantī gṛhāṇā́ṅgāny apve párehi, abhí préhi nír daha hṛtsú śókair andhénāmítrās támasā sacantām.* It is interesting to note that R. Müller uses this hymn to support his principal theory of disease in the *Ṛgveda*, i.e. fiery nature of disease is indicated by the burning in the heart; and the blind darkness into which the unfriendly ones are sent, is, according to him, the evil or dark fire ("Medizin im Ṛg-Veda," 357).

[2] See Macdonell-Keith, *Vedic Index*, 1: 27; Filliozat states that it cannot be identified with certainty (*La doctrine*, 106).

[3] *Der Rigveda*, 3: 321 n.

[4] "Altpers. *afuvāyā*," *Corolla Linguistica: Festschrift Ferdinand Sammer*, ed. Hans Krahe (Wiesbaden: Otto Harrassowitz, 1955), 82 and *Aufsätze*, 1: 208ff.

omatopoeic sound of flatulence, *kāhābāha*. Because of the suggestion that the disease-entities should be expelled from the anus, one might speculate that the charm was recited during the administration of a purgative. The most auspicious time for performing such a healing rite appears to have been early morning, when the sun begins to rise (verse 22).

The later ritual practice is purely symbolic and rather short, offering little insight into the original rite and no indication of therapeutics: The healer first touches the patient (presumably on the head) while muttering the charm; and then with the last two verses, he worships the sun.[5]

9.8

We charm out of you every head-disease: headache, pain in the head, earache [and] *vilohitá*. 1.

We charm out of you every head-disease: the earache [and] the *visálpaka* (cutaneous swelling) from your two ears, from your *káṅkūṣas*. 2.

We charm out of you every head-disease; because of that, the *yákṣma* flows forth from the ear, from the mouth. 3.

We charm out of you every head-disease: [him] who makes a man *pramóta* (deaf, mute?), [him who] makes [him] blind. 4.

We charm out of you every head-disease: [the *yákṣma* who causes] cutting pain [and] fever in the limbs [and] the *visálpaka* (cutaneous swelling) who affects all the limbs. 5.

We charm out of [you] the *takmán* who recurs every autumn [and] whose awful aspect makes man tremble. 6.

We charm out from within your limbs the *yákṣma* who crawls along the two thighs and enters the two *gavīnikās* (ureters?). 7.

If [he] arises out of desire, out of abhorrence [or] from the heart, [then] we charm away the *balā́sa* from [your] heart [and] limbs. 8.

We charm the causer of *yákṣma* out from within your self, the yellowness (jaundice) out of your limbs, Apvā from within [your] stomach 9.

Let the *balā́sa* become ash; let the pain-causing one become urine. [For] I have exorcised from you the poison of all the *yákṣmas*. 10.

Let [him] stream forth out of the (anal) orifice, out of the stomach, [sounding like] *kāhābāha*. [For] I have exorcised from you the poison of all the *yákṣmas*. 11.

I have exorcised from you the poisons of all the *yákṣmas*—from your stomach, lung[s], navel [and] heart. 12.

Let the throbbings in the head, who rip apart the crown, stream forth, harmless [and] without causing pain, out of the (anal) orifice. 13.

---

[5] KauśS 32.18–19: 18. *śīrṣaktim ity abhimṛśati; 19. uttamābhyām ādityam upatiṣṭhate.* Cf. Bloomfield, *Hymns*, 600 and Caland, AZ, 106.

Let [those], who surge on to the heart [and who] extend along the vertebrae, stream forth, harmless [and] without causing pain, out of the (anal) orifice. 14.

Let [those], who surge on to the flanks [and who] bore along ribs, stream forth, harmless [and] without causing pain, out of the (anal) orifice. 15.

Let the pangs, who surge across your chest, stream forth, harmless [and] without causing pain, out of the (anal) orifice. 16.

Let [those], who crawl about the intestines and perplex the bowels, stream forth, harmless [and] without causing pain, out of the (anal) orifice. 17.

Let [those], who suck out the marrow and rip apart the joints, stream forth, harmless [and] without causing pain, out of the (anal) orifice. 18.

I have exorcised from you the poison of all the *yákṣmas*—your pain-causing *yákṣmas* who intoxicate the limbs. 19.

I have exorcised from you the poison of all the *yákṣmas*, of the *visalpá* (cutaneous swelling), of the *vidradhá* (abscess), of the *vātīkārá* or of the *alají* (small abscess or boil). 20.

I have destroyed the pangs from your feet, knees, hips, *bháṃsas*, spine [and] nape of the neck, [and] the affliction from [your] head. 21.

Sound are the skull-bones and the heart-palpitation (?). [For] you, O Āditya, arising, have destroyed the head-disease with [your] rays [and] have appeased [the *yákṣma* who causes] the disintegration of the limbs. 22.

B. Internal Diseases not closely related to yákṣma *and/or* takmán

10: *ÁMĪVĀ*

One of the disease entities most frequently encountered in both the *Ṛg* and *Atharva-Vedas* is *ámīvā* (feminine). The word is related to the verb *āmáyati,* 'to ache,' 'to cause pain,' from the root *am,* 'to seize.' As R. Emmerick notices, it probably originally had the meaning, 'seizure by a god.' [1]

From the Vedic hymns, we notice that she was conceived as a definite evil; and in some cases, she almost becomes, as Grassmann suggests, a personification of disease or unhealthy states.[2] She is often found in connection with the nocturnal demons, the *rákṣas*-s.[3] Likewise, she occurs with a host of other evil or demonic elements.[4] Other references indicate that she was associated with the committed sins which are attached to the body[5] and perhaps also with the sins which lead one astray.[6] She is described as a domestic demon[7] and is found in relation to *ánirā,* or lack of nourishment.[8] We see, therefore, that to the ancient Indian, *ámīvā* was a feminine demon who perhaps, as Emmerick suggests, attacked her victim by seizing his body, bringing about a general state of malnutrition characterized, among other things, by bodily decay. In another aspect as an evil-named flesh-eater, she indicates a demon which attacks unborn children causing abortion or stillbirth.[9] Her causes seem to have included sin; and most importantly, she seems to have been a domestic demon. It is impossible, however, to determine the exact disease which the poets were describing.

---

[1] "Indo-Iranian concepts of disease and cure," 12; see also J. Narten, "Ved. *āmáyati* und *āmayāvín,*" St. II, 5/6: 165 and Mayrhofer, Wb, 1: 44.

[2] Wb, col. 93.

[3] See, in particular, ṚV 1.35.9–10; 3.15.1; 7.38.7; 8.35.16–18; 9.85.1 and 10.98.12. The compound *amīvacā̆tana,* 'dispeller of *ámīvā,*' is found along with *rakṣohán,* 'destroyer of the *rákṣas*-demons' at ṚV 7.8.6; 10.97.6; AVS 8.2.28; 19.44.7. R. Müller goes as far as to say that ". . . *ámīvā* wird in dieser Bedeutung [i.e. Krankheitsbegriff] nicht selten in einer wörtlichen Verbindung mit den Dämonen Rakṣás gebracht . . ." ("Medizin im Ṛg-Veda," 347).

[4] See, in particular, ṚV 1.35.9–10; 1.189.2–3; 2.33.2; 3.15.1; 6.74.2; 7.1.7; 7.38.7; 8.18.10; 9.97.43; 10.37.4; 10.63.12; 10.98.12; AVŚ 7.42(43).1.

[5] ṚV 6.74.2, 3; AVŚ 7.42(43).1–2 (cf. P 1.109.1, 4).

[6] ṚV 1.189.1, 3.

[7] ṚV 6.74.2 [cf. also AVŚ 7.42(43).1], *ámīvā yā́ no gáyam āvivéśa;* cf. ṚV 7.46.2, 54.1, 55.1.

[8] ṚV 7.71.2; 8.48.11 and 10.37.4.

[9] Cf. the connections with the belly illustrated by J. Narten, St. II, 5/6, 153–54, 155.

Her opposite, *anamīvā́*, is very auspicious, indicating a healthy and sound bodily condition.[10] She is associated with the greatest (*várṣiṣṭha*) wealth (*raí*)[11] and is related to long life.[12] She is connected with the dawn (Uṣas);[13] and food (*íṣas*) is requested to be without *ámīvā*.[14] Not only in humans, but also in cows the condition of *anamīvā́* is desired.[15]

Treatment

In order to make the body free from *ámīvā*, a state said to be given by Yama's two dogs,[16] the Vedic Indians relied on various means. Ointment (*ā́ñjana*), referred to as *ámīvā*-dispelling and *rákṣas*-destroying was called on to destroy *ámīvā* and to banish apparitions.[17] The plant *pūtúdru* is said to be capable of, among other things, dispelling *ámīvā*,[18] and a shell (*śaṅkhá*)-amulet is stated as being able to overcome *ámīvā* and *ámati* (indigence).[19] Likewise, the *jaṅgiḍá*-amulet and an amulet of plants and material derived from a tiger (i.e. its claw or tooth?) were worn to ward off *ámīvā*.[20] Her most predominant dispeller, however, appears to have been water.[21] We learn that the healer who held medical herbs in his hand was considered to be a dispeller of *ámīvā* and a destroyer of the *rákṣas*-demons.[22] Primarily in the *Ṛgveda*, various divinities are said to remove *ámīvā*.[23]

Association with malnutrition

As we have seen, *ámīvā* is found in connection with lack of nourishment (*ánirā*) and indigence or poverty (*ámati*), both of which are associated with hunger (*kṣúdh*). Hunger is found along with *ánirā* at ṚV 8.60.20. In two Ṛgvedic hymns, Indra is requested to release worshippers from both *kṣúdh* and *ámati*.[24] At ṚV 10.42.10 [cf. AVŚ 7.50(52).7], he is invoked to help his worshippers overcome malignant indigence (*ámatiṃ durévāṃ*) by means

---

[10] See ṚV 3.59.3; 7.46.2 and 7.54.1 (both of which refer to the domestic situation); 10.14.11 and 10.18.7 (occurring in the funeral rites); 10.98.3; AVŚ 2.30.3; 11.1.22; 12.1.62; 12.2.26 (cf. ṚV 10.53.8; VS 35.10 and TĀ 6.3.2); 12.2.32 (=18.3.57; cf. ṚV 10.18.7 and TĀ 6.10.2).

[11] ṚV 3.16.3; following Renou, EVP, 12: 61; cf. however, Geldner, *Der Rigveda*, 1: 352: ". . . auf die höchste, . . . gesund . . . ist." This offers no solution to the problem. See also Oldenberg, *Vedic Hymns*, 2: 273–74.

[12] ṚV 10.37.7.

[13] ṚV 10.35.6.

[14] ṚV 3.22.4; 3.62.14 and 10.17.8.

[15] AVŚ 3.14.3.

[16] AVŚ 18.2.12.

[17] AVŚ 19.44.7.

[18] AVŚ 8.2.28.

[19] AVŚ 4.10.3.

[20] AVŚ 19.34.9; 8.7.14.

[21] ṚV 10.137.6; AVŚ 3.7.5; 6.91.3; P 5.18.9; 19.18.9.

[22] ṚV 10.97.6.

[23] The Aśvins at 7.71.2; 8.35.16–18; Agni at 1.12.7; 1.28.1; 1.189.3; 3.15.1; 7.1.7; 10.98.12; Agni and Soma at 9.85.1; Soma at 1.91.12; 8.48.11; 9.97.48; Soma and Rudra at 6.74.2; Savitṛ at 1.35.9; 10.100.8; Sūrya at 10.37.4; Ādityas at 8.18.10; Viśvedevas at 10.63.12; the magical words (*vácas*) at 7.8.6; the race horses at 7.38.7; Uṣas at 10.35.6; Rudra at 2.33.4, 7.46.2 and Brahmaṇaspati at 1.18.2.

[24] ṚV 8.66.14 and 10.43.3.

of cows and to satisfy their entire hunger (*kṣúdham . . . víśvām*) with barley; and at ṚV 1.104.7, he is asked to give food and drink to the hungry (*kṣúdhyadbhyas*). Likewise, Agni is requested not to give up the worshipper to the *rákṣas*-demon or to hunger.[25] The gods, without showing preference for social or economic status, inflict hunger as a punishment.[26] These connections with the morbid bodily conditions caused by poverty and hunger suggest symptoms of malnutrition manifested by one thought to be seized by the demonic *ámīvā*. It is perhaps no coincidence therefore that *ámīvā* is often described as a domestic demon.

We notice that cows—probably a reference to dairy products—were used to cure the worst kind of poverty (i.e. that involving hunger); and barley, considered along with rice to be a medicine,[27] was employed to cure hunger. In addition to these, an amulet fashioned with the *udumbára*-tree was worn to force away poverty and hunger.[28] The *jaṅgiḍá*-amulet also wards off poverty.[29] Similarly, the *apāmārgá*-plant was employed to remove death by hunger and death by thirst.[30]

Evil-named flesh-eater: ṚV 10.162

In addition to the symptoms of malnutrition, *ámīvā* was also conceived to be one of the principal characteristics of an evil-named flesh-eater who destroyed the embryo, causing an abortion or a stillborn child. From the parallels of this hymn found at AVŚ 8.6,[31] we notice that this evil-named flesh-eater is described as hairy and as consuming raw meat, human flesh, and embryos.[32] He is an excessive licker who crawls down between women's thighs and separates them with what appears to have been a hand-held horn.[33] Likewise, he sleeps with the woman and attacks at night.[34] The remedies against this type of demon were the *bajá*- and *piṅgá*-plants which, perhaps in the form of an amulet, were to be worn in the undergarments.[35] Likewise, AVŚ 2.25[36] is a charm against an embryo-consuming, blood-

---

[25] ṚV 7.1.19.

[26] ṚV 10.117.1; see also Geldner, *Der Rigveda*, 3: 342 n, and Renou, *Hymnes spéculatifs du Véda*, 113, 251.

[27] AVŚ 8.2.18; 8.7.20; cf. ṚV 10.100.10 and 175.2.

[28] AVŚ 19.31.11.

[29] AVŚ 19.34.3.

[30] AVŚ 4.17.6, 7; on the inauspiciousness of hunger and thirst, cf. AVŚ 7.60(62).4.

[31] KauśS 35.20 prescribes that this hymn should be recited at the *sīmanta* ('parting of the hair') rite, in which an amulet of *bajá* and *piṅgá* (white and yellow mustard?) is bound to a pregnant woman (*yau te māteti mantroktau badhnāti;* Dārila specifies that the woman should be in her eighth month: *aṣṭame māsi karma kuryāt;* see also Caland, AZ, 117).

[32] AVŚ 8.6.23.

[33] AVŚ 8.6.3, 6, 14.

[34] AVŚ 8.6.7, 8, 19; cf. ṚV 10.162.4–5.

[35] AVŚ 8.6.20.

[36] Sāyaṇa alludes to its occurrence in the series of hymns devoted to the exorcising of demons (*cātanagaṇa*), found at KauśS 8.25 and to its use in the rites for the curing of all diseases beginning with skin disease (*kuṣṭhādisarvarogabhaisajyakarmaṇi*) at KauśS 26.33–40. According to Dārila, it is specifically referred to at KauśS 26.36, which states that the plant

sucking demon called *káṇva*,[37] who is also classed as among the evil-named flesh-eaters.[38] The principal remedy against this demon was the *pṛśniparṇī*-plant.[39]

Nowhere in these Atharvavedic charms is such a demon characterized as *ámīvā*. It is only in the Ṛgvedic hymn that the male, evil-named flesh-eater is referred to as *ámīvā*. In the mind of the poet, the disease-entity *ámīvā* would be an apt description of a demon who entered the domestic abode, who attacked at night during copulation, and who caused bodily destruction in the form of a dead fetus. The means for destroying such a demon involved exorcism by a hymn or spell which invoked Agni. There is no mention of a plant or plants used as amulets.

The later ritual tradition mentions this hymn's use in a rite to secure the successful birth of a child which otherwise may have been aborted:

> A woman whose fetus might be aborted should [, while reciting ṚV 10.162,] pour a burnt-offering, with ghee, into the fire, in accordance with the ritual prescription. Then the pregnant woman, having anointed herself with the dregs of ghee, should bring forth her child; she should drink the dregs: [for then] her child will be born alive. And if [her childen] should be born dead, she, having prepared ghee which has been consecrated and having offered it [with the hymn], should pour out the dregs of ghee on an amulet (*maṇi*); then on a threefold thread, she should clothe the amulet with a garment and with the sheath of the Indian fig (*nyagrodha*); thereupon [it is] wrapped in white and red. Then, having consecrated it. . . . , the pregnant woman, being ritually pure, should carry [the amulet] on her head; in the third month of her pregnancy, she should fasten it [to her body]. When she has had her [first] menses [after giving birth], the woman, together with her suckling, should live for a year like a cow with calf, with much to eat and drink. When a boy has been born, she should fasten the amulet to his neck; and having previously prepared the dregs of ghee, she should anoint the little boy with them. . . .[40]

It is remarkable that a rite so characteristic of the *Atharvaveda* should find a place in the *Ṛgveda:* abortions and stillbirths must have been quite common in ancient India.

---

mentioned in the hymn (i.e. *pṛśniparṇī*) is mixed with the dregs of ghee and smeared on to the patient [*dvitīyena* (i.e. AVŚ 2.25.1) *mantroktasya saṃpātavatānulimpati;* cf. Bloomfield, *Hymns,* 302 and Caland, *AZ,* 79–80].

[37] AVŚ 2.25.3.

[38] AVŚ 2.25.2, 5.

[39] AVŚ 2.25.1–4. At SuŚāSth 10.61, *pṛśniparṇī* is listed along with many other remedies for use with milk during the first seven months of pregnancy in the case of a threatened miscarriage or abortion.

[40] *Ṛgvidhāna* 4.17–18: 17.1. *yasyā garbhaḥ pramīyate tatrāgnau juhuyād dhaviḥ, brahmaṇāgniḥ saṃ vidāna ity ājyena yathāvidhi;* 17.2. *ājyaśeṣeṇa cābhyajya garbhiṇī prasavet tataḥ, pibed evājyaśeṣaṃ tu jīvaṃs tasyāḥ prajāyate;* 17.3. *jātāni cet pramīyerann ājyaṃ kṛtvānumantritaṃ, brahmaṇāgnir iti, hutvā sampātān ninayed maṇau;* 17.4. *maṇiṃ tu triyṛti sūtre vāsayed vāsasā saha, nyagrodhaśuṅgayā tatra śuklalohitaveṣṭitaṃ;* 17.5. . . . *anumantrya* . . . ; 18.2. *śirasā dhārayen nārī prayatā garbhiṇī satī, tṛtīye garbhamāse tu maṇim etaṃ samāsajet;* 18.3. *puṣpyantī śaradaṃ nārī gauḥ savatsā vased yathā, bahupānīyayavasā vatsena pibatā saha;* 18.4. *jātasya tu kumārasya kaṇṭhe tam maṇim āsajet, ājyaśeṣaṃ puraskṛtya tam abhyajya kumārakaṃ;* . . . . Cf. also Gonda, *The Ṛgvidhāna,* 113–14 and notes.

One of the important points to be noted in ṚV 10.162 is the allusion to gross stages of embryonic development. It appears that the Vedic Indians distinguished two basic phases, culminating in birth: 1. copulation, when the sperm flies into the womb and settles with the fertilization of the egg; 2. the period when the fetus begins to kick and move about, leading finally to the birth of the child.

ṚV 10.162

Let Agni, the slayer of the *rákṣas*-demons, in conformity with the spell, expel from here [him] who, [as] *ámīvā,* is situated in your embryo [and, as] the evil-named one, in [your] womb. 1.

Agni, together with the spell, has utterly destroyed that flesh-eater who, [as] *ámīvā,* is situated in your embryo [and, as] the evil-named one, in [your] womb. 2.

We make him, who slays [the embryo] leaping and settled [in the womb], who [slays it when it is] moving about [in the womb], who tries to kill your [new]born [child], perish from here. 3.

We make him, who separates your thighs, who is situated between husband and wife [and] who licks inside the womb, perish from here. 4.

We make him, who, after having become [as] a brother, a husband [or] a lover, lies down with you [and] tries to kill your offspring, perish from here. 5.

We make him, who, after having confounded [you] with a dream [and] with darkness, lies down with you [and] tries to kill your offspring, perish from here. 6.

11: *VÍṢKANDHA-SÁṂSKANDHA* (TETANUS?)

AVŚ 2.4; 3.9; 19.34, 35 are charms primarily devoted to the consecration of the amulet, *jaṅgiḍá,* which is particularly efficacious in destroying *víṣkandha* (neuter) and in protecting individuals from it as well as other demonic forces. An exact determination of the malady, which *víṣkandha* represents, is troublesome. Sāyaṇa considered it to be an impediment (*vighna*), a problem which causes the body to dry up or even the name of a great wind-type disease which brought about the dislocation of the shoulders.[1] Bloomfield thought it was a demon.[2] Weber[3] and Griffith[4] speculated, on etymological grounds (*vi-skandha,* 'tearing apart of the shoulders'), that it might be identified as rheumatism. Filliozat, more cautiously, stated that its exact meaning cannot be determined.[5] Karambelkar has recently argued that it can in fact be identified as "wasting palsy, progressive muscular atrophy." [6] With such widely differing views on its exact nature, any statement about its definition must be viewed discreetly.

Unlike the internal disease-demons *yákṣma, rápas, takmán,* etc., *víṣkandha* is not said to reside inside the body. Nor does it exhibit any of the characteristics of those demonic diseases. It does, however, appear to have been considered demonic in nature, for it is often found associated with other demons and evils,[7] and there are said to have been 101 (an inauspicious number) of them scattered over the earth.[8]

Likewise, it appears to have been regarded as causing a morbid bodily condition. At AVŚ 2.4.2, it is mentioned in a list of four physical disabilities which cause great pain.[9] Similarly at P 1.46.3 it is said to be a malady from which one suffers when wounded;[10] and at TS 7.3.11.1 the term is used to describe the desired condition of a foe's body.[11] Finally, it is mentioned along with *sáṃskandha* which, etymologically, would suggest its opposite,

---

[1] See notes to AVŚ 2.4.1 and 19.34.5 below, 171, 180–81.

[2] *Hymns,* 282–83.

[3] IS, 13: 141. See also Macdonell-Keith, *Vedic Index,* 2: 314.

[4] *Hymns of the Atharvaveda,* 1: 20, 45, 91, etc.

[5] *La doctrine,* 106–107.

[6] *The Atharva-Veda and the Āyur-Veda,* 267, 276–77.

[7] See AVŚ 1.16.3; 2.4.3, 4; 3.9.3–5.

[8] AVŚ 3.9.6.

[9] I.e. *jambhá,* 'lock-jaw'; *viśará,* 'tearing or contorting pain'; and *abhiśócana,* 'burning or scorching pain.'

[10] Following Bh: *dānaṃ tṛṣṇāyāḥ pari pātu viddhaṃ (!) dānaṃ kṣudho dānavideva mṛtyoḥ, aviṣkandho bhavatu yo dadātyā pyāyate papurir dakṣiṇayā* (cf. also vss. 1, 5, 6 and Renou, JA, 252: 439).

[11] Here the commentator Sāyaṇa describes it as a condition of the body in which the limbs, beginning with the shoulders, are deformed (*virūpāḥ skandhādyavayavā . . .*).

but about which, unfortunately, nothing more is known.[12] From this evidence, it would appear that *víṣkandha* was conceived to be a demonic force which rendered the body unhealthy. The exact way in which this was accomplished is uncertain. We do notice, however, that both *víṣkandha* and its opposite, *sáṃskandha,* were deemed to be injurious to the body. Perhaps, after all, an etymological evaluation of the two words *víṣkandha* and *sáṃskandha* can help us gain an insight into the particular disease being described: *víṣkandha,* as we noticed, suggests 'tearing the shoulders apart,' while *sáṃskandha* implies 'the forcing together of the shoulders.' In this way, the Vedic poet-healer could have been describing the spasmodic contortions of the body of one suffering from the internal disease commonly known as tetanus or lockjaw. Such a serious condition was first characterized by Hippocrates (5th–4th centuries B.C.) who made the connection between wounds and the spasms of tetanus.[13] The association with the open flesh-wound is likewise attested at P 1.46.3;[14] and among the painful conditions listed along with *víṣkandha* at AVŚ 2.4.2, there is *jambhá* which points to 'lockjaw,' the ordinary name for tetanus, and *viśará,* which reflects a 'tearing or contorting pain.' At AVŚ 19.34.10, the principal remedy for *víṣkandha* is said to destroy the following symptoms: *ā́sarīka,* perhaps 'a pain which wrenches the body together,' *víśarīka,* 'a pain which wrenches the body apart' and *pṛṣṭyāmayá,* 'rib-pain,' or 'pain along the sides.'

Among the remedies for *víṣkandha* and the protections against it, a lead (*sī́sa*)-amulet is mentioned as expelling it[15] and *ā́ñjana* (ointment) is said to protect one from its attacks.[16] The most important protector and destroyer of the demonically caused malady, however, was the *jaṅgiḍá*-plant,[17] which appears to have been a cultivated tree[18] used as an amulet.

jaṅgiḍá is specifically given the epithet of the *víṣkandha*-ruining amulet;[19] yet, being called the 'medicine for all [diseases],'[20] it was also effective against *balā́sa* and *takmán*[21] as well as the devouring demons, distress,[22] the *rákṣas*-demons,[23] witchcraft, enemies,[24] evil-eye,[25] all *ámīvās,*[26] and *ṛṣṇús*

[12] AVS 19.34.5.

[13] See Charles Singer and E. A. Underwood, *A Short History of Medicine* (Oxford: Clarendon Press, 1962, second edition), 37.

[14] Cf. also P 1.46, a charm to Soma for the healing of a donor, vss. 1, 2, 4–6, where there are strong suggestions that the donor was a warrior who had suffered arrow-inflicted wounds incurred in battle (see Renou, JA, 252: 439–40).

[15] AVŚ 1.16.3.

[16] AVŚ 4.9.5.

[17] It is called an herb (*óṣadhi*) and lord of the forest (i.e. tree) (*vanaspatí*) at AVŚ 19.34.9; cf. also 19.34.7. It may also be equated with the plant *arjuna* (see AVŚ 2.4.1 n, 172 below).

[18] AVŚ 2.4.5; 19.34.6.

[19] AVŚ 2.4.1; 3.9.6; cf. 2.4.4; 19.34.5, where it is said to have conquered both *víṣkandha* and *sáṃskandha.*

[20] AVŚ 2.4.3; 19.35.5.

[21] AVŚ 19.34.10.

[22] AVŚ 2.4.3.

[23] AVŚ 2.4.4; 19.34.9.

[24] AVŚ 2.4.6; 19.34.2–4; 19.35.2.

[25] AVŚ 19.35.3.

[26] AVŚ 19.34.9.

and others who remain (?).[27] It was considered to be delightful,[28] auspicious, having boundless strength,[29] possessed of a thousand eyes[30] and a thousand powers,[31] and divinely created or produced. We also have fragments of a mythology surrounding its origin from divinities: It is said to have been originally created or produced three times, selected and given by the gods.[32] It was known as "Aṅgiras" by ancient Brāhmaṇas;[33] and the seers are said to have presented it to man while reciting the auspicious name of Indra.[34] As *upadāna* (?), its energy may have been sapped by a powerful female but restored by Indra.[35] These mythological references and others as well seem to have been used to consecrate the talisman and to increase its overall potency and effectiveness.

There is a suggestion, at AVŚ 3.9, that more than one vegetal amulet may have been effective both against *víṣkandha* and against an obscure demonic disease called *kābavá*. The *karśaphá* and *viśaphá*[36] may also be divinely produced amulets (verse 1) and appear to have been originally bound without ties (verse 2). There is also the *khṛ́gala*, a stick or stock, perhaps of *jaṅgiḍá*, which was, however, bound by men with a red thread (verse 3). These, then, were effective against *kābavá* (verses 3–5). For the destruction of *víṣkandha*, however, the gods preferred and selected the *víṣkandha*-ruining, *jaṅgiḍá*-amulet which was also bound, but with hemp which grew in the wild.[37]

Those, who were not harmed and who were always able to do so, wore the consecrated amulet to protect themselves from *víṣkandha* and other evils and diseases, and to insure long life and abundant joy.[38] It is not stated who wore it. One would presume, however, that they would have been warriors and others who could have afforded to do so.

The ritual tradition gives us very little information about the curative practices surrounding the disease. In the *Kauśika Sūtra*, AVŚ 2.4 and 3.9 are mentioned rather in the sections treating oracles (*vijñānakarmāṇi*), a ritual in which there is the binding of the *jaṅgiḍa*-amulet to ruin witchcraft, to protect oneself and to remove impediments.[39] AVŚ 19.34 and 35 are found in another ritual text, the *Śāntikalpa* (17.4 and 19.6), and are employed during the binding of the *jaṅgiḍa*-amulet in the ceremony of the great consecration called, 'wind' (*vāyu*). Evidently an amulet fashioned from the

---

[27] AVŚ 19.35.5.
[28] AVŚ 2.4.4.
[29] AVŚ 19.34.8.
[30] AVŚ 19.35.3.
[31] AVŚ 2.4.2.
[32] AVŚ 2.4.4; 3.9.6; 19.35.1.
[33] AVŚ 19.34.6; 19.35.2.
[34] AVŚ 19.35.1.
[35] AVŚ 19.34.8–9.
[36] See AVŚ 3.9.1 n, below, 174.
[37] AVŚ 2.4.5.
[38] AVŚ 2.4.1, 2, 3, 5, 6; 19.34.1, 4, 5, 7; 19.35.2, 3, 4.
[39] KauśS 42.23 and 43.1–2.

jaṅgiḍa-plant was considered auspicious for a variety of occasions in ancient India, indicating that it functioned generally as a prophylactic and a bringer of luck and good fortune.

2.4

For long life [and] for abundant joy, we, who are not harmed [and] who are always able to do so, wear the *víṣkandha*-ruining *jaṅgiḍá*-amulet. 1.
Let the *jaṅgiḍá*-amulet, with [its] thousand powers, protect us on all sides from *jambhá, viśará, víṣkandha* [and] *abhiśócana.* 2.
This [amulet] overpowers the *víṣkandha* [and] it expels the demons which devour. [Therefore,] let this *jaṅgiḍá* [-amulet], the medicine for all [diseases], protect us from distress. 3.
By means of the delightful *jaṅgiḍá*-amulet, given by the gods, we overcome in struggle *víṣkandha* [and] all the *rákṣas*-demons. 4.
Let both the hemp [-cord] and the *jaṅgiḍá* [-amulet] protect us from *víṣkandha.* The one is procured from the forest, the other from the essences of cultivation. 5.
Therefore, may this powerful witchcraft-ruining and enemy-ruining *jaṅgiḍá*-amulet prolong our lives. 6.

3.9

Of the *karśaphá* [and] of the *viśaphá,* heaven [is] the father; earth, the mother. Just as you, O gods, have [in the past] produced [them], so also you must [now] again prepare [them]. 1.
[Those] devoid of fasteners held tight; so it was performed by Manu. Like a gelder of bulls, I make *víṣkandha* impotent. 2.
The performers of the rite tie the *khṛ́gala* (stick?) on to the reddish thread. [Therefore,] let bound (amulets) render the fleeting [and] inflamed *kābavá* impotent. 3.
Whereby, O fleeting ones, you wander about, like gods under the influence of demonic magic, and, as the monkey is of the dogs, so is the bound (amulet) the ruin of the *kābavá.* 4.
Indeed, for the sake of ruining, I will bind you [, O amulet, and] I will ruin *kābavá.* Together with the curses, you will go forth like speedy chariots. 5.
A hundred and one *víṣkandha* [are] scattered over the earth. Of these [amulets], (the gods) originally selected you, the *víṣkandha*-ruining amulet. 6.

19.34

You, the *jaṅgiḍá,* are *jaṅgiḍá;* you, the *jaṅgiḍá,* are a protector. [Therefore,] let the *jaṅgiḍá* protect our whole [property, consisting of] bipeds [and] quadrupeds. 1.

Let *jaṅgiḍá* separate all the clever ones who number fifty-three and the practitioners of witchcraft who number a hundred from [their] efficacy; and may [it] make [them] powerless. 2.

[May it make] the deceitful sound powerless [and] the seven debilities powerless. [For,] as an archer [his] arrow, you, O *jaṅgiḍá,* dispel indigence far away from here. 3.

Therefore, may this powerful witchcraft-ruining and enemy-ruining *jaṅgiḍá* prolong our lives. 4.

Let *jaṅgiḍá*'s greatness, with which [it] has conquered *víṣkandha, sáṃskandha* [and] the [evil] power with [its] own power, protect us on all sides. 5.

Thrice the gods created you who are fixed in the earth; and also, the ancient Brāhmaṇas knew you as "the Aṅgiras." 6.

Neither the old, nor the new herbs surpass you. [For] *jaṅgiḍá* [is] a powerful expeller, a protector [and] a bringer of success. 7.

Moreover, at first a powerful female partook of you, O *upadāna,* O auspicious *jaṅgiḍá* whose strength is boundless; [but then,] Indra gave [you back your] strength. 8.

To be sure, powerful Indra granted energy to you, O lord of the forest. [Therefore,] O herb, you, dispelling all *ámīvās*, kill the *rákṣas*-demons. 9.

May *jaṅgiḍá* make *ā̆sarīka, víśarīka, balā̆sa,* rib-pain [and] the *takmán* who recurs every autumn, powerless. 10.

19.35

[While] taking Indra's name, the seers presented [to man] *jaṅgiḍá* which the gods formerly made [as] the *víṣkandha*-ruining medicine. 1.

Let the *jaṅgiḍá,* which the gods [and] the Brāhmaṇas have made [as] an enemy-killing protector, protect us as a treasurer [protects] the treasures. 2.

The very terrible eye of the enemy, the approaching [of that] which has done evil—those destroy in [your] vigilance, O you of a thousand eyes. 3.

May *jaṅgiḍá* protect me from heaven, from earth, from midspace, from the plants, from the past and from the future, [all of] us in all directions. 4.

Let *jaṅgiḍá,* which is the medicine for all [diseases], make powerless all those *ṛṣṇús* who are divinely made and also another who has remained. 5.

12: ASCITES

In the Vedic *saṃhitās* there are no specific hymns or charms which in themselves are devoted to the cure of ascites, which only in the later medical literature is included under the general category of diseases of the abdomen, called *udara.*[1] All we have are scattered references to an abnormal bodily condition which seems to suggest ascites.

At ṚV 7.89, a hymn to Varuṇa requesting his forgiveness for a transgression committed against him and his moral order,[2] there are two verses which offer evidence of a morbid bodily state:

> verse 2: If I go, as it were, quivering like an inflated leather water-bag,
> O lord of the mountains, forgive, good ruler, be gracious.[3]
>
> verse 4: Thirst found the singer who stood in the midst of the waters;
> forgive, good ruler, be gracious.[4]

More evidence can be gathered from the *Atharvaveda.* At AVŚ 4.16, a hymn to various gods, verse 7, is addressed to Varuṇa:

> O Varuṇa envelop him with a hundred bonds; [and], O watcher of men, do not let the speaker of lies escape. Let the scoundrel sit, causing [his] belly to fall asunder, like an unbound vessel being cut open all around.[5]

AVŚ 1.10 and 7.83(88) are two hymns to Varuṇa which tradition has prescribed for use in a rite to cure dropsy (*jalodara*).[6] AVŚ 7.83(88) presents only the slightest indication of a malady: verses 3, 4 request Varuṇa to loosen various bonds, of which the midmost may refer to that affecting the stomach. It does, however, hint at Varuṇa's domination over the waters. In verse 1, his golden house is said to be constructed in the waters;[7] and

---

[1] See CaCiSth 13 and SuNiSth 7, CiSth 14; cf. also J. Jolly, *Medecin* (Strassburg: Karl J. Trübner, 1901), 80.

[2] See Geldner, *Der Rigveda,* 2: 179, 290.

[3] *yád émi prasphuránn iva dṛ́tir ná dhmātó adrivaḥ, mṛḷā́ sukṣatra mṛḷáya.*

[4] *apā́m mádhye tasthivā́ṃsaṃ tṛ́ṣṇāvidaj jaritā́ram, mṛḷā́ sukṣatra mṛḷáya.*

[5] *śaténa pā́śair abhí dhehi varuṇainaṃ mā́ te mocy anṛtavā́n nṛcakṣaḥ, ā́stāṃ jālmá udáraṃ śraṃśayitvā́ kóśa ivābandhráḥ parikṛtyámānaḥ.* On *śraṃśayitvā́,* see Whitney-Lanman, Pt. 1, 179; Sāyaṇa reads *sraṃsayitvā́* and glosses: "making fallen by means of ascites (water-belly)" (. . . *jalodararogeṇa srastaṃ kṛtvā* . . .).

[6] For AVŚ 1.10, Keśava states: *atha jalodarabhaiṣajyam ucyate,* Sāyaṇa: *jalodararoganivṛttaye,* at KauśS 25.37. For AVŚ 7.83(88), Keśava prescribes: *jalodare varuṇagṛhīte bhaiṣajyam ucyate* Sāyaṇa: *jalodarabhaiṣajyārthaṃ,* and Dārila: *varuṇagṛhītam,* at KauśS 32.14–16.

[7] *apsú te rājan varuṇa gṛhó hiraṇyáyo mitáḥ* [Sāyaṇa: *mitháḥ* (?); see Whitney-Lanman, Pt. 1, 150].

in verse 2, the waters are praised along with Varuṇa.[8] AVŚ 1.10.4 mentions only a great deluge (*arṇavā̃n mahatás*) from which the victim is requested to be released.[9] It does, however, allude to a myth expressed in greater detail in the AB. We render 2*cd:* "I urge a thousand others, jointly, [to you], so that this your [man] may live a hundred autumns." [10] As Sāyaṇa and others following him have suggested,[11] this passage seems to refer to AB 7.15.7 where a hundred victims are substituted so that one may be redeemed.[12] In this same Śunaḥśepa-legend, at AB 7.15.1, there is a passage which states that Varuṇa seized the descendant of Ikṣvāku and his belly swelled up;[13] and at AB 7.16.12–13, it is said that with the reciting of various auspicious verses, the bonds around the belly of Ikṣvāku's descendant became loosened, his stomach began to shrink, and when the last bond was loosened, he was released and became free of the disease.[14]

These are the earliest references which the traditional commentators and Western scholars[15] have utilized to identify Varuṇa's seizure (*váruṇagṛhīta*) as dropsy or, more particularly, ascites. Although the textual evidence is meager, there are parallels from the later tradition of Indian medicine which suggest that ascites may have in fact been a malady which the ancient Indians considered to have been sent by Varuṇa because of a breach of certain taboos. As we have seen, the earliest passages from the *Ṛgveda* and *Atharvaveda* describe the victim as looking like a quivering, inflated waterbag when he walks; and when he sits, his belly hangs and falls about like a vessel when it has been unbound. He is also described as experiencing thirst while being surrounded by water. The AB informed us that Varuṇa sent a disease which caused the stomach of Ikṣvāku's descendant to swell; and when the bonds of disease were released, his abdomen began to shrink, until it was normal size. In both the *Caraka-*[16] and *Suśruta-*[17]*Saṃhitās*, an

---

[8] . . . *ā̃po . . . íti váruṇéti* . . . Cf. also AVŚ 4.16.3c where the two oceans are said to be the two half-bellies of Varuṇa (*utó samudráu váruṇasya kukṣī̃* . . .).

[9] Cf. Henry: "Cette phrase est la seule allusion—et combien détournée!—au principal symptôme de la maladie que conjure le guérisseur: sans elle, et même avec elle, l'hymne pourrait aisément passer, si le Sūtra n'en précisait l'emploi, pour une pieuse et humble adjuration en vue de la rémission des péchés" (*La magie,* 210).

[10] *sahásram anyā̃n prá suvāmi sākáṃ śatáṃ jīvāti śarádas távāyám.*

[11] See, in particular, Bloomfield, *Hymns,* 241 and Whitney-Lanman, Pt. 1, 10.

[12] *taṃ hovāca: ṛṣe 'haṃ te śataṃ dadāmy, aham eṣām ekenātmānaṃ niṣkrīṇā iti.*

[13] *atha haikṣvākaṃ varuṇo jagrāha, tasya hodaraṃ jajñe.*

[14] *sa uṣasaṃ tuṣṭāvāta uttareṇa tṛcena* (ṚV 1.30.20–22) *tasya ha smarcyṛcy uktāyāṃ vi pāśo mumuce, kanīya aikṣvākasyodaram bhavaty; uttamasyām evarcy uktāyāṃ vi pāśo mumuce, 'gada aikṣvāka āsa.*

[15] See, in particular, Zimmer, *Leben,* 392; A. Hillebrandt, trans. *Lieder des Ṛgveda* (Göttingen: Vandenhoeck and Ruprecht, 1913), 79; Geldner, *Der Rigveda,* 2:260; Bloomfield, *Hymns,* 11, 241. Filliozat has gone into great detail explaining the connection between Varuṇa and dropsy and Varuṇa and the waters, and maintaining the often expressed notion that dropsy was the special disease of Varuṇa, the lord of the waters, which he inflicted upon a person as a result of an infringement against the moral order or norm (*ṛtá*). This, then, forms the basis for his theory of disease in the Vedic literature (*La doctrine,* 78–80).

[16] CiSth 13.45–48.

[17] NiSth 7.21–24.

udara-condition called either *dakodara,* or *udakodara* (water-belly) is described. It is said to be caused by the drinking of cold water at the wrong time, or by the drinking of oil;[18] and the afflicted patient's abdomen enlarges, resembling a fully inflated water-bag which fluctuates under pressure. The patient is also said to suffer from thirst. These symptoms bear a rather close resemblance to those found in the Vedic literature. One may, therefore, be reasonably confident that ascites was a disease from which the early Indians suffered when seized by Varuṇa.

Unlike the cure mentioned in the Vedas, which requires the propitiation of the god Varuṇa, the āyurvedic texts prescribed, among other things, a laparotomy in order to release the water. The water must, however, be released slowly so that complications do not set in.[19]

---

[18] It is interesting to note that at TS 6.4.2.3–4 one is implored not to partake of non-moving or stagnant waters because Varuṇa has seized them; for, if one were to partake of them, one would cause his sacrifice to be seized by Varuṇa [*ná sthāvarāṇām gṛhṇīyād, vāruṇagṛhītā(!) vai sthāvarā̄; yát sthāvarā̄ṇāṃ gṛhṇīyāt, váruṇenāsya yajñáṃ grāhayed;* cf. Keith, VBYS, Pt. 2, 529]. Cf. also ŚB 4.4.5.11.

[19] See CaCiSth 14.18.

13: INSANITY

AVŚ 6.111 is a charm against insanity. There are two types of insanity or madness mentioned in the charm: *únmadita* which implies the demented state brought on by the patient himself as a result of his infringement of certain divine mores or taboos; and *únmatta* which suggests an abnormal mental state caused by possession by demons, such as the *rákṣas*-s (verse 3). To the ancient Indian, insanity, like death, was considered to be a state when the mind leaves the body (verse 2). Likewise the patient exhibited the distinctive symptom of uttering nonsense (verse 1).

In order to cure such a condition, the healer had to return the mind to the body (verse 4). He did this primarily by making offerings to the gods in order to appease them, in the case of *únmadita*-madness (verse 1). He also prepared medicines, perhaps to calm the patient, and to drive away the evil forces invading his body, in the case of *únmatta*-madness (verses 2, 3). There is also the suggestion that a victim of madness was restrained, perhaps in a sort of straightjacket, presumably so that he could not harm anyone (verse 1).

In the ritual literature, the charm is not specifically mentioned in the section on healing; it is, however, at KauśS 8.24, characterized as one of the three hymns containing the names of the mothers (*mātṛnāman* or *mātṛgaṇa*), which are included in a rite for curing one possessed by demons. The ritual practice is, as Bloomfield points out, purely symbolic, with the emphasis placed on purification and on the expulsion of the demon:

> Having offered, with the two *mātṛnāman*-hymns (which are not specified), various fragrant powders anointed [with ghee], [the healer] smears [the patient] with the remainder; and at a crossroad, [the fragrant powders], anointed [with ghee], [are offered] over a coal in a bowl, [which has been placed] in a wicker-basket made of *darbha*-grass [and situated] on the [patient's] head; going into a stream against the current, [the patient] scatters [the fragrant powder] from a sieve [into the water], while someone sprinkles [him] from behind; having thrown [more of the fragrant powders] into an unburned vessel, having wet [them and having placed the vessel] in [a sling of] three strands made of *muñja*-grass, he binds [it] in a tree with a bird's nest.[1]

In later Indian medicine, insanity or madness is termed *unmatta* or *unmāda* and is classified into various types on the basis of the *doṣa*-theory.[2] The

[1]KauśS 26.29-32: 29. *mātṛnāmnoḥ sarvasurabhicūrṇāny anvaktāni hutvā śeṣeṇa pralimpati;* 30. *catuṣpathe ca śirasi darbheṇḍve 'ṅgārakapāle 'nvaktāni;* 31. *titauni pratīpaṃ gāhamāno vapatītaro 'vasiñcati paścāt;* 32. *āmapātra opyāsicya mauñje tripāde vayoniveśane prabadhnāti.* Cf. Bloomfield, *Hymns*, 518–19 and especially, Caland, AZ, 79.

[2] See Jolly, *Medicin*, 121.

most severe forms of insanity are included under the category of *bhūtonmāda*, 'insanity caused by demons,' which corresponds most closely to the type of insanity mentioned in this charm. The remedies prescribed for one suffering from *bhūtonmāda* include medicines to be taken internally, to be given as ointments, as nasal-therapy, and as fumigants. The treatment, however, also necessitated the appeasement of the demons by worship and the presentation of oblations, etc.[3] We do notice, however, that in cases of insanity arising from lust (*rati*) and the desire for worship (*abhyaracana*),[4] in cases of insanity due to external causes (*āgantu*)[5] and in cases of insanity caused by gods (*devas*), sages (*ṛṣis*), fathers (*pitṛs*) and Gandharvas,[6] magical healing rites, involving the recitation of (Vedic) charms, the use of simples and the execution of various sacrificial, religious, ascetic and propitiatory observances, are employed.

6.111

O Agni, for me, release this man who, bound [and] well-restrained, utters nonsense. Hence, he shall make an offering to you when he becomes sane. 1.

If your mind is agitated, let Agni quieten [it] down for you. [For] I, being skilled, prepare the medicine, so that you may become sane. 2.

I, being skilled, prepare the medicine so that he, insane because of a curse of the gods and demented because of the *rákṣas*-demons, may become sane. 3.

Let the Apsarases return you; let Indra [and] Bhaga re[turn you; in fact,] let all the gods return you so that you may become sane. 4.

---

[3] Ibid., 122.
[4] CaNiSth 7.15–16, CiSth 9.23.
[5] CaCiSth 9.33, 93–94.
[6] CaCiSth 9.88–90.

14: *KRÍMI* (WORMS)

AVŚ 2.31 and 5.23 are charms against *krími* or worms, vermin, etc. The former is a general incantation against worms; while the latter is specifically directed to worms in children. AVŚ 2.32 is also a charm for worms. Since it is for the eradication of worms in cows, however, it pertains more to veterinary medicine and has, therefore, been excluded.[1]

Worm-disease is historically important because it provides an unbroken continunity from the very early Vedic texts down to the classical medical treatises of Caraka and Suśruta. Supportive evidence is uniquely gained from archaeology; and parallels are noticed in the Germanic tradition. Worms and other parasites which live in man have plagued him from time immemorial. Their eradication was initially effected by magical means and later by a more empirically based method of surgery.

Definition

The word *krími* (*kṛ́mi*)[2] does not occur in the *Ṛgveda.*[3] In the *Atharvaveda,* it designates any type of parasitic and crawling vermin which enters either man or animal.[4] As in the case of the native flora, the Vedic Indian presented detailed descriptions of this class of fauna. Sometimes the characterizations of these vermin border on the mythical; mostly, however, they appear to be quite plausible. The *krími*s are divided into two basic types: those which are seen, i.e. visible, diurnal, and those which are unseen, i.e. invisible, nocturnal.[5] They can be black, red, dark-brown eared,[6] black with white arms, variegated with white underparts,[7] and some seem to possess a poison-sac.[8] In a more mythical vein, some worms are described as being spotted and whitish with three heads and three horns;[9] others are said to

---

[1] Because it exhibits variants to AVŚ 5.23, it is included in the notes to that charm.

[2] On the use of *krimi* or *kṛ́mi* in the *Atharvaveda,* see Whitney-Lanman, Pt. 1, 73. In the later texts, it is almost always written as *kṛmi,* a form closer to the original (see Mayrhofer, Wb. 1:261–62).

[3] See Macdonell-Keith, *Vedic Index,* 1: 179–80, and R. Müller, "Indische Würmerkrankheiten," 14–16.

[4] Sāyana to AVŚ 2.31.1 defines them as 'all small animals which have gone inside the body' (*śarīrāntargatān sarvān kṣudrajantūn*). Cf. also Yāska who states: A worm (*krimi*) is that which grows fat on a decaying corpse; or it could be from the root *kram,* 'to creep,' or from the root *krām,* 'to crawl' (Nir. 6.12: *krimiḥ kravye medyati. kramater vā syāt. saraṇakarmaṇaḥ. krāmater vā*) and Kuhn, "Indische und germanische Segenssprüche," KZ, 13: 136–37.

[5] AVŚ 2.31.2; 5.23.6.

[6] AVŚ 5.23.4.

[7] AVŚ 5.23.5.

[8] AVŚ 2.32.6; see AVŚ 5.23.13 n, 194.

[9] AVŚ 5.23.9, cf. 2.32.2 and 5.23.9 n, 193.

be vulture(-like) and wolf(-like).[10] They are called by a variety of names, the meanings of which are obscure: *kurū̃ru, algáṇḍu, śalúna, avaskavá, vyadhvará,*[11] *yévāṣa, káṣkaṣa, ejatká, śipavitnuká* and *nadanimán.*[12] The ancient Indian seems also to have been able to distinguish the sex of these creatures[13] and spoke of them in terms of a society, with a chief, his subjects and their dependents.[14] There is a strong suggestion that one type was a maggot which is said to feed upon the decaying corpse.[15]

These various types of *krími*s were known to have become most active during the early rainy season[16] and to have resided in mountains, in forests, in plants, in domestic animals, in the waters and, most importantly, in the body.[17] The bodily *krími*s were located in the entrails, in the ribs and in the head, which included the eyes, nostrils and teeth.[18]

Treatment

The means for the removal of these *krími*s consisted of ritually crushing and grinding them with a stone-slab and burning them. In the rite, the healer identified himself with the serpent-killer *par excellence,* Indra with his great weapon, the *vájra* or thunderbolt.[19] Since such procedures could hardly have been performed on the worms while they were in the body, we are led to believe that a symbolical rite took place in which worms were smashed and burned outside of the body. Sympathetically, the action outside the body affected the inside as well. Agastya's charm was recited to overpower and ensure the death of the demonic *krími*s.[20] There is a suggestion that the most auspicious time for the rite was at sunrise, when the sun's rays exposed the invisible *krími*s and aided in the destruction of all noxious vermin with their heat.[21]

kṛmi in the later traditions

In the ritual literature of the *Kauśika Sūtra* we notice a merging of the purely symbolical and sympathetic measures of treatment, reminiscent of the *Atharvaveda,* with more empirical and therapeutic means, perhaps anticipating those found in the āyurvedic tradition. At KauśS 27.14–20, the healer is first instructed to make an oblation consisting of *alāṇḍu* (*algaṇḍu*) and *hanana* worms along with black chick-peas mixed with ghee. He then

---

[10] AVŚ 5.23.4; these names suggest perhaps the voraciousness of the creatures.
[11] AVŚ 2.31.2–4.
[12] AVŚ 5.23.7–8.
[13] AVŚ 5.23.13.
[14] AVŚ 5.23.11–12; cf. 2.32.4–5.
[15] AVŚ 11.9.10: . . . *tṛpyatu krímiḥ páuruṣeyé 'bhi kúṇape.* . . , cf. also Sāyaṇa: . . . *māṃseṣu jīrṇeṣu jāyamānaḥ prāṇī,* 'a being which is born in decayed flesh,' and AVŚ 2.31.4n, 189–90.
[16] AVŚ 12.1.46: *krímir jínvat pṛthivi yádyad éjati prāvṛ́ṣi,* . . .
[17] AVŚ 2.31.5.
[18] AVŚ 2.31.4; 5.23.3.
[19] AVŚ 2.31.1–4; 5.23.1, 5, 8, 9, 13.
[20] AVŚ 5.23.10; cf. 2.31.3–4; 32.3.
[21] AVŚ 5.23.6–7; cf.2.32.1.

winds the tail-hair (of a cow)[22] around a black-spotted arrow, from right to left, and smashes it (with a stone). He heats (the pieces) over the fire and lays them in the fire (while inhaling the smoke). The rite continues with the healer throwing up dust with his left hand, while facing south, and scattering it over the patient who then grinds it up. Finally, the healer puts ordinary wood on the fire (and the patient is made to inhale its smoke).[23] At KauśS 29.20–26, the actions in a rite against worms in children, initially symbolical, quickly become more empirically based, suggesting an actual therapeutic application: Utilizing a root from the *karīra*-plant and dust from the village the medicine-man follows the procedure prescribed at KauśS 27.14–20. He then places (the child with worms) on the lap of its mother to the west of the fire and warms the palate of the child by pressing on it three times with the bottom of a pestle smeared with fresh butter. He smears it with the seeds of the *śigru*-plant mixed with fresh butter. He then takes twenty-one roots of the *uśīra*-plant and consecrates them with AVŚ 5.23.13*cd*, performing the action mentioned there (i.e. according to Keśava: mashing the roots and burning their surfaces with fire). He gives these roots (to the patient) and pours water along with the twenty-one (roots over the patient).[24]

In the āyurvedic medical texts, we find a concern for worm-caused diseases and, moreover, a continuation of the detailed descriptions and classification of worms, initiated in the *Atharvaveda*. There are twenty kinds of external and internal worms mentioned in the *Caraka-* and *Suśruta-Saṃhitās*.[25] Of these, the only worms or *kṛmis*, which seem to be similar to those referred to in the *Atharvaveda*, are the *dantāda*-worms, i.e. those which eat the teeth.[26] SuUtt 3.9 and 14.9–11 also mention a disease known as *kṛmigranthi* which is a worm-caused cyst on the eyelids. In this case, the *kṛmis* are found to inhabit the region of the eye.[27] These texts also speak of the diseases created by worms which have infested the head.[28]

---

[22] Following Keśava-Sāyaṇa and Caland who reads: *vālān* (AZ, 84n). Bloomfield, following Dārila, reads: *bālān*, 'young worm' (*Hymns*, 314).

[23] 27.14: . . . *khalvaṅgān alāṇḍūn hananān ghṛtamiśrān juhoti.* 15: *vālān (bālān) kalmāṣe kāṇḍe savyaṃ pariveṣṭya saṃbhinatti.* 16: *pratapati.* 17: *ādadhāti.* 18: *savyena dakṣiṇāmukhaḥ pāṃsūn upamathya parikirati.* 19: *saṃmṛdnāti.* 20: *ādadhāti*; cf. also Bloomfield, *Hymns*, 314 and especially Caland, AZ, 84.

[24] 29.20: . . . *karīramūlaṃ kāṇḍenaikadeśam.* 21: *grāmāt pāṃsūn.* 22: *paścād agner māturupasthe musalabudhnena navanītānvaktena triḥ pratīhāraṃ tāluni tāpayati.* 23: *śigrubhir navanītamiśraiḥ pradegdhi* 24: *ekaviṃśatim uśīrāṇi bhinadmīti mantroktam.* 25: *uśīrāṇi prāyacchati.* 26: *ekaviṃśatyā sahāplāvayati*; cf. Bloomfield, *Hymns*, 452–53, and Caland, AZ, 94.

[25] See CaSūSth 19.4 and ViSth 7.9; SuUtt 54.7 and Jolly, *Medicin*, 81–82; cf. also R. Müller, "Indische Würmerkrankheiten," *Gesnerus*, 21: 17–22, and Meulenbeld, *The Mādhavanidāna*, 291–92.

[26] See CaSūSth 19.9 and ViSth 7.9–32 and SuUtt 54.37; cf. Bloomfield, *Hymns*, 454.

[27] Cf. also CaViSth 7.11 where certain "blood-born worms" (*śoṇitajakṛmi*) are said to be destructive of eyelashes and SuUtt 54.12–14 where certain "phlegm-born worms" (*kaphajakṛmi*) are said to bore into the eyeballs.

[28] See in particular CaCiSth 26.118, 184–187, ViSth 7.20 and SuUtt 25. 10b–11a; 26.26b–30a and 54.34.

In the case of external worms, they are removed by hand or by the use of suitable instruments. Where the worms are found to be internal, the texts prescribe four basic types of therapies for their eradication: head-purgation, vomiting, purgation and corrective type of enema.[29] For a worm-caused head disease, the *śirovirecana* or head-purgation and nasal-therapy are prescribed.[30]

Jīvaka and the worm-caused head-disease

As we noticed above, the Vedic healer recognized that the head was one of the principal residences of harmful worms. In the story of the physician Jīvaka Komārabhacca, found in the eighth chapter of the *Mahāvagga* of the Buddhists' *Vinaya Piṭaka,* there is an interesting account of a treatment he performed on a citizen of Rājagṛha for a head-disease caused by worms. The technique involved what appears to have been a trepanation.[31] The essential part of the operation has been reported as follows:

> Now as the story goes, Jīvaka Komārabhacca made the householder lie down on the couch [and] bound him to it. Having cut away the skin of the head, [and] twisted open a suture [of the skull], he extracted two living beings and showed them to the crowd of people, [saying]: "Do you see these living beings, one small and one large. . . ?" . . . Then he closed the suture, sewed back the skin of the head and applied ointment.[32]

The classical texts of *āyurveda,* as we have noted, also mentioned a similar disease but prescribed quite a different treatment, involving rather nasal-therapy and head-purgation than surgery.

The *Mahāvagga* account of the story of Jīvaka is the earliest literary account of such a surgical procedure to be found in India. We also have corroborative evidence for the treatment in archaeological data, which suggests that it may have been practiced at a very early date in India, at a time at least as old as the Atharvavedic tradition. The most probable example of a trepanned skull has been unearthed at Timargarha in West Pakistan, dating from about the ninth to the middle of the sixth century B.C.[33] Other, apparently trepanned skulls, have been excavated from the

---

[29] CaViSth 7.15; cf. also SuUtt 54.21–38.

[30] See references in note 28 above.

[31] See my article "Studies in traditional Indian medicine in the Pāli Canon: Jīvaka and Āyurveda," *The Journal of the International Association of Buddhist Studies,* 5 (1982): 70–86. Cf. also R. Müller, "Schädeleröffnungen nach indischen Sagen," *Centaurus,* 6 (1959): 68–81. A similar technique appears in the *Bhojaprabandha,* by Ballāla; see Louis Gray, trans., *The Narrative of Bhoja (Bhojaprabandha), by Ballāla of Benares* (New Haven, Conn.: American Oriental Society, 1950), 93–95.

[32] *Mahāvagga* 8.1.18: *atha kho Jīvaka Komārabhacco seṭṭhiṃ gahapatiṃ mañcake nipajjāpetvā mañcake sambandhitvā sīsacchaviṃ upphāletvā sibbiniṃ vināmetvā dve pāṇake* (!) *nīharitvā janassa dassesi-passeyyātha* (or: *passath'ayyo*) *ime dve pāṇake ekaṃ khuddakaṃ ekaṃ mahallakaṃ. . . , sibbiniṃ sampaṭipādetvā* (or: *sampaṭicchādetvā*) *sīsacchaviṃ sibbetvā ālepaṃ adāsi.*

[33] See A. H. Dani, ed., "Timargarha and The Gandhara Grave Culture," *Ancient Pakistan,* 3 (1967): 48, 100, 240, and Wolfram Bernhard, "Human Skeletal Remains from the Cemetery of Timargarha," ibid., 368–69.

chalcolithic sites of Harappā[34] and Kalibangan in Northern Rajasthan,[35] dating from about 2000 B.C. and from the neolithic site of Burzahom in Kashmir, which dates from about 1800 B.C.[36] These latter examples, however, have not been confirmed as exhibiting definite signs of trepanation.

We notice, therefore, that the concern with bodily worms or vermin, especially those which infest the head, dates from an early period in ancient India and that various means for their eradication were employed. In the Atharvavedic tradition, the healing rite of removal appears to have been purely symbolic; while in the later traditions the symbolic procedures of the *Atharvaveda* merge with the developing empirical tradition of *āyurveda*, in which the more therapeutic techniques of nasal-therapy and head-purgation are the predominant means of treatment. Likewise, in the later period, we have evidence of another method for the elimination of worms from the head, trepanation. Although recorded later than the *Atharvaveda*, it may have been practiced at a time contemporaneous with that tradition, if not prior to it.

Worms in the Germanic tradition

It was not only among the peoples of ancient India that worms were considered to be an important cause of disease. In the Germanic tradition also, worms or vermin were looked upon as harmful to the bodies of both men and animals. A. Kuhn has examined the charms from both of these traditions and has noticed some interesting similarities between them: 1. in both traditions the worm was considered to be a disease; 2. there was a common belief in the color of worms; and 3. the notion of the toothworm (Zahnwurm) is recorded in both.[37] He concludes by stating rather boldly: "Das alles zeigt, dass sich für die Vorstellungen von den Krankheiten als Würmern bereits bestimmte Formen in der Sprache ausgebildet hatten und dass sie daher unzweifelhaft als altes Gemeingut anzusehen sind."[38] Whether the Atharvavedic and Germanic notions about worm-disease were derived from a common source is a debatable question.[39] In both traditions, as Kuhn has rightly demonstrated, there is, nevertheless, a rich storehouse of literature and folk-belief surrounding worms (*krími*, Würmer) and the diseases associated with them.

2.31

With that which is Indra's great stone-slab, the crusher of every worm, I grind together the worms as the *khálva*-grains [are ground] with an [ordinary] stone-slab. 1.

---

[34] See A. K. Roy Chowdhury, "Trepanation in Ancient India," *Asiatic Society of Calcutta*, Communications, 25 (1973): 203–206.

[35] See A. K. Sharma, "Kalibangan Human Skeletal Remains—an Osteoarchaeological approach," JOIB, 19 (1969): 109–14.

[36] See A. K. Sharma, "Neolithic human burials from Burzahom, Kashmir," JOIB, 16 (1967): 239, 247.

[37] "Indische und germanische Segenssprüche," 135–51.

[38] Ibid., 150.

[39] See in particular, Bloomfield, *Hymns*, 313–14.

I have crushed the seen and the unseen ones; I have also crushed the *kurū́ru*. With the charm, we grind up all the *algáṇḍu* and *śalúna* [types of] worms. 2.
With the great weapon, I kill the *algáṇḍus*. [Both] the burned [and] the unburned have become powerless. With the charm, I overpower [both] the remaining [and] the unremaining ones, so that not one of the worms may be left. 3.
With the charm, we grind up the worms: [the one] in the entrails, in the head and in the ribs, [as well as] the *avaskavá* and the *vyadhvará* worms. 4.
I kill that entire race of worms: those which are in the mountains, in the forests, in the plants, in the domestic animals, in the waters [and] those which have entered our body. 5.

5.23

Heaven and earth have been invoked for (by?) me, the goddess Sarasvatī has been invoked; [and] both Indra and Agni have been invoked for (by) me. [Thus, I say,] "let those two crush the worm." 1.
All the enemies have been destroyed by my powerful spell; [so now,] you, O Indra, lord of wealth, destroy this boy's worms. 2.
We crush that worm which crawls about the eyes, which crawls about the nostrils [or] which goes in amongst the teeth. 3.
The two with a similar appearance, the two with a different appearance, the two black ones, the two red ones, the dark-brown one and the one with dark-brown ears, the vulture(-like) one and the wolf(-like) one have [all] been destroyed. 4.
We crush those worms which have white underparts, which are black with white arms and whichever ones are variegated. 5.
In the east, the sun rises, seeing all, the destroyer of the unseen. It destroys both the seen and unseen and crushes all worms. 6.
Let both the seen and the unseen worm—the *yévāṣas*, the *káṣkaṣas*, the *ejatkás* [and] the *śipavitnukás*—be destroyed. 7.
Of the worms, the *yévāṣa* has been destroyed; likewise, the *nadanimán* has been destroyed; [for] I have ground down to a powder all [worms], like *khálva*-grains with a stone-slab. 8.
I crush the ribs [and] cut off the head of this spotted [and] whitish worm with three heads [and] three horns. 9.
Like Atri, like Kaṇva [and] like Jamadagni, I destroy you, O worms; [and] with Agastya's spell, I grind together the worms. 10.
The king of the worms has been destroyed and also their local headman has been destroyed; the worm, whose mother, brother and sister have been destroyed, has [also] been destroyed. 11.
His subjects have been destroyed; [and so] have their dependents been destroyed. Likewise, all those worms, which are so very small, have been destroyed. 12.
With a stone, I split the head of all the male and female worms; [and] with fire, I burn [their] face[s]. 13.

15: URINE-RETENTION (AND CONSTIPATION)

AVŚ 1.3 is a charm primarily against the retention of urine. It is unique because it is the only hymn of its type found either in the *Ṛgveda* or in the *Atharvaveda.*

The waste-matter, we learn, was known to be blocked in the bowels, in the two *gavīnīs* (ureters ?) and in the bladder (verse 6). As urine does not normally become obstructed in the bowels, we are led to assume that the hymn may have also been used in cases of constipation. This receives support from the *Kauśika Sūtra* (see below); likewise, in later Indian medicine, there is a class of diseases known as *udāvarta,* which is characterized, among other things, by constipation, retention of flatus and retention of urine.[1] The emphasis in this charm, however, is quite clearly on the retention of urine.

The means of liberating the obstructed flow of urine involved the breaching of the urethra and the probing of the bladder-orifice (verses 7, 8) with what appears to have been an arrow-like reed. It has been suggested that this reed was a primitive type of catheter, called *vasti-yantra* in later Indian medicine.[2] Filliozat, seeing difficulties with the hollowing out of a thin reed to be used as a catheter, suggests rather that its use was probably symbolic.[3] Although an arrow made from a reed is symbolic in verse 9, it does not imply that the mention of the reed throughout the hymn is to be understood in this way. It seems quite possible that a reed was originally employed in the treatment of urine-retention, to be replaced later by a more sturdy metal catheter. It points to an advanced technique of surgery encountered only rarely in these early hymns. The repetition of the refrain throughout adds to the archaic and magical quality of the charm: the nonsense sound, "*bāl,*" onomatopoeic for discharging water, would have helped to direct the purpose of the hymn and, in addition, would have had the psychological effect of aiding the patient to relax his bladder and to let the urine flow freely.

Crucial to a complete understanding of this disease and its treatment is the practice outlined in the later ritual which, like the charm itself, incorporates elements of both magical and empirical medicine. The passages are plagued with obscure readings; nevertheless, we can obtain a fairly accurate view of a healing procedure not too different from that which was originally performed:

---

[1] CaCiSth 26.6–25; SuUtt 55; cf. also AHSūSth 4.

[2] See Whitney-Lanman, *Atharva-veda-saṃhitā,* Pt. 1, 3; cf. also Caland, AZ, 69–70 n7, Henry, *La magie,* 208, and G. N. Mukhopādhyāya, *Surgical Instruments of the Hindus,* 2 vols. (Calcutta: Calcutta University, 1913–14), 1: 137.

[3] *La doctrine,* 111–12; cf. also R. Müller, "Die Sagen vom Katheterisieren der Inder bei Harnverhaltung," *Sudhoffs Archiv für Geschichte der Medizin und der Naturwissenschaften,* 42 (1958): 377–84.

With AVŚ 1.3, [the healer] binds [to the patient an amulet] which promotes urination; he gives [him] a concoction of [dirt from] a mole-hill, *pūtīka*-plant, curded milk, dried *pramanda*-plant, with [some] twigs, to drink; with the last two verses, [he] makes [the patient] sit at ease and [administers an oily enema through a funnel—commentator]; he makes [him] mount a vehicle; he launches an arrow; he splits open the urethra and releases [the urine in] the bladder [by means of a copper instrument—commentator]; having poured twenty-one barley-grains with water into a milk-pail, having secured a bow (or an axe) at the pudenda (?), he pours [the water and grains] down the member (?); he gives [the patient] a decoction of *āla*-plant (wheat), lotus-stalk (*bisa*) and *ula* to drink; [this treatment can] also [be employed] in cases of retention of excrements (*udāvarta*).[4]

1.3

We know the father of the reed, Parjanya, whose potency is a hun-
dredfold. With that I shall make your body healthy. On to the
earth let your outflowing be, out of you, [sounding like] "*bā̆l.*" 1.
We know the father of the reed, Mitra, whose potency is a hun-
dredfold. With that I shall make your body healthy. On to the
earth let your outflowing be, out of you, [sounding like] "*bā̆l.*" 2.
We know the father of the reed, Varuṇa, whose potency is a hun-
dredfold. With that I shall make your body healthy. On to the
earth let your outflowing be, out of you, [sounding like] "*bā̆l.*" 3.
We know the father of the reed, Candra (the moon), whose potency
is a hundredfold. With that I shall make your body healthy. On
to the earth let your outflowing be, out of you, [sounding like]
"*bā̆l.*" 4.
We know the father of the reed, Sūrya (the sun), whose potency is
a hundredfold. With that I shall make your body healthy. On to
the earth let your outflowing be, out of you, [sounding like]
"*bā̆l.*" 5.
That which has been blocked in the bowels, in the two *gavīnīs* (ure-
ters?) [and] in the bladder—thus may your urine be released en-
tirely, [sounding like] "*bā̆l.*" 6.
I breach your urethra as the dike of a lake [is breached]. Thus, may
your urine be released entirely, [sounding like] "*bā̆l.*" 7.
Released is your bladder-orifice as [the orifice] of a water-holding
ocean. Thus, may your urine be released entirely, [sounding like]
"*bā̆l.*" 8.
As an arrow flies forth [when] released from a bow, so also may your
urine be released entirely, [sounding like] "*bā̆l.*" 9.

---

[4] KauśS 25.10–19: 10. *vidmā śarasyeti pramehaṇaṃ badhnāti;* 11. *ākhukiripūtīka-mathitajaratpramandasāvraskān pāyayati;* 12. *uttamābhyām āsthāpayati;* 13. *yānam ārohayati;* 14. *iṣuṃ visṛjati;* 15 (16). *vartiṃ bibhetti;* 16 (15). *vastiṃ viṣyati;* 17. *ekaviṃśatiṃ yavān dohanyām adbhir ānīya drughnīṃ jaghane saṃstabhya phalato 'vasiñcati;* 18. *ālabisolaṃ phāṇṭaṃ pāyayati;* 19. *udāvartine ca.* Cf. Bloomfield, *Hymns,* 236 and Caland, AZ, 69–70. Based on the hymn and a logical progression of events, *sūtras* 15 and 16 have been reversed. On *ula,* see Meulenbeld, The *Mādhavanidāna,* 448–49; perhaps it is the same as *okula,* lightly fried wheat.

II. EXTERNAL DISEASES

Unlike the internal diseases which are characterized as entering and residing in the body of their victims, the external diseases are less precisely defined but are quite naturally distinguished as those afflictions which affect the exterior of the body. They include broken limbs and flesh wounds, blood-loss, perhaps due to excessive menstrual discharge, and skin disorders, such as discoloration of the skin (leukoderma), rash with pustules, and loss of hair.

16: BROKEN LIMBS AND FLESH WOUNDS

This chapter will be divided into two sections: 1. charms to cure broken bones and wounds (AVŚ 4.12; 5.5); 2. charms to cure flesh wounds characterized by bleeding (AVŚ 2.3; 6.44; 6.109).

In both instances, the principal remedy appears to have been plants or their products; while in the case of bleeding wounds, water was also used. The vegetal part of the treatment is significant, as it involved the healing plant-goddess and protectress Arundhatī who, being multiformed,[1] was invoked in her various forms in order to make the remedy, in this case the simples, more efficacious.[2] The mere mention of her name or one of her epithets would have had the effect of deifying the plant which the healer was to use in the healing rite.

Broken bones, fractures and wounds

AVŚ 4.12 is a charm against a common external injury suffered by both men and animals, the broken bone (*asthnáḥ chinnásya,* verse 1) which was caused by falling into a hole or by being struck by a rock (verse 7). The principal cure for such an injury is said to be the plant *róhaṇī,* made efficacious through its association with the goddess Arundhatī (verse 1).

Perhaps the most interesting aspect of this charm is its close linguistic parallel to the Germanic incantations which are based on the tenth-century Merseburg spell. A. Kuhn has presented these spells and analyzed their similarities, concluding that this Atharvan charm which prescribed the use of a healing plant, like that from Merseburg, may have originally been part of a healing rite for an injured horse.[3] Bloomfield, however, dismisses such a supposition by saying: "Any kind of genetic connection between the

---

[1] AVŚ 6.59.3.

[2] See chapter 21, below, 96f.

[3] "Indische und germanische Segenssprüche," 51–63, 151–54.

Hindu and the German charm is none too certain, since the situation may have suggested the same expressions independently."[4] To posit any direct connection between these two charms is indeed risky; but one should not indiscriminately reject a valuable clue to the understanding of this Atharvan charm. To be sure, we may present some evidence which points to the fact that it may have originally been recited during the healing of a horse's broken limb. At P 4.15.2, we notice that the sinew (*snāvan*) is added to the list of parts of the limb to be rejoined.[5] In almost all the versions of the Merseburg spell presented by Kuhn, the sinew was reckoned as such a part.[6] More importantly, the evidence contained in the charm itself suggests that a horse may be meant. With the rendering of verse 6 (see also notes on 200–201, below) according to the printed text, we have what appears to be an incantation recited by the healer, imploring a horse to stand up, boldly and strongly, and to proceed to its chariot which, for its benefit, has been fitted out with strong and sturdy parts. Likewise, at verse 7, falling into a hole and being struck by a rock suggest accidental injuries which a horse, rather than a man, would be more likely to incur.

These few pieces of evidence in no way prove that this charm was originally intended for a horse, nor do they confirm any connection with the German spells. In fact, the tradition employs it for an injury suffered by a man.[7] They do, however, raise some interesting points which, in the past, would have been brushed aside as ridiculous.

AVŚ 5.5 is a charm devoted to the cure of a very similar injury, the fracture (*rúta*)[8] or wound (*árus*) caused by a club, an arrow or a flame (verses 4, 6). The remedy employed to mend the injury was *lākṣā̄* or *silācī̄*. Controversy surrounds the exact meaning of these words. Early translators considered them to be plants, perhaps parasitic in nature,[9] while more recent examiners of this charm understand them to refer to a resin or exudation. Filliozat and Vishva Bandhu view *lākṣā̄* as such a substance, which is commonly called lac, an āyurvedic medicine.[10] Likewise, K. N. Dave has understood it to mean lac and has even noticed in the charm the process of the production of lac from the so-called lac-insect.[11] There is no

---

[4] *Hymns*, 386. More recently, this same view has been propounded by B. Schlerath in his article "Zu den Merseburg Zaubersprüchen," *Innsbrucker Beiträge zur Kulturwissenschaft*, Sonderheft, 15 (1962): 139–43.

[5] It should be kept in mind, however, that this P charm exhibits evidence of being late.

[6] KZ, 1 3: 51–57, 151–54.

[7] See KauśS 28.4, and Caland, AZ, 89.

[8] Words from the root *ru*, 'to break,' occur four times in the *Ṛgveda* and at each place they suggest a bodily injury involving a smashed or broken limb, or fracture [see ṚV 10.39.3; 10.86.5; 10.105.7 and 9.112.1 where the healer (*bhisáj*) is characterized as the one who desires a fracture (to cure)].

[9] See Macdonell-Keith, *Vedic Index*, 2: 450, and Weber, IS, 18: 182.

[10] Filliozat, *La doctrine*, 109–11; Vishva Bandhu, VIJ, 9: 1–3. On both the medicinal and non-medicinal uses of lac, see Dutt and King, *Materia Medica*, 277–78.

[11] "Lac and the Lac-insect in the Atharva-Veda," *International Academy of Indian Culture* (Nagpur, 1950), 1–16; see also S. L. Hora's excellent summary: "Lac and the Lac-insect in the Atharva-Veda," JASB, 18 (1952): 13–15.

question that there are strong indications that the poet-healer was, on occasion, describing something that resembles resin (verses 2, 3, 5, 8, 9). It is unlikely, however, that he was aware of the fact that lac was not a product of the plant, but the result of the activities of an insect. It is more reasonable to assume that *lākṣā̆* (*silācī̆*) was a substance derived from auspicious plants and that both were divine aspects of the plant-goddess Arundhatī. In other words, in the poet's mind, the plant and its product were looked upon as possessing the same divine characteristics which were given to it through its association with Arundhatī.[12]

In addition to the numerous mythological references to the goddess, we have at least one which hints at the fact that she was to be drunk, perhaps in a potion, in order to save the patient and to promote his well-being (verse 2). This receives support from the later ritual practice which, being largely therapeutic with elements of symbolism and no reference to the use of plants, suggests a more recent attitude toward healing (the rite incorporates both hymns):

> With 4.12, [the healer] sprinkles [the wound] with water at the time when the stars begin to fade away (i.e. at dawn); he gives [the patient] a mixture of ghee and milk to drink [and] anoints [the wound with the same mixture]. With the verses characterized with the word *lākṣā* [AVŚ 5.5 (and 4.12-commentator)], [the healer] gives [to the patient] a decoction [of *lākṣā*] in milk to drink.[13]

4.12

You, the *róhaṇī*, are *róhaṇī*, the healer of the severed bone. [Therefore,]
make this [limb] grow, O Arundhatī. 1.
Let Dhātṛ propitiously reunite, joint with joint, whatever broken bone
[or] inflamed piece of flesh [is] in your body. 2.
Let your marrow be united with marrow and [let] your joint [be]
united with joint. Let your torn [piece] of flesh and [your] bone
grow together. 3.
Let the marrow be united with marrow; let the skin grow with skin;
let your blood grow with blood [and] let flesh grow with flesh. 4.
You, O herb, make hair join with hair, make skin join with skin.
Unite what is severed. Let bone grow forth with bone. 5.
You there stand up, advance, run along, [your] chariot [has] strong
wheels, rims [and] hubs. Stand erect firmly! 6.
If falling in a hole, [he] has been injured, or if a hurled rock has
struck [him, then] may [Dhātṛ] unite the limbs, joint with joint, as
Ṛbhu [the parts] of a chariot. 7.

---

[12] The charm itself suggests something similar: at vs. 8, the father of the *lākṣā̆* (*silācī̆*) is called what appears to be by the same name as the goddess; but, because it is the father and a son, it must be understood as a masculine divinity.

[13] KauśS 28. 5–6; 14: 6. *rohaṇīty avanakṣatre 'vasiñcati; 6. pṛṣātakaṃ prāyayaty abhyanakti; 14. lākṣāliṅgābhir dugdhe phāṇṭān pāyayati.* Cf. Bloomfield, *Hymns*, 285, and Caland, AZ, 88, 90.

5.5

The night [is] your mother, the cloud, your father [and] Yama, your grandfather. Indeed, you are *silācī́*, by name, [and] you are the sister of the gods. 1.

He who drinks you lives; you save the man; for you are the protectress of all and the refuge of the people. 2.

You, like a mannish young girl, mount each and every tree. Indeed, you are, by name, triumphant, steadfast and delivering. 3.

You are the mender of that wound which is inflicted by a club, by an arrow or by a flame. [Therefore,] mend this man. 4.

You, O Arundhatī, arise out of the auspicious *plakṣá, aśvatthá, khadirá* [and] *dhavá;* [likewise,] out of the auspicious *nyagródha* [and] *parṇá* [and] come to us. 5.

May you, O golden one, O auspicious one, O sun-colored one, O most beautiful one, go to the fracture; [for] you, O mender, are indeed mender by name. 6.

O golden one, O auspicious one, O fiery one, O hairy-sided one, O *lākṣā́*, you are the sister of the waters [and] your very self has become the wind. 7.

The young girl's son, *silācín* (?), by name, [is] your father; [and] you, O goat-brown one, were sprinkled with the blood of Yama's tawny horse. 8.

Having streamed from the horse's blood, she crept on to the trees. [So] having become [as] a winged stream, come to us, O Arundhatī. 9.

Flesh wounds characterized by bleeding

AVŚ 2.3, 6.44 and 6.109 are charms for the cure of a bodily affliction called *róga* (or *rogaṇa*). Etymologically, the word *róga* points to a breach of some part of the body, i.e., a flesh-wound or affliction,[1] which, at AVŚ 6.120.3, beings of the heavenly world are said to have abandoned. These divinities are also mentioned as being not lame in the limbs and being devoid of dislocated (limbs).[2] The affliction or wound appears to have been characterized by *āsrāvá*. According to the native commentators and most western interpreters, *āsrāvá* represented any bodily discharge or flux.[3] In the context of a flesh-wound, however, it seems to refer specifically to a discharge of blood. The cause for this bleeding wound is the infliction of

---

[1] See T. Chowdhury, JBORS, 17: 48. Later the word *roga* came to mean 'disease' or 'infirmity' (see Meulenheld, *The Mādhavanidāna*, 505).

[2] *yátrā suhā́rdaḥ sukŕ̥to mádanti vihā́ya rógaṃ tanvàḥ svā́yāḥ, áśloṇā áṅgair áhrutāḥ svargé tátra paśyema pitárau ca putrā́n* (cf. AVŚ 3.28.5).

[3] See KauśS 25.6 and its commentaries as well as Sāyaṇa to AVŚ 1.2.4 and 2.3.2, below in the notes, 207–208; Macdonell-Keith, *Vedic Index*, 1: 74; cf. also Bloomfield, AJPh, 7: 467–69; *Hymns*, 233; Filliozat, *La doctrine*, 101; and Chowdhury, JBORS, 17: 48.

a weapon.[4] Closely related to this bloody discharge is the morbid condition known as *vātīkṛta*, which, etymologically, suggests perhaps gastric problems and which may look back to the very beginnings of what later could have given rise to the *tridoṣa*-doctrine of classical *āyurveda*.[5]

The medicines used in the treatment of such a wound included water and herbs.[6] The water, called Rudra's urine,[7] is said to have come from the mountain streams and from the sea (*samudrá*).[8] At AVŚ 2.3.4, termites (*upajīkās*) are said to have taken up this type of water. A similar connection between termites and water occurs at AVŚ 6.100.2.[9] In this instance, however, the water is used against poison. Because termites are not normally connected with the salty water of the ocean, it would appear that the *samudrá*-water mentioned here refers to the fresh water of a large lake.

The other medicine, said to have come from the earth,[10] refers to the herbs or plants. They are called *viṣāṇakā́*, and *pippalī́*.[11] *viṣāṇakā́*, being etymologically connected to 'horn' (*viṣā́ṇa*), is, at AVŚ 6.44.3, called "the destroyer of *vātīkṛta*";[12] and at P 15.15.9, *arundhatī* is titled "medicine for *vātīkṛta*." This points to an ultimate connection of *viṣāṇakā́* and *pippalī́* with the medicinal plant-goddess Arundhatī. In an obscure mythical reference, the *ásuras* are said to have buried the "medicine-for-wounds" which is also the "medicine for *āsrāvá*" and the "medicine for *vātīkṛta*," i.e. *pippalī́*, deep below the earth[13] and the gods are said to have dug it up again.[14]

There is another plant, *múñja*-grass, which may also have been used in this healing rite. At AVŚ 1.2, a hymn primarily concerned with the protection from enemies' arrows,[15] verse 4 mentions *múñja* in relation to *róga* and *āsrāvá*: "As the *téjana* (perhaps a reference to the "sharp" arrow) stands between heaven and earth, so then let the *múñja*-grass stand between both the affliction and [its] (bloody) discharge."[16] The implication is that the

---

[4] AVŚ 6.109.1, 3; cf. AVŚ 2.3.6.

[5] See Filliozat, *La doctrine*, 140–41. The word *vātīkārá*, a variant of *vātīkṛta*, occurs at AVŚ 9.8.20 (47 above).

[6] AVŚ 2.3.6.

[7] AVŚ 6.4.4.3.

[8] AVŚ 2.3.1, 4.

[9] Cf. also MS 4.5.9; ŚB 14.1.18 and TĀ 5.1.4, where there is the association between termites or white ants and water.

[10] AVŚ 2.3.3, 5.

[11] AVŚ 6.44.3; 6.109.1, 2.

[12] It is interesting to note that the *pippalī́*-plant is utilized as a medicine in *āyurveda*. Its root and fruit are given internally for various ailments, many of which include gastric disorders (see Dutt and King, *Materia Medica*, 244–45, and P. N. V. Kurup, et al., *Handbook of Medicinal Plants* [New Delhi: Central Council for Research in Ayurveda and Siddha, 1979], 166).

[13] AVŚ 2.3.3; 6.109.3.

[14] AVŚ 2.3.4; 6.109.3.

[15] In the ritual literature, we find the hymn employed both as a battle charm at KauśS 14.7–13 and a medical charm at KauśS 25.6–9. The verses of the hymn itself point to an original usage as a battle charm.

[16] *yáthā dyā́ṃ ca pṛthivī́ṃ cāntás tíṣṭhati téjanam, evā́ rógaṃ cāsrāvā́ṃ cāntás tiṣṭhu múñja ít.* K 20.33.6 is a similar verse in which the notion of disease or discharge does not occur: *yathā dyāṃ ca pṛthivīṃ ca múñja it tiṣṭhaty antarā, asthād idaṃ viśvaṃ bhuvanam asthād vaco anusyavaḥ* (?, perhaps read as *anusravaḥ*), which may tentatively be rendered: "As indeed the *múñja*-grass stands between heaven and earth [so also] did this entire living world stand [and so]

múñja-grass was somehow used to prevent the bleeding which, from the context of the hymn, appears to be from an arrow-wound. It could be merely a reference to the symbolic use of the *múñja*-grass: just as the sharp reed-arrow (*śará*, verse 1) is the cause of the affliction, so also the pointed *múñja*-grass should be able to ward off the wounds caused by them. It may, however, point to the use of small bits of *múñja*-grass as a type of gauze-pad which, when applied to the bleeding wound, aided in stopping the blood-flow.[17]

The ritual mentioned in the *Kauśika Sūtra* for each of these hymns illustrates a combination of symbolism and actual therapeutics and shows very little connection with what is stated in the hymns:

With AVŚ 1.2 and 2.3, [the healer] binds [to the patient] the top of a stalk of *muñja*-grass by means of a cord [made from the grass]; having ground up pieces of the grass and the mud from a termite's nest (or an anthill), he gives [it to the patient] to drink; he anoints [him] with ghee and blows [through an opening in a piece of hide] upon [the affected areas]. While muttering AVŚ 6.44, [the healer makes the patient sip water] by means of a ghee-smeared, deciduous horn of a pining away cow(?) [and sprinkles him with it]. With AVŚ 6.109, [the healer] makes [the patient] eat pepper-corns.[18]

2.3

I prepare for you that medicine which runs down, flowing from the
mountain, so that you may be an effectual medicine. 1.
Then indeed, what then indeed! Of those which are your hundred
medicines, you are superior, without *āsrāvá* [and] without the afflic-
tion. 2.
The *ásuras* bury this great treatment-for-wounds deep below [the
earth]. It is the medicine for *āsrāvá* and it has destroyed the
affliction. 3.
The *upajīkās* (termites) take up the medicine from the sea. It is the
medicine for *āsrāvá* and it has destroyed the affliction. 4.
This great treatment-for-wounds has been taken up from the earth.
It is the medicine for *āsrāvá* and it has destroyed the affliction. 5.

---

did the after-flowing(?) of speech stand [between those two]." O reads similar to Śau, except in *cd*, it has *muñjas tiṣṭhaty antarā*. The next verse (7) in O is as follows: *asthād idaṃ viśvaṃ bhuvanam asthād vāto vanacyavaḥ, asthur vṛkṣā ūrdhvasvpnās tiṣṭhād rogo ayaṃ tava*, "The entire living world stood still; the wind shaking the forest stood still; the upright-sleeping trees stood still; [therefore] may this your affliction stand still (i.e. stop its discharge)" (cf. AVŚ 6.44.1).

[17] Cf., below, P 19.4.14 to AVŚ 1.17.4 (215–16 below) where a similar use of reeds (*śara*), along with sand, is mentioned.

[18] KauśS 25.6–9; 31.6; 26.38: 25.6. *vidmā śarasyādo yad iti muñjaśiro rajjvā badhnāti;* 7. *ākṛtiloṣṭavalmīkau parilikhya pāyayati;* 8. *sarpiṣālimpati;* 9. *apidhamati;* 31.6. *asthād dyaur ity apavātāyāḥ svayaṃsrastena gośṛṅgeṇa saṃpātavatā japan;* 26.38. *caturthenāśayati.* Cf. Bloomfield, *Hymns*, 234, 277–78, 481–82, 516; Caland, AZ, 68–69, 99–100, and 80; and Henry, *La magie*, 196. Bloomfield remarks that KauśS 31.6 is "another salient instance of the conscious employment of a hymn in a ritual in a secondary manner" (AJPh, 12: 427 n).

Let the water be healthy for us [and let] the herbs [be] auspicious [to us]. Let Indra's thunderbolt ward off the *rakṣás*-demons [and] let the released arrows of the *rakṣás*-demons fly into the distance. 6.

6.44

Heaven stood still; earth stood still; the entire living world stood still; the upright-sleeping trees stood still; [therefore] may this your affliction stand still. 1.

A hundred, a thousand of your medicines have been brought together, [of which you are] the best medicine for *āsrāvá* [and] the most excellent destroyer of the affliction. 2.

You are Rudra's urine [and] the navel of immortality. To be sure, you are *viṣāṇakā́*, by name, arisen from the fathers' root [and] the destroyer of *vātī́kṛta*. 3.

6.109

pippalī́ (pepper) is the medicine for [wounds from] missiles [and] the medicine for those pierced deeply [by weapons]. The gods thought of her [as] the one "capable of restoring life." 1.

Coming together just after their birth, the *pippalī́* (pepper)-plants conversed amongst themselves: "May that man, whom we should visit [and find] living, not be harmed." 2.

The *ásuras* buried you, the medicine for *vātīkṛta* and the medicine for [wounds from] missiles, [and] the gods dug you up again. 3.

17: BLOOD-LOSS

AVŚ 1. 17 is a charm to stop the flow of blood. Although it is not explicitly stated in the hymn, there is the implication, gathered from variant readings at P 19.4.15 and *Nirukta* 3.4 and from a comparison with AVŚ 7.35 (36).2 that the blood-flow was considered to be that characterized by an excessively heavy menstrual discharge.[1] The blood was believed to issue from two types of vessels, the *hirā́s* which are perhaps distinguished as being smaller (verses 1, 2) than the larger, *dhamánis* (verse 2). Both, however, were recognized as existing in large numbers in the body (verse 3).

The cure for this condition involved the recitation of incantations imploring the blood to stop its flow and the use of sand to surround the vessels and to inhibit the blood-loss. At P 1.94.4 (see 216, below) the healer is directed to sprinkle or to spread the sand on to the spot from which the blood is streaming. In this way, the sand acted as a kind of coagulant allowing the blood to clot and the bleeding to stop. If, however, we consider that the charm may have originally been used in a rite to stop excessive menstrual discharge, the reference to "the solid bow-like bank of sand" which was to have surrounded the vessels and to have brought about the cessation of the blood-flow, may point to an early kind of sanitary napkin.[2] In both explanations a more empirical attitude toward medical treatment is implied.

The ritual tradition prescribes the use of this hymn in the treatment of excessive blood-loss caused by menstruation and by wounds. The procedure is empirically based and reflects a close connection with the hymns, especially those of the Paippalāda recension:

> While muttering AVŚ 1.7, [the healer touches the site of the blood-flow] with a bamboo-staff containing five joints [and then] scatters sand and gravel around [the site]; he binds [to the patient] fragments from the site of ruins (or mud from a marsh?); he gives [the patient a solution of pulverized fragments in water] to drink [and also] a concoction of curded milk and ground sesame with four tips of *dūrvā*-grass to drink.[3]

In the later medical tradition, the disease, characterized by the excessive flow of blood during and after menses, was known as *asṛgdara;*[4] and the

[1]See notes to AVŚ 1.17.1,3, 214-15, below.

[2] Cf. P 19.4.14, where sand and reeds are mentioned, perhaps for the same purpose (215, below).

[3] KauśS 26.9(10)–13: 9(10). *amūryā iti pañcaparvaṇā pāṃsusikatābhiḥ parikirati;* 11. *armakapālikāṃ badhnāti;* 12. *pāyayati;* 13. *caturbhir dūrvāgrair dadhipalalaṃ pāyayati.* Cf. Bloomfield, *Hymns,* 257–58, and especially Caland, AZ, 74–75. See also Henry, *La magie,* 196.

[4] SuŚāSth 2.18–21; cf. also Jolly, *Medicin,* 50, and Kutumbiah, *Ancient Indian Medicine,* 179.

treatment for it was the same as that prescribed for a hemorrhage (*raktapitta*) mentioned at SuUtt 45.11–15.

1.17

Let those young women, the *hirā́*-[blood] vessels, clothed in red garments, who proceed as brotherless sisters, stop with their beauty drained. 1.

Stop, you lower one; stop, you upper one; and also stop, you middle one. And [since] the smallest one stops, indeed the *dhamáni*-[blood] vessel should [also] stop. 2.

Of the hundred *dhamáni*-[blood] vessels [and] of the thousand *hirā́*-[blood] vessels, these middle ones have indeed stopped. Jointly, the end ones have come to rest. 3.

The solid bow-like bank of sand has surrounded you [,O vessels?]. Stop, remain perfectly still. 4.

18: SKIN DISORDERS

kilā́sa (Discoloration of the Skin; Leukoderma)

AVŚ 1.23 and 24 are charms for what appear to be two kinds of skin disorders, *kilā́sa* and *pálita.* The latter term, means 'pale', and denotes in the *Suśruta Saṃhitā,* white hair caused by age and by pain.[1] In the *Atharvaveda,* however, the word indicates a white-colored spot on the skin, closely related to *kilā́sa,* and is perhaps merely a characterization of it (1.23.2). *kilā́sa,* on the other hand, is more problematic. Sayaṇa considers it to be a skin-disease characterized by cutaneous whiteness (*śvetakuṣṭha*); and most western interpreters view it as a type of "leprosy."[2] In classical Indian medicine, however, there are three types of *kilā́sa* which itself is a variety of *kuṣṭha* or 'skin-disease,' among which group leprosy is also found.[3] The symptoms of the Atharvavedic *kilā́sa* are cutaneous white marks or spots (1.23.2, 3, 4) which are said to arise from within the body and to be caused by a curse (1.23.4). Such a description suggests the general skin disorder known as leukoderma: "A condition of defective pigmentation of the skin, especially a congenital absence of pigment in patches or bands."[4] Unlike leprosy, therefore, leukoderma is less severe and does not produce skin-lesions.

In order to cure this condition, the healer uses a spell or spells, presumably AVŚ 1.23 and 24, and a dark, even-colored herb which appears to possess a dyeing or tincturing quality (1.23.1, 4; 1.24.4). Sympathetically, everything with a dark hue, connected with the herb, is mentioned in the charm. It is born at night (1.23.1), the soil in which it grows is dark and the environment in which it is found is also dark (1.23.3). To strengthen its effectiveness, the poet-healer presents a mythological episode in which a female *āsurá,* the first one to produce the medicine for *kilā́sa* and to bring about its destruction, was conquered in battle and gave the trees an eagle's gall-colored appearance. This *āsurī́* destroyed the *kilā́sa* and restored an even color to the skin (1.24.1, 2).[5] He goes on to recount the herb's lineage: both the

[1] See NiSth 13.32–33 and Filliozat, *La doctrine,* 102.

[2] See Macdonell-Keith, *Vedic Index,* 1: 158 and notes to AVŚ 1.23, 24, 217, below.

[3] See CaCiSth 7.173; SuNiSth 5.14 and Filliozat, *La doctrine,* 103.

[4] Normand L. Hoerr, and Arthur Osol, eds., *Blakiston's New Gould Medical Dictionary,* (New York: McGraw-Hill, 1956, second edition), 663. Filliozat, being more cautious, explains it as a "trouble de coloration de le peau dû à des maléfices . . ." (*La doctrine,* 104); cf. also Karambelkar, *The Atharva-Veda and the Āyur-Veda,* 185.

[5] *āsurī́* is traditionally equated with *rājasarṣapa* or the brown mustard (see AthPariś 35 and Karambelkar, *The Atharva-Veda and the Āyur-Veda,* 90).

mother and the father have the same name as the herb, i.e. 'even-colored' (1.24.3). Thereupon, the herb is requested to restore the skin to its natural evenness of color by staining it dark or gall-colored (1.24.3-4). There is also a hint that part of this healing ritual included uprooting the plant from the ground (1.24.4). Although the charm does not indicate how the herb was applied, one would assume that it was made into a decoction and rubbed on to the skin.

The ritual practice combines magical and empirical techniques; and since it follows the hymns closely, it reflects a quality of originality:

With AVŚ 1.23 and 1.24, [the healer], having scrubbed [the discolored patches] with (dried) cow-dung until they are red, anoints [them with the vegetal substances] mentioned in the hymn (i.e. *bhṛṅgarājā, haridrā, indravāruṇī* and *nīlī*—commentator); he pulls out the grey hairs; and, covered, [the healer performs] the rites to the Maruts[, which at KauśS 41.1–7 are for rain].[6]

1.23

You, O dim, black and dark herb, are born at night. O you colorer,
color him who is *kilā́sa* and pale. 1.
Make the spotted one, both the *kilā́sa* and the pale one, vanish from
here. Let your own [natural] color enter you. Make the white ones
fly away. 2.
Your bed [is] dark; your site [is] dark and you, O herb, are dark.
Make the spotted one vanish from here. 3.
By means of the spell, I have destroyed the cutaneous white mark
of *kilā́sa* born of the bone, of the body [and] caused by a curse. 4.

1.24

The eagle was the first born. You were his gall. Then, the *āsurī́* con-
quered in battle, gave the trees [their] appearance. 1.
The *āsurī́* was the first one to produce this medicine for *kilā́sa*, the
[means for the] destruction of *kilā́sa*. She destroyed *kilā́sa* [and]
made the skin even-colored. 2.
Even-colored, by name, [is] your mother; even-colored, by name, [is]
your father. [Since] you, O herb, are even-colored, [therefore] make
this [skin] even-colored. 3.
The dark one, who makes things even-colored, was taken up from
the earth. You must now quite properly accomplish this [end and]
restore [the skin's natural] colors. 4.

*apacít*s (Rash with Pustules)

AVŚ 6.25; 83; 7.74(78).1, 2 and 7.76(80).1, 2 are charms against the skin affliction known as *apacít* (feminine). This is a rather obscure malady be-

[6] KauśS 26.22–24: 22. *naktaṃjātā suparṇo jāta iti mantoktaṃ śakṛdā lohitaṃ praghṛṣyālimpati;* 23. *palitāny ācchidya;* 24. *mārutāny apihitaḥ.* Cf. Bloomfield, *Hymns,* 266–67; Caland, AZ, 76–77; and Henry, *La magie,* 190. See also notes to AVŚ 1.23.1, 217 below.

cause of its confounding characteristics. Sāyaṇa, however, has defined the word as *gaṇḍamālā*, or 'scrofulous swellings' which are often located about the neck.[1] Following along these lines, Bloomfield has pointed to the fact that *apacít* probably represents the disease *apacī* mentioned in the *Suśruta Saṃhitā* (NiSth 11.8–9),[2] which Filliozat has shown to be more particularly a case of adenopathy.[3]

The *apacít*s are characterized as raised bumps or pustules[4] called *gurvikā*[5] and *agrū* (a female demon).[6] There are types which are variegated, white, black and red.[7] The black color, as Filliozat suggests, may be a gangrenous tinge which the abscess assumes just before rupturing and the red color could be characteristic of the swelling before it reaches the abscessed stage.[8] There is also a barren *apacít*[9] who is called the black one's daughter. This may describe the state of the swelling before it suppurates or after it has done so, when the pus cannot be seen. The *apacít*s are associated with oozing boils or sores[10] and seem to be located amongst the hairs of the head.[11] They are also stated to be on the nape of the neck, about the neck, on the shoulders, the abdomen, along the sides and on the *vijā́man* (twin ?) joints beginning with the armpits and moving down the body, including perhaps the pudenda.[12] They seem to have occurred in large numbers, but were considered to have increased in number as they spread down the body,[13] suggesting perhaps a type of rash with pustules.[14]

The most puzzling qualities, which the *apacít*s are said to possess, include their ability to fly[15] and to make noise.[16] These characteristics led early translators to suggest that the *apacít*s represented some type of flying and buzzing insect.[17] Although the arguments of Bloomfield and Filliozat are quite convincing, the fact remains that these two traits do not correspond with the descriptions of the glandular swellings commonly known as ad-

---

[1] This view is also supported by Karambelkar, *The Atharva-Veda and The Āyur-Veda*, 170f.
[2] *Hymns*, 472, 503, 504, and cf. AJPh, 11: 327.
[3] *La doctrine*, 91–92; see also AHUtt 29.25; 30.13–41.
[4] See P 8.16.1–3 to AVŚ 6.25.1–3.
[5] P 1.59.3, see note 26, 84 below.
[6] Ibid.
[7] AVŚ 6.83.2, 3; 7.74(78).1.
[8] *La doctrine*, 91–92.
[9] AVŚ 6.83.3.
[10] AVŚ 6.83.3.
[11] AVŚ 6.83.1; cf. also P 1.59.1, 2. which reads: *yasmād aṅgāt saṃśusrāva* (*K manuscript: śuśrāva*) *yad babhūva galantyarśaḥ* (Bar: *galuntikā* or *kam*; Raghu Vira: *galattsva ?*), *gāvo vatsam iva jānānās tat paraitu* (K: *tad upaiti*) *yathāyatham*. Vs. 2: *nāsṛgasti* (K: *nāsṛgasya*) *pataṅgasya tardasya maśakādyāḥ, veṇoḥ pūtudror nāsty asṛṇi māsya glaur māpacid bhuvat* (see also Renou, JA, 252: 446).
[12] AVŚ 6.25.1–3; 7.74(78).2, 7.76(80).2 and P 8.16.3.
[13] AVŚ 6.25.1–3.
[14] Jean Mulholland, a Ph.D. student working in Thai traditional medicine, has informed me that a similar notion concerning the enumeration of the pustules occurs in the description of the disease "Birth *sāng*," found in the Thai medical text, *Khamphī pratham čhindā* of *Phāet-thayasāt songkhro*, vol. 1.
[15] AVŚ 6.83.1, 3; P 1.59.4 (see note 26, 84 below).
[16] AVŚ 6.25.1–3.
[17] See Macdonell-Keith, *Vedic Index*, 1: 24.

enopathies. It may be possible, however, to shed some light on this apparent contradiction. To the poet-healer, the swellings or pustules, which covered the body in great numbers from the nape of the neck down to the last twin joint, may have resembled the rash caused by the bites of noxious, parasitic insects which suck the blood of their host and whose wings make a sort of buzzing or humming noise.[18] It is conceivable that the ancient Indian looked on these noxious insects as the cause of his affliction. By making the pests fly away, vanish or more colloquially, "buzz-off,"[19] the healer would have effectively initiated a cure.

Like other flying vermin,[20] the *apacíts* were exposed and destroyed by the light from the sun,[21] suggesting that the rite was probably performed at dawn. More efficiently, however, the healer pricked them with the root of the divine medicine-man in order to cause the sores to suppurate and then cut them off level with the skin.[22] There is also the strong suggestion that one treatment involved the use of salt,[23] which will be discussed below. These cures, which incorporated lancing and the use of salt, point to a more empirical approach to medical treatment. The healer also employed techniques of healing which were more magical in nature and which occurred often in the medical charms. He appeased the *apacíts* in an effort to win them over by making an offering to them;[24] and by taking possession of or by knowing their names (i.e. characteristics), he was able to establish his superior power over them.[25] Found only at P 1.59.3, 4, the healer sent the *apacíts* to an undesirable victim, such as an enemy or a woman with a black neck;[26] and also found only at P 1.59.5–6, he requested the demons to depart to the ground.[27] The latter may simply be a more formulaic way of imploring the *apacíts* to drop off, as we noted above.

In the ritual text, which is obscure in places, there is, as in the hymn itself, a strong inclination toward empirical procedures for the removal of the pustules, implying a degree of originality in the rite:

With AVŚ 6.25, [the healer], with sticks, kindles fifty-five leaves of the *paraśu*-plant; he smears [their sap], which has bubbled forth in a cup, [on the pustules]

---

[18] It is important to note that at P 1.59.2, 4 insects, such as the *tarda*, 'grain-infesting insect,' and the mosquito (*maśaka*), are mentioned in relation to *apacíts* (see note 11, 83 above and note 26 below).

[19] At AVŚ 6.83.1, the request for the *apacíts* to fly forth as an eagle from its nest suggests the flight of insects from bodily hair.

[20] See in particular ṚV 1.191.

[21] AVŚ 6.83.1.

[22] AVŚ 7.74(78).1–2.

[23] AVŚ 7.76(80).1–2.

[24] AVŚ 6.83.4.

[25] AVŚ 6.83.3; P 1.59.3 (see next note).

[26] P 1.59.3, 4: Vs.3: *ahaṃ veda yathāsitha gurvikā nāma vā asi, amuṃ taṃ tvam ito gaccha yam ahaṃ dveṣmi pūruṣam.* Vs. 4: *tasyāpi madhya āsīda nīlagrīvāsu sīdatā, vātasyānu pravāṃ maśakasyānu saṃvidam* (cf. Renou, JA, 252: 446–47).

[27] P 1.59.5–6: *preto yantv agruvo nir ito yantv agruvaḥ, adharācīr itaḥ paraḥ.* Vs. 6: *prāhaṃ glāvam adhmāsaṃ nir ahaṃ glāvam adhmāsam, adharācīr itaḥ paraḥ* (note: K combines these two vss. into one vs. 4; cf. Renou, JA, 252: 447).

with a stick; [he smears the pustules] with crushed mussel or the saliva from dogs and makes leeches, house-flies, etc., bite [them] (?). With AVŚ 6.83 and 7.76(80), [the healer does as] in the case of the crushed mussel, etc. [above]; having crushed rock-salt into fine bits, [he puts it on the sores and] spits on [them]. With AVŚ 6.83.3cd, [the healer follows the same procedure as] at KauśS 31.11–15 (see 94 below). With AVŚ 6.83.4, after having sprinkled the sore of unknown origin with holy-water, he [makes an offering] with the dregs of ghee while contemplating [its source]. With AVŚ 7.74(78). 1–2, [the healer performs the action] mentioned in the hymn (i.e. pricking and cutting) with a bow [made] from the (*veṇu*) *dārbhūṣa*- tree(?) which has a bow-string fashioned from black wool and [three] black arrows with tufts of wool at their points. With the fourth verse [perhaps, AVŚ 7.76(80).2], he, having touched [a fourth arrow to the pustules], pierces [them]; [at dawn, he sprinkles the pustules] with [water] warmed by [burning] the bow-string and the tufts of wool.[28]

Of special interest is the use of salt which, as we have noticed, is prescribed in the ritual literature and is mentioned in the hymn at AVŚ 7.76(80).1. In an interesting passage found in the *Mahāvagga* of the Pāli Buddhist Canon, salt-crystal is recommended in the treatment of a sore which has stood up: The ripened pustule is to be cut off with the salt-crystal.[29] Such a description of a pustule closely resembles the etymological definition of *apa-cít* (root *ci* plus *ápa*), 'that which is heaped up (or increased in size).'[30] In the later medical literature, the treatment of *granthi*s, pustules very similar to *apacī,* involved lancing and the spreading of salt on them in order to make them suppurate.[31] The references to the general practices of lancing and especially to the use of salt in the treatment of such pustules, therefore, provides an unbroken continuity from the very earliest accounts and has helped to define more clearly the *apacít*s as pustules with an accompanying rash.

6.25

Let all those fifty-five, who accumulate on the nape of the neck,
vanish from here, like the words of the *apacít*s. 1.
Let all those seventy-seven, who accumulate all about the neck, van-
ish from here, like the words of the *apacít*s. 2.

---

[28] KauśS 30.14–16; 31.16–17; 31.20; 31.21; 32.8–10: 30.14. *pañca ca yā iti pañca pañcāśataṃ paraśuparṇān kāṣṭhair ādīpayati;* 15. *kapāle praśṛtaṃ kāṣṭenālimpati;* 16. *kiṃstyaśvajāmbīlodakarakṣikāmaśakādibhyāṃ daṃśayati;* 31.16. *apacita ā susrasa iti kiṃstyādīni;* 17. *lohitalavaṇaṃ saṃkṣudyābhiniṣṭhīvati;* 31.20 *glaur ity akṣatena;* 31.21. *vīhi svām ity ajñātāruḥ śāntyudakena samprokṣya manasā saṃpātavatā;* 32.8 *apacitām iti vaiṇavena dārbhyūṣeṇa kṛṣṇorṇājyena kālabundai stukāgrair iti mantroktam;* 9. *caturthyābhinidhāyābhividhyati;* 10. *jyāstukājvālena.* For detailed explanations of certain obscurities, see especially, Bloomfield, AJPh, 11: 325, 327–28; *Hymns,* 472, 504, 558; Caland, AZ, 96–98, 101–102, 104–105; cf. also, Henry, *La magie,* 193–94.

[29] 6.14.5: *vaṇamaṃsaṃ* (or *vaḍḍhamaṃsaṃ,* 'increased flesh,' found in some readings) *vuṭṭhāti. (bhagavato etam atthaṃ ārocesuṃ.) anujānāmi, bhikkhave, loṇasakkharikāya chindituṃ ti.* Cf. Buddhaghosa at *Samantapāsādikā,* (5, 1092): *vaḍḍhamaṃsaṃ ti adhikamaṃsaṃ āṇi viya uṭṭhahati.*

[30] Cf. the variant reading *upacít* at VS 12.97 to ṚV 10.97.2 n (248 below).

[31] See SuCiSth 18.6–24; AHUtt 30 (especially vs. 15) and *Yogaśataka,* 36–38.

Let all those ninety-nine, who accumulate on the shoulders, vanish from here, like the words of the *apacíts*. 3.

6.83

O *apacíts*, fly forth as an eagle from its nest. Let the sun effect the remedy; let the moon drive you off. 1.
One [*apacít* is] variegated; one, white, one, black [and] two [are] red. I have taken possession of all their names, [therefore,] let them depart without killing our heroes. 2.
The barren *apacít*, the black one's daughter, will fly forth; [likewise,] the *gláu* will fly forth. [Hence,] the *galuntá* (pus?) will be destroyed. 3.
When I make this [offering] with the mind, [saying:] "*svā́hā*," you, finding delight with the mind, accept your own oblation. 4.

7.74(78)

We have heard that the mother of the *apacíts* is black. With the root of the *múni* ("medicine-man"), the god, I prick them all. 1.
I prick their first one and I prick [their] midmost one; now, I cut off their hindmost one like a tuft [of wool]. 2.

7.76(80)

[These are the *apacíts*] who drop off more easily than the most easily dropping-off one, who are less existent than the non-existent one, who have less strength than the one devoid of spit, [and who] are more moist than the salt. 1.
The *apacíts*, who are about the neck, who are along the sides [and] who are on the *vijā́man* (twin ?) joint, fall off by themselves. 2.

Hair-loss

AVŚ 6.21; 136; 137 are charms for the strengthening of hair and for the promotion of its growth. We are informed that having it fall out naturally or having it pulled out either in battle or accidentally were the principal ways by which one lost one's hair.[1] The cure for such a condition involved the use of plants,[2] one of which appears to have been *nitatnī* which may have been concocted and ritually sprinkled over the head of the patient suffering from the loss of hair.[3]

AVŚ 6.21, being devoted primarily to the consecration of the plants to be used in the rite, focuses on their glorification. The healer begins by extolling the ground from which the plants have grown and from which

[1] AVŚ 6.136.3.
[2] AVŚ 6.21.
[3] AVŚ 6.136.3.

they have been collected, while symbolically associating it with the bodily integument from which hairs grow (verse 1). He continues by calling the plants auspicious names and by equating them with Soma, Bhaga and Varuṇa (verses 2, 3). AVŚ 6.136, 137 specify more clearly the herb *nitatnī́* ('the down-growing one'), perhaps a plant with narrow pendulous trailers or fronds, as the plant most beneficial for hair-growth. The healer, in order to strengthen the plant's efficacy, presents mythological episodes which recount the virtues of such a divine simple. Being a goddess born from the divine earth, she was first uprooted from the daughters of Varuṇa by Indra.[4] Another version relates how she was dug up by Jamadagni to promote the growth of his daughter's hair and was obtained by Vītahavya from the abode of Asita.[5] We are told that she increased the length of Jamadagni's daughter's hair from a finger's width to two arms' length.[6] Because of the marvellous results once formerly obtained from the use of this herb, the healer requests it to stimulate the growth of old hairs, to produce new ones and to make the existing ones long lasting,[7] to fasten the root, to protract the tip and to extend the length of the hairs.[8] In other words, the healer used the herb to produce a healthy crop of hair for his patient.

From the mythology surrounding the herb *nitatnī́*, it appears that these charms may have originally been employed in rites to restore the hair of women. Looking back to the *Ṛgveda,* we notice in the legend of Apālā that both bald-headed men and ugly women who lacked their pubic hair were regarded as unlucky: At ṚV 8.91(80), a young prepubescent girl named Apālā is said to have requested Indra to cover the head of her father, her abdomen and symbolically the field with hair and to beautify her skin. Indra answered her petition by putting her through the nave-hole of a chariot (-wheel), of a cart (-wheel) and finally through the opening of a yoke, making her "skin like (the color of) the sun."[9] In the later tradition of the *Brāhmaṇas,* an elaborated form of the story is recounted. At JB 1.221, we learn that it was on her pudenda (*upastha*) that she wished the hair to grow and that when Indra cleansed her skin by pulling her through the various openings, she became progressively more beautiful: first, she became as a lizard's skin, then, as a female chameleon and finally, like one

---

[4] P 1.67.2 (see notes to AVŚ 6.136.2, 232–33 below).

[5] AVŚ 6.137.1.

[6] AVŚ 6.137.2.

[7] AVŚ 6.137.2.

[8] AVŚ 6.137.3.

[9] Vs. 5: *imā́ni trī́ṇi viṣṭápā tā́nīndra ví rohaya, śíras tatásyorvárām ā́d idáṃ ma úpodáre.* Vs. 6: *asaú ca yā́ na urvárā́d imā́ṃ tanvàṃ máma, átho tatásya yác chíraḥ sárvā tā́ romaśā́ kṛdhi.* Vs. 7: *khé ráthasya khé nasaḥ khé yugásya śatakrato, apālā́m indra tríṣ pūtvy ákṛṇoḥ sū́ryatvacam.* For a recent reexamination and more plausible interpretation of this hymn, see Hanns-Peter Schmidt's lecture, "The affliction of Apālā (Ṛgveda 8.91)," in his *Some Women's Rites and Rights in the Veda* (Poona: Bhandarkar Oriental Research Institute, 1985). Cf. also J. Gonda, "The so-called secular, humorous and satirical Hymns of the Ṛgveda," *Selected Studies,* 3: 378, and Geldner, *Der Rigveda,* 2: 414. Note that in vs. 7, the openings seem to become progressively smaller (cf. Sāyaṇa and Geldner, 2: 414).

to be embraced (*saṃśliṣṭakā*).[10] Versions of the story with minor variants occur in the *Bṛhaddevatā* and the *Ṣaḍguruśiṣya,* in which Indra's cure of her father's baldness is omitted; and one version is told by Sāyaṇa in his introduction to ṚV 8.91(80). Sāyaṇa informs us that Apālā was to have been rejected by her husband because she had a skin-disease which caused the loss of hair to her pudenda and that when she was pulled through the first opening, her cast-off skin became a pangolin or monitor-lizard (*śalyaka*); after she was pulleu through the second opening, it became a varan (*godhā*); and finally when she was pulled through the third opening, her skin turned into a chameleon (*kṛkadāsa*).[11] In each of these accounts, hair-loss was a definite mark of inauspiciousness. By the time of the *Mānava Dharma Śāstra* (3.8), it became an ordinance that no man might marry a young girl who is hairless.[12]

It should be pointed out that the method used to beautify Apālā and to restore her hair is quite different from that recorded in the Atharvavedic charms. It does, however, bear a resemblance to a cure found in the Germanic tradition: it was believed that by making a patient creep through a gap in an oak-tree, in the earth, in a stone or under a horse, the disease from which the victim suffered would be transferred to the object through which he or she had passed.[13]

The ritual, being primarily therapeutic, follows the procedures implied in the hymns; in places, however, it adds its own symbolism with the color black and increases the vegetal ingredients:

With AVŚ 6.21, [the healer] sprinkles [the affected area] with [water] heated by the burning [of plants] growing on the ground [at the base] of trees; [he anoints the area] with a decoction of *akṣa*-nuts [and] *śīrṣa*(?); and with two [plants located] on the sides [of the tree] [or with two *nikaṭā*-plants(?)]. With AVŚ 6.136 and 137, at dawn, before the (black) crow flies on the new moon day, the healer, dressed in black and eating black food, sprinkles [the affected area with a decoction of] the fruit, from the plant mentioned in the hymn (i.e. *nitatnī*) and the plants, *jīvī* and *alākā*.[14]

6.21

The ground [is] indeed the best of these three earths; and from their
skin, I have collected the medicine. 1.

---

[10] See Schmidt, "The Affliction of Apālā"; cf. also H. Oertel, "Contributions from the *Jaiminīya Brāhmaṇa* to the History of the *Brāhmaṇa* Literature," JAOS, 18 (1897): 29–30.

[11] Ibid., 26–27; cf. also Geldner, *Der Rigveda,* 2: 413–14. On the identification of these animals, see Meulenbeld, *The Mādhavanidāna,* 508, 461–62 and 455–56, respectively.

[12] *nodvahet . . . kanyām . . . alomikaṃ. . . .*

[13] J. Grimm, *Teutonic Mythology,* trans. by J. S. Stallybrass (1883; rpt. Gloucester, Mass.: Peter Smith, 1976), 3: 1167; see also Julius von Negelein, "Das Pferd in der Volksmedizin," *Globus,* 80 (1901): 201–202.

[14] KauśS 30.8–10; 31.28: 30.8. *imā yāstisra iti vṛkṣabhūmau jātājvālenāvasiñcati;* 9. *śīrṣa phāṇṭākṣaiḥ;* 10. *nikaṭābhyām;* 31.28. *devī devyāṃ yāṃ jamadagnir iti mantroktāphalaṃ jīvyalākābhyām amāvāsyāyāṃ kṛṣṇavasanaḥ kṛṣṇabhakṣaḥ purā kākasaṃpātād avanakṣatre 'vasiñcati.* Cf. Bloomfield, *Hymns,* 470, 536–37, and Caland AZ, 96, 103.

You are the most excellent of the medicines [and] the best of the plants. [Likewise, you are] as Soma (the moon) [and] Bhaga (the sun) among the watches [and] as Varuṇa among the gods. 2.

You, O prosperous, unassailable [and] gracious [plants], be generous [to our hair; for] you are both hair-strengtheners and, indeed, promoters of hair-growth. 3.

6.136

You are a goddess, O herb, born from the divine earth. We uproot you, O *nitatnī* ('down growing one'), for the sake of strengthening the hair. 1.

Strengthen the old, beget the unborn and make the existing ones long lasting. 2.

With [a concoction made from] the plant, the medicine for all [diseases], I sprinkle over this your [cranial] hair which falls out [naturally] and which is pulled out by its roots. 3.

6.137

Vītahavya ('one whose offering is acceptable') fetched from Asita's dwelling that hair-promoting [herb] which Jamadagni uprooted for [his] daughter['s hair]. 1.

[Her hairs] were to be measured [at first only] by a finger-width; afterwards, they were to be measured by two arms' length. [Therefore,] let your black hairs grow like reeds all over your head. 2.

O herb, fasten the root, protract the tip [and] stretch out the middle [of the hairs]. [Therefore,] let your black hairs grow like reeds all over your head. 3.

III. MEDICINES

The word *bheṣajá*, 'medicine,' 'remedy,' is derived from *bhiṣáj*, 'healer,' and signifies that which belongs to the *bhiṣáj*. In other words, it refers to that which the healer uses in order to cure or heal.

Throughout our discussion of the internal and external diseases which plagued the Vedic Indians numerous medicines or remedies were encountered. Most of them, however, were either of a watery nature or of a vegetal origin. Our examination of medicines therefore will be divided into three chapters: 1. Waters; 2. *jālāṣá*; 3. Medicinal Herbs.

Other medicines included ointment (*ā̃ñjana*),[1] the mineral lead (*sī̃sa*)[2] and wind.[3] Elsewhere, we learn that the products derived from a cow were also considered to be medicinal.[4] The Vedic Indians considered all medicines to be derived from three sources: heaven, earth and the waters.[5]

19: WATER (*ÁP*)

Water was considered to be an important element of the cure of the internal diseases *kṣetriyá*, *rapás* and *ámīvā*. When employed in the healing rites, water was usually consecrated with the following formulaic verse:

> The waters [are] indeed medicinal; the waters [are] the *ámīvā*-dispellers [and] the waters [are] medicines for every [disease]. [Therefore,] let them make (be) medicine for you.[6]

Elsewhere, the waters are stated as being without *yákṣma* and *yákṣma*-expelling,[7] as being the medicine for dislocation (*āhrutabheṣajī́*).[8] The waters are said to protect the body[9] and carry away evil.[10] They are praised and as being more healing than the healers[11] and are said to contain the immortal medicine, brought by a chariot, known by Mātalī and put into them by

[1] See chapters on *jāyā̃nya*, 18, on *balā̃sa* 32, on *takmán* 34, on *hṛddyotá* (*hṛdrogá*) and *harimán* 29, on *ámīvā* 49 and on *víṣkandha-sáṃskandha*, 54.

[2] See chapters on *yákṣma*, 12, and on *viṣkandha-sāṃskandha*, 54.

[3] See chapter on *rápas*, 25, and ṚV 1.89.4; 10.186.1.

[4] See ṚV 10.100.10 and 10.175.2; cf. chapter on *ámīvā*, 49.

[5] ṚV 1.34.6 *ab: trír no aśvinā divyā̃ni bheṣajā̃ tríḥ pā̃rthivāni trír u dattam adbhyáḥ.*

[6] *ā̃pa íd vā̃ u bheṣajī̃r ā̃po amīvacā̃tanīḥ, ā̃paḥ sárvasya bheṣajī̃s tās te kṛṇvantu bheṣajám* (ṚV 10.137.6; AVŚ 6.91.3; P. 5.18.9; cf. also AVŚ 3.7.5; P 3.2.7 and P 19.18.9).

[7] AVŚ 3.12.9; 9.3.23; cf. 19.2.5.

[8] AVŚ 19.2.5, cf. ṚV 8.20.26.

[9] ṚV 1.23.21; cf. 10.9.7 and AVŚ 1.6.3.

[10] ṚV 1.23.22; cf. 10.9.8.

[11] AVŚ 19.2.3.

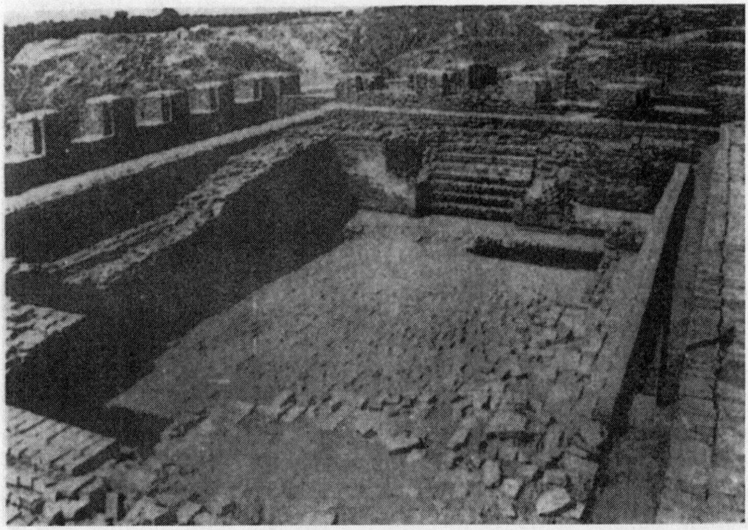

FIG. 3. The Great Bath at Mohenjo-Dāro. 3rd–2nd millennium B.C.

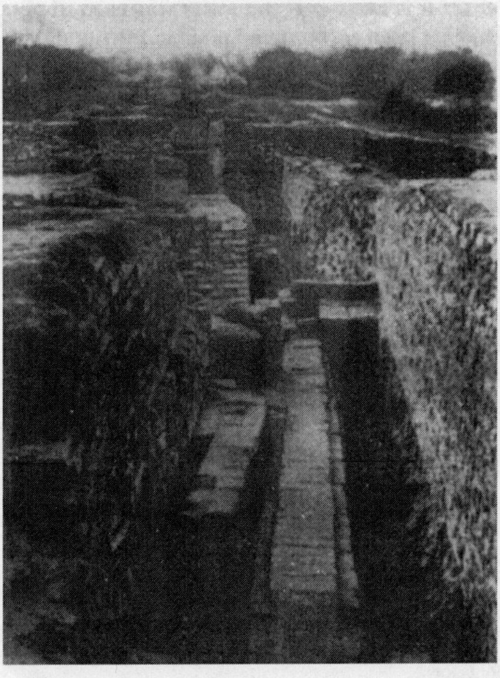

FIG. 4. A covered drain at Mohenjo-Dāro. 3rd–2nd millennium B.C.

Indra.[12] Soma also is declared to have stated that the waters are all medicines and medicines for every (disease).[13] The Maruts, the storm gods, are also connected with the medicinal quality of water, for their rain-water,[14] known as the Marut-medicine,[15] is said to be pure, most beneficial, comforting and the medicine chosen by father Manu.[16] It is said to be in the Sindhu, in the Asiknī-river and in the seas,[17] and to possess the ability to dispel *rápas* and to heal a dislocated (limb).[18] Being possessed of such valuable properties and having such an influence on the well-being of man, the waters are, therefore, requested to bestow their medicine.[19]

AVŚ 6.24 is the only complete charm in the *Atharvaveda* which focuses on the healing properties of water. It was recited primarily by the patient and its aim was the eradication of various internal diseases and symptoms, including *hṛddyotá* ('chest-pain, or perhaps angina pectoris) and all the demons which afflict him in the eyes, in the heels and in the front of the foot (i.e. the demonic *rápas*?) (verses 1–2).

The ritual *sūtras* prescribe merely a recipe for the purification of water, which surely goes back to a time immemorial: After he has drawn water from a stream along its current, [the healer should heat it] by means of burning thatch.[20] Although the *sūtra* is silent as to how the water was to be used, the commentator Keśava assumes that it was sprinkled over the patient (*avasiñcati*); while the commentator Sāyaṇa concludes that it was drunk, suggesting that the benefits mentioned in verse 3 of the hymn are in the form of nourishment.[21] It is likely that the water was used in both ways: the sprinkling of it having been encountered often in the ritual practices and the consumption of it being obviously quite natural.

6.24

Indeed may the divine waters, [which] flow forth from the Himavant
[and form] a confluence somewhere in the Sindhu, bestow on me
that medicine against *hṛddyotá* (chest-pain). 1.
May the waters, best healers among healers, eradicate all that which
has afflicted [me] in my two eyes, in [my] two heels and in the
front of [my] two feet. 2.
You, who are all the rivers which have Sindhu as husband and king
bestow on us the medicine for that [disease; and] by means of it,
may we gain your benefit. 3.

---

[12] AVŚ 11.6.23; cf. ṚV 1.23.19; AVŚ 1.4.4. Mātalī is commonly known as Indra's charioteer (cf. Sāyaṇa: . . . *indrasya sārathiḥ*; see also ṚV 10.14.3).

[13] ṚV 1.23.2; cf. 10.9.6 and AVŚ 1.6.2.

[14] ṚV 5.53.14.

[15] ṚV 8.20.23.

[16] ṚV 2.33.13.

[17] ṚV 8.20.25.

[18] ṚV 8.20.26.

[19] See in particular ṚV 10.9.5; AVŚ 1.5.4; cf. MS 4.9.27; TB 2.5.8.5 and TĀ 4.42.4.

[20] KauśS 30.13: *himavata iti syandamānād anvīpam āhārya valīkaiḥ*. Cf. Bloomfield, *Hymns*, 471 and Caland, AZ, 97.

[21] See notes to AVŚ 6.24:3, 236, below.

20: *JĀLĀṢÁ*, RUDRA'S MEDICINE AGAINST RUDRA'S DISEASE

Another important medicine (*bheṣajá*) is *jālāṣá* (ṚV: *jálāṣa*, as an adjective) which refers to Rudra's remedy.[1] Although it is impossible to know its precise meaning, it appears to have the qualities of a cooling, watery medicine.[2]

Bloomfield, based primarily on KauśS 31.11–15 and its commentaries (see below), has argued that it refers to urine;[3] while Geldner has maintained that it is rainwater conceived as cosmic urine.[4] Filliozat cites both explanations and concludes that it does not refer to any real remedy.[5]

From the few references to the word and its variants occurring in the *Ṛgveda* and in the *Atharvaveda*, we notice that it was considered to be Rudra's powerful, bright and very beneficial medicine, with the ability to promote long life and to incite heroes;[6] and, interestingly, it was thought to be connected with Rudra's hand which is said to possess valuable medicines as well as a pointed weapon.[7]

AVŚ 6.57 is a charm devoted principally to this medicine, used to cure the afflictions caused by Rudra's arrows. We do not know to what these afflictions refer. The tradition considers them to be sores, perhaps ones which have not ripened.[8] This interpretation receives some support from AVŚ 6.44.3, where Rudra's urine, perhaps referring to *jālāṣá*, is employed in the healing of bleeding flesh-wounds.[9] Rudra's weapons, as we have previously noticed, can also refer to the thunder and lightning associated with the internal disease-demon *takmán*.[10] At AVŚ 6.90.1, 2, however, an

[1] See ṚV 1. 43.4; AVŚ 2.27.6. Cf. also ṚV 2.33.12 and 7.35.6.
[2] Yāska at *Nighaṇṭu* 1. 12.100 states: . . . *jalāṣam* . . . *ity* . . . *udakanāmāni*. Cf. also Bloomfield, AJPh, 12(1891): 425. Pisani has suggested that *jálāṣa* could be derived from *jala-aśa* (root *aś*, 'to eat'), meaning 'to be taken with water' (review of Mayrhofer's Wb, *Paideia*, 20: 328). This interpretation, however, does not fit its prescribed use of being sprinkled on the affected area (AVŚ 6.57.2). Burrow, however, has noticed that it has the sense of 'cooling' ("Sanskrit *jálāṣa*" in *W. B. Henning Memorial Volume*, edited by Mary Boyce and Ilya Gershevitch [London: Lund Humphries, 1970], 89–97). Cf. also Mayrhofer, Wb, 1: 423, and 3: 709.
[3] AJPh, 12 (1891): 425–29.
[4] See Macdonell-Keith, *Vedic Index*, 1: 279–81.
[5] *La doctrine*, 109.
[6] ṚV 2.33.2, 4; 8.29.5 and AVŚ 6.57.2.
[7] See RV 1.114.5; 2.33.7; cf. RV 7.46.3, where Rudra is said to possess a thousand medicines.
[8] See KauśS 31.11, below; cf. Sāyaṇa to AVŚ 6.57: *mukharahitavraṇabhaiṣajyārtham*.
[9] See "Flesh Wounds Characterized by Bleeding," 75, above.
[10] See chapter on *takmán*, 34, above.

arrow, called all-pervading, was shot at a victim's limbs and heart; and the poisons from that arrow entered the hundred *dhamáni*-vessels and spread along the limbs.[11] As we have noted, the arrow was said to be held in Rudra's hand; and from AVŚ 6.57.2, we learn that it was single-shafted with a hundred points. Rudra is also identified with Agni and is the father of the storm-gods, the Maruts; and his weapons are frequently described in terms of lightning and thunderbolts.[12] Both Rudra's weapons and arrows, therefore, appear in this context to refer to the lightning flashes which carry down from heaven diseases which can take the form of *takmán* or poison. The poison appears to have been the cause of an external condition characterized by sores in the flesh. This brings to mind the symptoms *balā́sa* (swelling) and *harimán* (jaundice), noticed in a victim of *takmán*.

The cure for this, Rudra's disease, was Rudra's medicine which, we are told, was sprinkled on and about the affected area (AVŚ 6.57.2). Because of the prescribed treatment, we are led further to believe that Rudra's disease involved sores, wounds, or more generally swellings, spread about the limbs and exposed parts of the body and that Rudra's medicine, *jālāṣá*, was a real remedy. That this medicine was, like his weapon or arrow, held in Rudra's hand and was of a cooling, watery nature suggests rainwater. The connection with Rudra's urine is, therefore, purely metaphorical.

The ritual tradition, however, makes a concrete connection between Rudra's medicine, *jālāṣá*, and Rudra's urine (*mūtra*) and has, therefore, incorporated the hymn secondarily into a cure for a boil which has yet to suppurate (*akṣata*):

> With AVŚ 6.57, [the healer], after having wet a non-suppurating boil with foam of [human or bovine] urine, splashes [it with the urine] and [eventually] rinses [it with the remainder of the urine]; he [then] smears on plaque (from teeth) and pollen from tufts of (*garī*-) grass.[13]

It is difficult to conceive that the fresh urine prescribed in the rite could be cooling. Urine, mostly from animals, is a common āyurvedic remedy for, among other things, jaundice, leprosy and various skin diseases[14] and appears rather to be more a part of the materia medica of the later tradition, suggesting that the ritual of the *sūtra* is probably more recent than that implied in the hymn itself.

---

[11] Vs. 1: *yā́ṃ te rudrá íṣum ā́syad áṅgebhyo hṛ́dayāya ca, idáṃ* (P 19.18.2: *imāṃ*) *tā́m adyá tvád* (P 19.18.2: *te*) *vayáṃ víṣūcīṃ ví vṛhāmasi.* Vs. 2: *yā́s te śataṃ́* (P. 19.18.1: *hirā*) *dhamánayó 'ṅgāny ánu víṣṭhitāḥ, tā́sāṃ te sárvāsāṃ vayáṃ* (P 19.18.1: *sākaṃ*) *nír viṣā́ṇi hvayāmasi.* Cf. also AVŚ 11.2.26 where poison (*viṣá*) is included as one of Rudra's inflictions.

[12] See A. A. Macdonell, *Vedic Mythology* (1898; rpt. Delhi: Motilal Banarsidass, 1971), 74-76.

76.

[13] KauśS 31.11–15: 11. *idam id vā ity akṣataṃ mūtraphenenābhyudya;* 12. *prakṣipati;* 13. *prakṣālayati;* 14. *dantarajasāvadegdhi;* 15. *stambarajasā.* Cf. Bloomfield, *Hymns*, 488–89, and Caland, AZ, 100–101. See also Henry, *La magie*, 193.

[14] See Dutt and King, *Materia Medica*, 285–87.

6.57

To be sure, this, indeed, is a medicine; it is Rudra's medicine, with which one may exorcise the single-shafted, hundred-pointed arrow. 1.

You sprinkle [the affected area] with *jālāṣá* [and likewise] sprinkle around [it] with *jālāṣá*. *jālāṣá* [is your] powerful medicine. With it, [O Rudra,] spare us, so that we may live. 2.

[Let there be] both benefit and pleasure for us and let nothing at all injure us. To the ground [let our] *rápas* go; let there be each and every medicine for us. 3.

21: SIMPLES

Medicinal plants and herbs (*vīrúdh, óṣadhi*)[1] were always a part of the healer's materia medica. This keen interest in the beneficial properties of the native flora led to the development of a rather large pharmacopoeia. The manner in which the plants were described points to the early stages of Indian scientific thought: in addition to the explanation of the healing virtues of the different plants and herbs, which were distinguished from each other and from trees (*vánaspáti*), the healer often included ecological and taxonomical distinctions. This is best illustrated in two hymns, ṚV 10.97 and AVŚ 8.7, devoted to the glorification and praise of simples. Because of their length (twenty-three and twenty-eight verses, respectively), it is unlikely that they were employed to cure any specific disease; rather, they were used generally in the healing rituals to consecrate the various plants of the healer's materia medica. That both hymns were employed for the same purpose is evidenced from the first verse of each, in which the healer states that he is now considering or addressing the numerous types of plants of which he has knowledge.

From the point of view of the practitioner, three stages, through which the plants pass on their way to becoming used as medicines, can be ascertained from the texts themselves.

Acquisition

The simples were either brought from great distances and traded or they were collected by the healer-apothecary himself: the healer invoked various herbs which he knew were spread all over the earth.[2] Many of these had to be brought to him from great distances,[3] most notably from the Aṅgiras, people who lived in the mountains.[4] Elsewhere, we noticed that the mountain-grown *kúṣṭha*-plant was brought and traded.[5] Likewise, the *gulgulú* (*gúggulu*)-plant was known to have been transported by sea.[6] In addition to the acquisition of herbs by trade, the healer also engaged in the uprooting and collection of auspicious plants from his local flora which, from the context, appears to have been in the plains.[7] During this collecting process,

---

[1] See Mayrhofer, Wb, 3: 77–78, and 1: 133, 561.

[2] ṚV 10.97.19; AVŚ 8.7.2, 6, 7, 10, 11, 23.

[3] AVŚ 8.7.16, 25.

[4] AVŚ 8.7.17, 24.

[5] AVŚ 5.4.2, 8; cf. also 4.7.6, where the *madā̆vatī* ('intoxicating' plant) is bartered.

[6] AVŚ 19.38.2(3).

[7] ṚV 10.97.20; VS 12.98, 100 (to ṚV 10.97.23n); cf. AVŚ 1.24.4; 2.3.5; 4.7.5, 6; 5.5.4; 6.21.1, 109.3, 136.1, 137.1; 10.4.14; P 1.67.2; 1.93.4 and VS 12.98 where harmful and beneficial plants are gathered by uprooting. See also *Ṛgvidhāna*, 4.1.2.

he propitiated the herbs, because of the harm he caused to them by uprooting them, indicating an early example of the later doctrine of nonviolence (*ahiṃsā*) to all living things.[8]

An integral part of the acquisition of plants from various places was the ancient Indian's knowledge of them according to a primitive system of classification based on gross morphology and habitat, which is fully appreciated in the Atharvavedic and Ṛgvedic hymns.[9]

Preparation

The plants which had been collected were then combined (often pulverized) and made (decocted or concocted) into medicines[10] or fashioned into amulets[11] as "companions of the charm"[12] or in order to "help the charm."[13] In fact, the healer (*bhiṣáj*) is characterized as a shaker (*vípra*) who knows both the preparation of the medicines from the plants and the correct recitation of the healing words.[14]

Employment

Often, as we have noticed, extracts or other preparations of the plants were drunk in a solution. The dominant form in which the natural plants were used, however, was as an amulet or a talisman. We have also documented their occasional employment as important ingredients in poultices or compresses. There is also evidence that they were held in the hand of the healer, perhaps as a type of amulet, and ritually waved over the patient in order to drive away his affliction which in turn was carried away by birds, or expelled with the passing of wind from the anus.[15]

An important point, which is apparent from these charms, especially ṚV 10.97, is that the *óṣadhi* or herb was personified, divinized and looked upon as a general luck-bringer.[16] One of the most auspicious *óṣudhi*s we have encountered is Arundhatī whose various forms were considered extremely efficacious in the treatment of broken limbs and flesh wounds. Because of her profound ability to bring about the cure of such infirmities, a mythology evolved, surrounding her and her various forms, which may be summarized as follows: She is described as a perennial, harmless, life-giving herb with a saving honey-sweet flower;[17] and as *sahádevī*, she is said to protect quad-

---

[8] The earliest reference to *ahiṃsā* in relation to plants is found at MS 3.9.3 and TS 6.3.3.2. For a discussion of the general notion of *ahiṃsā* in the early texts, see Hanns-Peter Schmidt, "The origin of Ahiṃsā," *Mélanges d' Indianisme* (Paris: Editions E. de Boccard, 1968), 626–55.

[9] See AVŚ 8.7.4, 9, 13, 20, 23, 27; ṚV 10.97.2, 3, 5, 7, 9, 15, 18, 19, 21.

[10] AVŚ 8.7.5, 18, 22; ṚV 10.97.21.

[11] AVŚ 8.7.14.

[12] AVŚ 8.7.7.

[13] ṚV 10.97.14.

[14] ṚV 10.97.6, 22.

[15] ṚV 10.97.11–13; see also chapters on *rápas* and on the General Removal of Internal Diseases Related to *yákṣma* and *takmán*, 25 and 46, above.

[16] See, in particular, ṚV 10.97.4, 5, 6, 8, 17; AVŚ 8.7.2, 19, 20.

[17] AVŚ 8.7.6.

rupeds (especially domestic ones), men and (small) birds from *yákṣma* and from harm.[18] As *róhaṇī,* she is the healer of the severed bone.[19] In her form as *silācī,* she is called the gods' sister whose mother is the night, father, the cloud and grandfather, Yama[20] and is given the epithets: triumphant, steadfast, delivering and mender.[21] As *lākṣā,* she is called the sister of the waters whose self has become the wind and is described as hairy-sided.[22] As *silācī* and *lākṣā,* she is said to be very beautiful, golden, sun- and fire-colored and goat-brown,[23] to be born from the blood of Yama's tawny horse[24] and to be arising out of, mounting and creeping on trees.[25] In the form of *viṣāṇakā,* she is said to have arisen from the fathers' root;[26] and as *pippalī,* she is mentioned as having been buried by the *ásuras*[27] and dug up again by the gods.[28]

There is little doubt that the ancient Indians had a high esteem for their flora. The admiration, even reverence, seems also to have been represented in their early iconography. Looking back to the Indus Valley Civilization, we find seals and sealings which depict a type of female tree- or plant-divinity.[29] In one particular seal, there is represented a female who resides in the branches of a pīpal tree and who is being worshipped by eight devotees.[30] Later this tree-goddess appears to have been stylized as the Cūlakoka Devatā at Bharhūt or the Yakṣī or Vṛkṣakā on the pillars at Sañci.[31] Finally, in a Jaina cave at Udayagiri (Orissa), there is an interesting panel which appears to show a sequential story in which a goddess standing or (sitting ?) in a tree instructs a man in the virtues of nonviolence (*ahiṃsā*).[32] Both in the literature and in the archaeology, therefore, we find evidence of female plant-divinities who were worshipped and who bestowed great benefits on their devotees.

In the later ritual practice, ṚV 10.97 is, according to *Ṛgvidhāna* 3.42.8–4.1.3, to be muttered for six months in constant praise of herbs. In the autumn, Rudra and the herbs are worshipped so that one does not suffer from disease or any kind of indigestion; and in order to find and acquire

---

[18] AVŚ 6.59.1–3.
[19] AVŚ 4.12.1.
[20] AVŚ 5.5.1.
[21] AVŚ 5.5.3, 5, 6.
[22] AVŚ 5.5.7.
[23] AVŚ 5.5.6, 7, 8.
[24] AVŚ 5.5.8, 9.
[25] AVŚ 5.5.3, 5, 9.
[26] AVŚ 6.44.3.
[27] AVŚ 2.3.3; 6.109.3.
[28] AVŚ 6.109.3; 2.3.5.
[29] See in particular, Walter A. Fairservis Jr., *The Roots of Ancient India* (Chicago: University of Chicago Press, 1975), 277, pls. 23–25.
[30] See fig. 9, 220 below.
[31] See Ananda K. Coomaraswamy, *History of Indian and Indonesian Art* (1927; rpt. New York: Dover Publications, 1975), 64–66, and figs. 39, 53, 54, 75.
[32] For access to photographs of this panel and for its interpretation, I thank Professor A. L. Basham.

herbs, the *vipra* observes the rite seven times a week (i.e. once a day) and worships Varuṇa in his own region.[33] It is significant that emphasis was placed on the acquisition of the plants, for it reflects a continuation of the practice mentioned in the hymns; and the elaborate manuals of materia medica and the *nighaṇṭus* (or word-glossaries) of more recent origin are testimonies that the activity has survived and developed throughout the ages. In the *Śatapatha Brāhmaṇa* (7.2.4), a version of the hymn found at VS 12.75ff. is used more symbolically in a rite devoted to the construction of the fire altar and to the healing of Agni. In particular, it is recited while preparing, by ploughing, by sprinkling with water and by sowing, the ground on which the altar is to be constructed.[34] In a doubtful healing rite at KauśS 26.40, AVŚ 8.7 is to be recited while the healer binds to the patient an amulet fashioned from the chips of ten different types of sacred wood.[35] The commentator, Dārila, however, has a different reading for this *sūtra: upottamena śālam,* 'With the penultimate hymn (which in this sequence is AVŚ 6.127), [the healer should bind to the patient an amulet fashioned from] the *śāla*-tree.' We can see therefore that there is some question as to the use of the hymn in the actual therapeutic part of a healing rite, lending further support to the assumption that the hymns were employed during the consecration of the plants.

ṚV 10.97

I shall now consider those hundred and seven kinds of brown herbs born formerly, three ages before the gods. 1.

Your kinds, O mama! [are] a hundredfold and your sprouts, a thousandfold. [Therefore,] you, O one whose powers are a hundredfold, make this [man] healthy for me. 2.

You, flowering [and] bud-bearing herbs, rejoice. [For] like victorious steeds [are] the plants leading one to safety. 3.

O mothers called herbs, I beg this of you, O goddesses: "May I gain a horse, a cow, a garment [and], O man, your ownself (life?)." 4.

Your dwelling is made in the *aśvatthá*-tree [and] your abode, in the *parṇá*-tree. If you could gain the man's [self(life?)], then, by all means, you [too] would be entitled to cows. 5.

---

[33] 3.42.8: *yā oṣadhīḥ svastyayanaṃ japeta niyatavrataḥ, oṣadhīś ca yajen nityaṃ ṣaṇ māsān eva nityaśaḥ.* 4.1.1: *iṣṭvā śaradi vai rudram oṣadhīś ca yajet tathā, tasyāmayā na bhavanti tathā 'jīrṇāni yāni ca.* 4.1.2: *kriyāṃ tu saptarātreṇa saptakṛtvo 'bhyaset tataḥ, prapadyetauṣadhīṃ vipraḥ sūktam etaj japant sadā.* 4.1.3: . . . *svakṣetre varuṇam iṣṭvā, vindate bhiṣag oṣadhīḥ;* cf. Gonda, *The Ṛgvidhāna,* 100–101.

[34] See J. Eggeling, trans., *The Śatapatha-Brāhmaṇa according to the Text of the Mādhyandina School,* 5 vols. (1882-1899; rpt. Delhi: Motilal Banarsidass, 1963), 3: 335-41. A version of this rite is found at TS 5.2.5 (see Keith, VBYS, Pt. 2, 409); cf. also KS 16.13–14; MS 2.7.13–14, KapS 25.4–5, ĀpŚS, 16.20.5–13 and BŚS 10.26, where only 14 vss. are found. See also MŚS 6.16 and KŚS 17.2.11–16.

[35] *uttamena śākalam.* Cf. Bloomfield, *Hymns,* 578; Caland, AZ, 80–81, and Henry, *Le livre VIII,* 58.

When these herbs have come together like kings at the council, [then] that healer, the destroyer of the *rákṣas*-demons [and] dispeller of *ámīvā*, is called shaker (*vípra*). 6.

So that this [man] may be unharmed, I have procured all the herbs: the one having the power of horses, the one containing Soma, the invigorating one [and] the one increasing the vital energy. 7.

The powers of the herbs, which cause to bestow a gift to your own self, O man, go forth as cows from a cow-pen. 8.

Your mother, by name, [is] eradicator, therefore, you are eradicators; you are [as] winged streams [and] what ails [that] you eradicate. 9.

The herbs have surmounted all barriers as a robber [the walls of] the fold [and] have removed every kind of bodily *rápas*. 10.

When I, causing to strengthen [the patient], hold these herbs in my hand, the essence of the *yákṣma* perishes as [life] in the presence of a beast of prey. 11.

You, O herb, like an impartial law-enforcer, drive away the *yákṣma* from him into whose every limb [and] every joint you creep. 12.

Fly away, O *yákṣma*, together with the *cā̄ṣa* [and] the *kikidīví*, perish with the force of the wind, together with the *nihā̄kā*. 13.

Let one of you help another; you must help one another. All of you [herbs], in unison, must help this my charm. 14.

Let those Bṛhaspati-produced [herbs], who bear fruit and those who do not, who bear flowers and who do not, free us from distress. 15.

Let [the herbs] release me from (the effects of an infringement) of the vow and indeed from Varuṇa's (bond), likewise, from Yama's foot-fetter and from every offence against the gods. 16.

Descending from heaven, the herbs announced: "May that man, whom we should visit [and find] living, not be harmed." 17.

Among those herbs whose king is Soma, who are many [and] who have a hundred skills, you are the choicest, suitable for [fulfilling my] desires [and] auspicious to the heart. 18.

You Bṛhaspati-produced herbs, whose king is Soma [and] who are scattered over the earth, bestow strength on her. 19.

Let your uprooter not be harmed; likewise, [let him] for whom I uproot you [not be harmed]. [Indeed,] let all our bipeds [and] quadrupeds be free from suffering. 20.

O plants, let all [the herbs], both [those] who listen closely to this [charm] and [those] who have departed into the distance [and do not listen closely to the charm], having assembled, bestow strength on her. 21.

The herbs converse with [their] king, Soma: "We, O king, rescue him for whom the Brāhmaṇa performs [his special craft]." 22.

You, O herb are the choicest; [indeed], trees are your inferiors. [Therefore,] may he, who bears ill-will toward us, be our inferior. 23.

AVŚ 8.7

We address all the herbs who are brown, white, red, spotted, black and dark blue. 1.

Let the plants whose father was heaven, whose mother was the earth [and] whose root was the ocean, rescue this man from the divinely sent *yákṣma.* 2.

In the beginning, the waters [fulfilled the function of] heavenly herbs. They destroyed from each and every limb your sin-caused *yákṣma.* 3.

I speak to the herbs who spread forth, who are clumpy, who have a single bud [and] who are bushy; I summon for you fibrous, segmented [and] branched plants who [are] related to the Viśvedevas, who are powerful [and] who bring life to man. 4.

Through that which [is] your power, O vanquishing [ones], [your] energy and which [is] your strength, release this man from *yákṣma,* O herbs. Therefore, I make the medicine. 5.

In order that this [man] may be unharmed, I invoke here the vigorous, harmless, life-giving herb, the saving honey-sweet flower, Arundhatī. 6.

Let the prudent companions of my charm come here, so that we may rescue this man from difficulty. 7.

Agni's food, the water's embryo, who grows up new again—let [those] fixed, thousand-named medicinal [herbs] be brought here. 8.

Let the sharp-horned herbs, whose envelope is the *ávakā* [and] whose essence is water, push aside difficulty. 9.

Let those herbs who liberate, who release [one] from Varuṇa's [bond], who are powerful [and] poison-destroying, likewise, [those] who are *balā́sa*-destroying and witchcraft-destroying, come here. 10.

Let the very powerful plants, who have been brought [and] who are extolled, rescue, in this clan, the cow, the horse, the man [and] the domestic beast. 11.

The root of these plants has become sweet, sweet [their] apex, sweet [their] middle, sweet [their] leaf [and] sweet their flower. [Since they] are possessed of honey [and are] the drink of immortality, let them yield ghee [and] food which has cow's milk as [its] principal [ingredient]. 12.

However many herbs [there] are on the earth, let those with a thousand leaves release me from death [and] from distress. 13.

Let the amulet, derived from a tiger [and composed] of plants, which rescues [and] guards against curses, repel far away from us all *ámīvā*s [and] the *rákṣas*-demons. 14.

They spring away in fear as from a lion's roar; as from fire, they dart from the [plants] brought here. [Therefore,] let the cows' [and] the

men's *yákṣma,* impelled by the plants, enter the navigable streams [and be carried away by them]. 15.
You plants, being released from Agni Vaiśvānara, [you] whose king is the forest tree (*vánaspáti*), go, spreading over the earth. 16.
Let those auspicious [and] sappy herbs, who, belonging to the Aṅgiras, grow on the mountains and in the plains, be beneficial to our heart. 17.
The plants whom I know, whom I observe with [my] eyes, who are unknown [but with whom] we are familiar and from whom we know [what] has been prepared— 18.
Let all [those] herbs heed my words, so that we may rescue this man from difficulty. 19.
Among the plants [there is] the *aśvatthá,* the *darbhá;* [likewise, there is] king Soma, the immortal oblation [and] the two medicines, rice and barley, the two immortal sons of heaven. 20.
When, with [his] semen, Parjanya promotes you, O children of the spotted one (Pṛśni), [then], O herbs, sprout up; [for] it thunders [and] roars. 21.
We give this man the strength of this nectar to drink; and now I prepare the medicine, so that he may live a hundred years. 22.
The boar knows the plant; the mongoose knows the medicinal [herb]. I summon to this [man] for help those [herbs] whom the snakes [and] the Gandharvas know. 23.
I summon to this [man] for help these herbs belonging to the Aṅgiras, whom the eagles [and] the heavenly *ragháṭs* know, whom the (small) birds, [and] geese know [and] whom all winged birds know. 24.
Let however many herbs, whom the oxen, cows, goats and sheep consume, provide protection to you, [when] brought here. 25.
In as many [herbs] as the human physicians know a medicine, that many, who are medicines for all [diseases], I bring to you. 26.
Let the flowering [and] shoot-bearing [herbs] as well as [those] who bear fruit [and those] who do not, as it were, having the same mother, yield [their] milky sap, so that this [man] may be unharmed. 27.
I have rescued you from that having five *śalás*, from that having ten *śalás*, from Yama's foot-fetter and also from every offence against the gods. 28.

TEXTUAL ANNOTATIONS

Notes to AVŚ 2.33

Most authorities agree that AVŚ 2.33, with its repetition at AVŚ 20.96.17–22 and its variant at ṚV 10.163, is a charm against *yákṣma,* commonly considered to be tuberculosis or consumption.[1] Sāyaṇa prescribes 2.33 for use "in a rite for the curing of the diseases arising in all bodily members beginning with the eye, nose, ear, head, tongue, and nape of the neck"[2] at KauśS 27.27–28.[3] He also includes it at KauśS. 54.11 in a list of hymns devoted to the removal of distress,[4] and mentions its occurrence at VaitS 38.1 in a rite for the curing of the sacrificer in the sacrifices beginning with the *aśvamedha* (horse-sacrifice).[5] It is also listed, at KauśS 54.11, among the hymns destined to bestow long life (*āyuṣyagaṇa*)[6] and a version of verse 1 is employed at *Pāraskara Gṛhya Sūtra* 3.7 for the cure of head-disease.[7] In the introduction to 20.96, the editor (or Sāyaṇa?) prescribes, at VaitS 34.20, that the entire hymn be recited in the *mahāvrata* at the midday pressing of Soma.[8] Based on the *Sarvānukramaṇī,* Sāyaṇa explains that ṚV 10.163 has as its *ṛṣi,* Vivṛhan ('the exorcist') who was born of the Kaśyapa-clan. He goes on to mention that the deity addressed throughout the hymn is *yakṣma* and that the hymn is for the removing of *yakṣma.*[9] BD 8.66 also mentions that it is "destructive of *yakṣma*";[10] and *Ṛgvidhāna* 4.19.3–5 prescribes its use in a rite devoted to the releasing of one from *yakṣma* or to the destruction of it. Likewise, at ĀpGS 3.9.10 (ĀpMB 1.17.1) it is mentioned in connection with the healing

---

[1] Kuhn: "Gegen des Schwinden (Against tuberculosis)," "Indische und germanische Segenssprüche," KZ, 13 (1864), 63; Weber: "Gegen *yakṣma* (schwund) [Against *yakṣma* (tuberculosis)]," IS, 13: 205; Griffith: ". . . a charm against *Yakṣma,* Phthisis pulmonalis or consumption . . . ," *Hymns of the Atharvaveda,* 1: 74; cf. 2: 412; Bloomfield: "Charm to secure perfect health," *Hymns,* 44, 321; Whitney-Lanman: "For the expulsion of *yákṣma* from all parts of the body," *Atharva-veda-saṃhitā,* Pt. 1, 76. Among the translators of ṚV 10.163, Geldner entitles it: "Gegen Auszehrung (Against consumption)," *Der Rigveda,* 3: 390, and Renou, "contre la consomption," EVP, 16: 174.

[2] *akṣināsākarṇaśirojihvāgrīvādisarvāvayavajarogabhaiṣajyakarmaṇi;* cf. Keśava: *sarvavyādhibhaiṣajyam ucyate.*

[3] See Caland, AZ, 85, and Bloomfield, *Hymns,* 327.

[4] *aṃholiṅgagaṇe.* But according to *AthPariś* 32.4, it is not found in that list (see also Bloomfield, *Hymns,* 321).

[5] *aśvamedhādiṣu dīkṣāvato yajamānasya bhaiṣajyakarmaṇi.* Cf. Whitney-Lanman, who state it is only in the *puruṣamedha* (human sacrifice). *Atharva-veda-saṃhitā,* Pt. 1, 76.

[6] See Bloomfield, *Hymns,* 321, and Whitney-Lanman, *Atharva-veda-saṃhitā,* Pt. 1, 76.

[7] *śīrṣarogabheṣajam;* cf. H. Oldenberg and M. Müller., *The Gṛhya-Sūtras Rules of Vedic Domestic Ceremonies,* 2 vols. (1886–92; rpt. Delhi: Motilal Banarsidass, 1967), 1, 350, where it is 3.6.

[8] *mahāvrate mādhyaṃdine savane.*

[9] *kaśypagotrotpanno vivṛhā nāmarṣiḥ. yakṣmanāśanapratipādyatvāt taddevatākaṃ kṛtsnaṃ sūktam. Anukramaṇī: akṣībhyāṃ vivṛhā kāśyapo yakṣmaghnam.*

[10] *akṣībhyāṃ yakṣmanāśanam.*

of a wife suffering from *yakṣma.*[11] At ŚŚS 16.13.3–4, it is used, along with ṚV 10.137, 10.161 and 10.186, in a rite to cure the sacrificer of what the commentary states is an infirmity caused by snakebite, etc.[12] Finally at ŚGS 1.21.3 it is employed along with ṚV 10.162 in the *garbharakṣaṇa* (ceremony performed in the fourth month for the protection of the fetus).[13]

We can see, from its repetition three times in the *Ṛg-* and *Atharva-vedas*, and by its extensive use in the ritual literature, that it was considered very popular and perhaps also very effective.

R. Müller considers that there is close relationship between the Ṛgvedic version of the hymn and *Vendīdād* 8.35–72, which also presents an enumeration of bodily parts beginning with the head and ending with the feet. On this basis, he concludes that the Avestan *drug-nasu*, 'the demonic fire,' which resides in these various anatomical parts and is expelled from them by water, corresponds to the Vedic *yákṣma.*[14]

Jean Filliozat, on the other hand, has quite convincingly demonstrated that the Avestan *drug* is not fiery in nature, but rather appears in the form of hideous insects which, at *Vendīdād* 8.35–72, take the form of flies surrounding a corpse. He concludes: "Le fait qu'on expulse rituellement la *yákṣma* et la *drug* de toutes les parties du corps successivement ne saurait établir leur communauté d'origine; on en use ainsi à l'égard de toute imprégnation funeste et non pas seulement dans l'Inde et dans l'Iran."[15] He has, however, noticed a similarity between the *drugs*, in the plural, and *yákṣmas*: they are both sin-related demons or evils which attack man; but he points out that the *drug* is the cause of the disease, while the *yákṣma* is both the cause and the disease itself.[16]

VERSE 1

In *b,* P 4.7.1 has *āsyād uta,* "and from the mouth," and in *d, lalāṭād vi vṛhāmasi,* "from the forehead, we tear away."

VERSE 2

In *d,* P 4.7.2 has *urasto vi vṛhāmasi,* "from [your] breast, we tear away." Why *grīvābhyas* and *uṣṇíhābhyaḥ* are plural is difficult to explain. Sāyaṇa states that the first refers to the fourteen small bones located in the neck (. . . *grīvāśabdena tadavayavabhūtāni caturdaśa sūkṣmāṇy asthīni ucyante bahuvacananirdeśāt*), quoting ŚB 12.2.4.10 as support. The second he ex-

---

[11] *yakṣma* . . . , cf. Oldenberg and Müller, *The Gṛhya-Sūtras,* 2: 270.

[12] See W. Caland, trans. and L. Chandra, *The Śāṅkhāyana-Śrautasūtra, being a major yājñika text of the Ṛgveda* (Nagpur: International Academy of Indian Culture, 1953), 456; Commentary of Varadattasuta Ānartīya: *athānantaram ṛtvijo yajamānaṃ bhiṣajyanti. . . . tṛṇābhyām upamārjayanti sarpadaṣṭādau darśanāt.*

[13] See Oldenberg and Müller, *The Gṛhya-Sūtras,* 1: 47.

[14] "Medizin im Ṛg-Veda," 357; see also Johannes Hertel, "Nachtrag zu Ṛgveda X.163, Vendidad VIII 35–72," *Asia Major,* 6: 377–85.

[15] *La doctrine,* 41.

[16] Ibid., 42, 80.

plains as vessels, which are smooth in the upper part or which have emerged (or protruded) with blood etc. (*ūrdhvaṃ snigdhābhyaḥ raktādinā utsnātābhyo vā nāḍībhyaḥ*). However, at ṚV 10.163.2, he glosses *grīvā́bhyas* as (blood) vessels in the throat (*galagatābhyo dhamanībhyaḥ*) and *uṣṇíhābhyaḥ* as tendons which are either smooth near the upper part or which have emerged (or protruded) (*ūrdhavābhimukhaṃ snigdhābhya utsnātābhyo vā snāyubhyaḥ*). Although it is clear that Sāyaṇa is merely guessing at the significance of the plurals, it seems possible that they could refer collectively to the various anatomical parts of the neck and the nape of the neck, which our rendering implies. Cf. Filliozat, *La doctrine,* 122, 123.

VERSE 3

For *ab,* ṚV 10.163.3 has a variant of verse 4*ab* (see below) and in *cd,* it reads: *yaknáḥ plāśíbhyo ví vṛhāmi te,* "from [your] liver, from [your] *plāśí* (see below, verse 4), I tear away for you. . . ." In *ab,* P 4.7.3 has: *klomnas te hṛdayyābhyo halīkṣṇāt* (Raghu Vira: *hṛdayād adhi halīkṣmāt*), "from your lungs, from [your] hearts, from [your] *halīkṣṇa.*" Here again notice the unexpected plural *hṛdayyābhyo,* which Raghu Vira emends to a singular. The exact meaning of *hálīkṣṇa* is unclear. Sāyaṇa explains it as 'a kind of fleshy lump connected to the lungs' (. . . *tat*[*klomán*] *saṃbandhād māṃsapiṇḍa-viśeṣāt*). Weber understands it to be that which appears (*īkṣaṇa*) yellow (*hari*) and translates 'gall' (206). Bloomfield suggests that it may be related to *hirā́,* canal,' 'vein,' and renders, "viscera" (45, 322). Whitney-Lanman leave the word untranslated and quotes Sāyaṇa for a possible explanation (76). Filliozat is unsure of its meaning, but points out that at TS 5.7.23 it refers to the name of an animal (*La doctrine,* 127). Kuhn leaves the word untranslated (68). Cf. also Macdonell-Keith, *Vedic Index,* 2: 500. Sāyaṇa explains the difficult *mátasnābhyāṃ* as 'the two kidneys connected to the two sides or the two receptacles of bile situated near them' (*ubhayapārśva-saṃbandhābhyāṃ vṛkyābhyāṃ tatsamīpasthapittādhārapātrābhyāṃ vā;* cf. to ṚV 10.163.3: *pārśvayor vartamānāv āmraphalākṛtī vṛkkau,* 'the two kidneys existing on either side of the body and having the shape of mango fruits'; Geldner follows this, *Der Rigveda,* 3: 390). Mahīdhara to VS 25.8 explains the word as 'two bones situated on either side of the heart and adhering to the part below the neck' (*grīvādhastād bhāgasthitahṛdayobhayapārśvasthe asthinī*). Kuhn, basing himself on Mahīdhara, renders 'the ribs near the heart' (Herzrippen, 67). Grassmann suggests 'the lungs' (Wb, col. 947). Weber (206) and Bloomfield (45) follow Sāyaṇa and translate it as 'kidneys'; while Whitney-Lanman leave it untranslated (76). Filliozat states that they are 'viscère non identifié' (*La doctriné,* 125).

VERSE 4

In *b,* ṚV 10.163.3 has *hṛ́dayād ádhi,* 'from [your] heart,' and P 4.7.4 reads *uta* at the end. In *cd,* ṚV is similar to verse 3*cd* above and P is a variant of verse 6 below. For *kukṣíbhyāṃ,* we follow Filliozat (*La doctrine,* 123) who seems to have based himself on Sāyaṇa, i.e. 'the right and left parts of the abdomen' (*dakṣiṇottarābhyām udarabhāgābhyāṃ*). Cf. also Weber (207) and Bloomfield (45): 'belly'; Whitney-Lanman: '(two) paunches' (76) and Kuhn: 'abdominal cavity' (68). An exact meaning for the word *plāśér* is wanting. Sāyaṇa glosses it: 'The large holed receptacle of feces' (*bahucchidrāt malapātrāt*). At ṚV 10.163.3 where the form *plāśíbhyo* occurs, he glosses 'lungs, spleen, etc.' (*klomaplīhādisaṃjñebhyaḥ*). The plural of the word (*plāśáyaḥ*) is found at VS 25.8 where Mahīdhara explains it as 'tubes at the root of the penis' (*śiśnamūlanāḍyaḥ*) and at VS 19.87 he glosses the singular *plāśír* as 'penis' (*śiśnaḥ*). Grassman, basing himself on Sāyaṇa, suggests that it may be the spleen or other entrails (Wb, col. 895). Weber (207) and Geldner (*Der Rigveda*, 3: 390) render it more generally as 'mesentery'; Bloomfield: 'guts' (45). Kuhn, to the ṚV (67) and Whitney-Lanman (76) leave it untranslated; but Kuhn to the AVŚ offers 'limbs' (68). Filliozat, who bases himself primarily on Mahīdhara, suggests that in the singular it may mean 'urèthre, pénis?' and in the plural, 'canaux spermatiques et urèthre (les canaux excréteurs)' (*La doctrine*, 125). Cf. also Mayrhofer, who proposes the meaning, 'a particular part of the intestines' and suggests a root-connection with the word *plīhā́*, 'spleen' (Wb, 2: 385) and A. Sharma, who notes that the form *plāśí* found at TB. 2.6.4.4. is secondary (*Beit. z. Ved. Lex.*, 209).

VERSE 5

In *c*, ṚV 10.163.4 omits *bhasadyàm* and reads *bhā́sadād*. P 4.7.6. deletes *bhā́sadaṃ* in *d*. The tradition, therefore, seems to suggest that *bhasadyà* and *bhā́sada* are equivalent, which lends further support to arguments of Weber (207), Kuhn (68) and Whitney-Lanman (77), who do not translate *bhā́sadaṃ* (cf. Bloomfield who does see justification for it, and, following Sāyaṇa, includes it in his rendering as a type of intensifier). *bháṃsaso* is uncertain. Sāyaṇa glosses it as 'the visible, secret place' [*bhāsamānād guhyasthānād;* likewise at ṚV: *bhāsadāt. bhasat kaṭipradeśaḥ tatsaṃbandhāt . . . bhāsamānāt pāyoḥ . . .* "from the connection with *bhā́sadād* (*bhasat*, 'private-parts'), it is the visible anus"]. Grassmann also suggests 'anus' (Wb, col. 921); Macdonell-Keith proposes 'pubic bone' (*Vedic Index*, 2: 360). Filliozat, taking these two views into account suggests, 'anus? pubis' (*La doctrine*, 125). Cf. also Mayrhofer, who states that it may be a particular part of the abdomen, perhaps the "private parts," but also points out that since the exact meaning of the word cannot be determined, a connection between *bhasát* (*bhā́sada*) and *bháṃsas*, likewise, cannot be demonstrated (Wb, 2: 456). According to the Viśveśvarānanda edition, *Āpastamba Mantrapāṭha* 1.17.1 reads *dhváṃsaso*(?).

VERSE 6

ṚV 10.163.5 has an entirely different verse: *méhanād vanaṃkáraṇāl lómabhyas te nakhébhyaḥ, yákṣmaṃ sárvasmād ātmánas tám idáṃ ví vṛhāmi te,*

"From [your] urethra, from [your] *vanaṃkárana*, from your hair, from [your] nails, from [your] entire body, I tear away for you this *yákṣma.*" *vanaṃkáraṇa* is unclear. Sāyaṇa considers it to be adjectival to *méhanād* ('urethra') in the sense of 'the penis by which the bodily water [*vanam* = *udakaṃ śārīram*] is discharged' (*tat kriyate visṛjyate yena tadvanaṃkaraṇam. tasmāt mehanāt meḍhrāt* . . .), so also Haradatta to ĀpMB. 1.17.5 (see Sharma, *Beit. z. Ved. Lex.,* 251–52). Kuhn takes *vánam* to mean 'joy' rather than 'water' and proposes the translation "joy-bringer (Wonnebringer)" (67) which, in the present anatomical context of the hymn, may be regarded as a euphemism for "penis." Mayrhofer supports Sāyaṇa (Wb, 3: 39), and Filliozat, likewise, suggests 'organe de la défécation' (*La doctrine,* 126. Cf. Oldenberg, *Noten,* 2: 361). In *a,* P 4.7.5*a* has *māṃsebhyaḥ,* 'from [your] flesh.' In *c,* P 4.7.4*c* reads: *yakṣmaṃ pāṇyor aṅgulibhyo* (Raghu Vira: *aṅgalibhyo*?), 'from [your] fingers on the two hands' and in *d,* P 4.7.4*d* has *vi vṛhāmasi,* 'we tear away.' Sāyaṇa considers *snā̆vabhyo,* which has the common meaning 'from the tendons, sinews' (see also Filliozat, *La doctrine,* 127), as 'small blood vessels' (*sūkṣmās sirāḥ snāvaśabdena ucyante*) as opposed to *dhamánibhyaḥ* which are large (*dhamaniśabdena sthūlāḥ*).

VERSE 7

ṚV 10.163.6 reads: *áṅgād-aṅgāl lómno-lomno jātáṃ párvaṇi-parvaṇi, yákṣmaṃ sárvasmād ātmánas tám idáṃ ví vṛhāmi te:* "From every limb, from every hair, from the entire body, I tear away for you this *yákṣma* born in every joint." *ātmánas* here and in ṚV 10.163.5 (see previous note) has the sense of 'from the body' (see Renou, EVP, 16: 174). In *a,* P 4.7.7 reads as ṚV; in *b,* it has *baddhaṃ parvaṇi-parvaṇi,* '[the *yákṣma*] attached to every joint'; and in *cd,* it reads: *vayaṃ viṣvañcaṃ vi vṛhāmasi,* 'we tear completely away.' *víṣvañcaṃ* is here rendered adverbially to intensify the notion of the verb (cf. Whitney-Lanman, 77). Sāyaṇa, however, explains it as "that one born of disease who has spread through every member beginning with the eye" (*cakṣurādisarvāvayavavyāptaṃ rogajātaṃ*) which in turn refers to the *yákṣma.* Thus, following Sāyaṇa, another possibility could be to take *víṣvañcaṃ* as adjectival to *yákṣmaṃ,* i.e. 'the all pervasive *yákṣma.*' Because of its proximity to the verb, however, one would favor the adverbial usage. *vībarhéṇa,* being from the root *bṛh,* 'to tear' plus *ví,* means literally, 'by the tearing,' i.e. by the exorcising, a pun on the verb *vívṛhāmasi.* Sāyaṇa suggests that the "hymn exorcises [the *yákṣma*] 'by means of the exorcism of the great *ṛṣi* Kaśyapa' " (. . . *kaśyapasya maharṣer* . . . *vivṛhatyaneneti vivarhaṃ sūktam*) and goes on to explain: "Now the fruitful power of the *mantra,* which is indeed being employed in the ritual, is indicated by the praise of the *ṛṣi* who revealed the *mantra*" (*mantradraṣṭur maharṣeḥ saṃkīrtanena idānīṃ prayujyamānasyāpi mantrasya amoghavīryatvaṃ sūcitaṃ bhavati*). He clearly indicates that Kaśyapa is the author of this spell. At AVŚ 1.14.4 there is a specific reference to the *bráhman* (spell) of Kaśyapa and at ṚV 9.114.2 he is mentioned as a *ṛṣi* and an author of a hymn of praise. It is likely, therefore, that *vībarhéṇa* refers to Kaśyapa's "exorcising spell," which is this charm itself (cf. Bloomfield, 322, 408). For other references to the beneficial qualities of Kaśyapa, cf. AVŚ 5.28.5; 8.5.13–14; 17.1.27–38; 18.3.15 and 19.53.10, where he is stated as being born from Kāla ('time'). See also TĀ 1.7.1; 1.8.8. P 4.7 adds another verse (8), not found in K: *aṅgād-aṅgād ahaṃ (vayaṃ?) tava paruṣaḥ paruṣas pari, kaśyapasya vi vṛheṇa yakṣmante (yakṣmaṃ te) vi vṛhāmasi.* The suggested emendations are mine.

Notes to AVŚ 6.85

Translators are in agreement that AVŚ 6.85 is a charm against *yákṣma.*[17] Sāyaṇa prescribes its use "in a rite for the healing of disease beginning with *rājayakṣma*"[18] at KauśS 26.37. At KauśS 26.33, it is mentioned in a list of hymns for various medical purposes;[19] and at AthPariś 32.7, verse 2 is reckoned in the list of hymns for the destruction of *takmán.*[20]

VERSE 1

This verse is also found at AVŚ 10.3.5. P(K) 19.6.1, although fragmented, has been emended to read as Śau. In *a,* P 16.63.5 has *varaṇo* (K manuscript *varuṇo*); in *b: idaṃ devo vṛhaspatiḥ;* and in *cd,* it reads: *yakṣmaḥ pratiṣṭhā yo 'smin tam u devā avīvaran,* "the gods also have checked that *yakṣma* who resides in this [man]." At AVŚ 10.3 (cf. P 16.63), we learn that the *varaṇá*-tree is called an enemy-destroying, powerful amulet (. . . *varaṇó maṇíḥ sapatnakṣáyaṇo vṛ́ṣā,* verse 1) and that the amulet is the medicine for all [diseases], thousand-eyed, yellow and gold (. . . *maṇír varaṇó viśvábheṣajaḥ sahasrākṣó hárito hiraṇyáyaḥ,* verse 3). Sāyaṇa, following KauśS 26.37, understands that a piece of the *varaṇa*-tree was formed into an amulet which removes the disease beginning with *rājayakṣma* (*varaṇavṛkṣanirmito maṇiḥ . . . rājayakṣmādirogaṃ . . . nivartayatu*). It is likely, therefore, that an amulet of *varaṇá* is to be understood here. On *varaṇó* and *varaṇā vatī,* cf. AVS 4.7.1 and its notes in Witney-Lanman, Pt. 1: 154.

VERSE 2

P(K) 19.6.2 reads as Śau. Sāyaṇa glosses *vácasā:* 'by the word having the form of a command' (*ājñārūpeṇa vākyena*); and Bloomfield thus renders it as 'command' (39–40). On spells attributed to various divinities, cf. AVŚ 2.32.3, 5.23.10, where the spell or a *ṛṣi* is mentioned.

---

[17] Griffith: "A charm against Consumption or Decline," *Hymns of the Atharvaveda,* 1: 292; Bloomfield: "Exorcism of a disease by means of an amulet from the *varaṇa*-tree," *Hymns,* 39, 505, and Whitney-Lanman: "For relief from *yákṣma,*" *Atharva-veda-saṃhitā,* Pt. 1, 344.

[18] *rājayakṣmādirogabhaiṣajyakarmaṇi;* cf. Keśava: *rājayakṣmādibhaiṣajyam ucyate.*

[19] See Caland, AZ, 78, and cf. AthPariś, 34.24.

[20] *takmanāśanagaṇa;* vs. 2*ab* also occurs at KauśS 6.17 (see Bloomfield, *Hymns,* 506; cf. Whitney-Lanman, Pt. 1, 344).

VERSE 3

In *b*, P(K) 19.6.3 has *viśvádhāyasaḥ* (accented), 'all-sustaining.' Sāyaṇa, on similar lines, reads *viśvádhāyanīḥ* and explains it as "the nourisher of the entire world characterized by sentient and non-sentient beings" (. . . *kṛtsnasya sthāvarajaṅgamātmakasya jagataḥ poṣayitrīḥ* . . .). Note the reference to the mythological episode in which the demon Vṛtra restrained the water. By using this in the simile, the healer, equating himself with the demon, gains access to his domain and, with the help of Agni Vaiśvānara, is better able to ward off the patient's affliction. From the theological point of view, it is interesting to note that Vṛtra, along with Indra, his destroyer in verse 2 is looked upon as being beneficent. His holding back of the waters which is generally considered to be an evil act is in this verse compared to the checking of a disease-demon.

Notes to 19.36

Translators consider AVŚ 19.36 to be a charm involving the amulet called *śatávāra*.[21] Sāyaṇa mentions that it is found at *Śāntikalpa* 17.4 and 19.6 in the *mahāśānti*, 'great consecration,' called *saṃtati*, 'progeny,' where the *śatávāra*-amulet is employed.[22] From its context it appears that the charm was originally recited during the consecration and binding of this particular vegetal amulet which was worn to protect the individual from various evils, including, in particular, the internal disease-demon *yákṣma*.

VERSE 1

P 2.27.1 reads as Śau, except, in *d*, Raghu Vira reads: *maṇiṃ durṇāmacātanam*. Sāyaṇa understands *śatávāro* to be either a hundred *vāras*, roots or awns of grain; or else it averts (root *vṛ*) a hundred diseases, i.e. because it is subsequently heard (verse 6) that it wards off a hundred diseases, it is a type of herb (*śataṃ vāra mūlāni śūkā vā yasya sa śatavārah. yadvā śatasaṃkhyākān rogān nivārayatīti śatavāraḥ 'śatavāreṇa vāraye' iti uttaratra śatasaṃkhyākarogavāraṇaśravaṇād oṣadhiviśeṣaḥ*). Sāyaṇa's first explanation seems to be based on the meaning of *vā́ra* as 'tail-hair of animal' and, therefore, is forced. His second suggestion appears more likely because of the pun on the word found at verse 6. Whitney-Lanman offer yet another possibility: "possessing a hundred choice things" (root *vṛ*, 'to choose,' thus, choice'). No interpretation, however, is entirely satisfactory. In *c*, Sāyaṇa considers *āróhan*, 'ascending,' to refer to the raising [of the amulet] to the region of the body beginning with the man's arm (*puruṣasya bhujādipradeśam adhitiṣṭhan*), so also Griffith (294 n; cf. Whitney-Lanman, 955). Such

---

[21] Griffith: "A charm against disease and evil spirits," *Hymns of the Atharvaveda*, 2: 294; and Whitney-Lanman: "With a *śatávāra*-amulet: for protection, etc.," *Atharva-veda-saṃhitā*, Pt. 2, 955.

[22] . . . *vihitāyāṃ saṃtatyākhyāyāṃ mahāśāntau śatavāraṃ maṇim abhimantrya badhnīyāt*; cf. Whitney-Lanman, ibid.

an interpretation is likely because, like the charms involving the *jaṅgiḍá*-amulet (AVŚ 2.4, 3.9, 19.34,35), this hymn appears to have been recited during the ritualistic binding of the talisman; in which case, "ascending with brilliance" could be a description of it radiating while being elevated during the tying process. In *d,* Sāyaṇa glosses *durṇāma-* as a skin disease (*tvagdoṣaḥ*).

VERSE 2

In *d,* Roth-Whitney emend *tatrati* to *tarati.* P 2.27.2 has *tatrati;* but Barret and Raghu Vira, following Roth-Whitney, emend to *tarati.* Bh., however, reads: *pāpmādhi tatrati.* Sāyaṇa also reads *tatrati* and explains it, in Pāṇinian terms, as from the root *tṝ,* 'to cross,' 'to pass through,' with the affixes *ślu* (third class affix, which according to Pāṇ. 6.1.10 causes reduplication in a root which is not normally reduplicated) and *śa* (affix of the sixth class, to which the root *tṝ* belongs) (*tṝ plavanasaṃtaraṇayoḥ, śluḥ śaś ceti vikaraṇa-dvayam*). He glosses it as 'overcome' (*atikrāmati*). Such a form from the root *tṝ* is indeed unusual; and for this reason, Roth-Whitney's emendation would be justified; but P supports Sāyaṇa, which is perhaps the correct reading. By *mádhyena,* Sāyaṇa understands, 'with the stem' (*kāṇḍena*). It is possible that the poet-healer is describing an amulet which was fashioned from an entire plant whose stem bifurcates near the top. In this way, the two horns could be analogous to its forked head, the middle to its stem, and the root to the part under the ground. Cf. AVŚ 9.4.17 where two bulls' horns are said to push away the *rákṣas*-demon (*śṛṅgābhyāṃ rákṣa ṛṣaty . . .*).

VERSE 3

In *c,* Roth-Whitney read: *sárvān durṇāmahā́.* P 2.27.3 reads as Śau; but for *śabdínaḥ* in *b,* K has *śapathinaḥ,* 'cursing' (?). Sāyaṇa understands there to be three types of *yákṣmas* or diseases in *ab:* those which are newly produced, those fully grown and those possessing sound, i.e. making noise or possessing sound means 'difficult to cure' (. . . *aprarūḍhā utpannamātrā . . . yakṣmā rogāḥ santi ye ca . . . abhivṛddhā yakṣmāḥ . . . śabdavantaḥ ete duścikitsā iti śabdyamānāḥ śabdavanto vā . . .*). Sāyaṇa's explanation of these *yákṣmas* is mere guesswork. It would appear syntactically that there are only two categories: the *arbhakā́,* 'small/childish,' and the *mahā́nto . . . śabdínah,* 'large/adult, which are vocal or speak.' It is, however, difficult to understand to what exactly these descriptions may refer. Perhaps, as Griffith suggests, they indicate a mild and severe case of the bodily affliction (284); or better, they may signify the demon's victims. In other words, there were small, childish *yákṣmas* who attacked children and large, adult-speaking *yákṣmas* who assailed the grown-ups. Cf. AVŚ 6.25, where the disease-entities *apacíts* are said to make noise.

VERSE 4

In *a*, Roth-Whitney read: *vīrā́m̐* for *vīrā́n*. P(O) 2.27.4 reads as Śau, except for *apa* for *ava* in *d*. K has *śataṃ vīryāṇi janayañ śataṃ* (Raghu Vira: *vīryāṇy ajanayac chataṃ*) *yakṣmān apāvapat, durṇāmaḥ sarvāṃs tṛḍhvāpa rakṣāṃsy apākramīt* (Raghu Vira: *akramīt*). P(K) *cd* is a slight variant (*apa* for *ava* in *d*), of AVŚ 19.36.5*cd*. The notion of *vīrya*, 'strength,' 'power,' makes better sense than *vīra*, 'heroes,' which Sāyaṇa, nevertheless, understands as 'sons' (*putrāḥ*), i.e. "Let this carved amulet produce, bring about, impart them" (*ayaṃ dhāryamāṇo maṇiḥ . . . tān . . . janayatu utpādayatu prayacchatu*).

VERSE 5

ab is wanting in K; but, for *cd*, cf. P(K) 2.27.4 (above). P(O) has the entire verse (P 2.27.5) which reads as Śau, except *tṛḍḍhvā apa* occurs in *cd* (cf. Whitney-Lanman, 955–67). Sāyaṇa considers *híraṇyaśṛṅga* to be 'that whose tip appears like gold, i.e. it is the upper part of the *śatavāra*' (. . . . .*yasyāgraṃ hiraṇyavad avabhāsate sa hiraṇyaśṛṅgaḥ. śatavārasyāgram evaṃ bhavati*) and *ṛṣabháḥ* as 'the best of herbs' (*oṣadhīnāṃ śreṣṭhaḥ*). Griffith suggests that the bull is "the potent charm" (294 n). It seems rather that the poet-healer is describing the upper, forked part of the plant as golden in color and implicitly comparing its branches to the horns of the horned bull whose efficacy destroys the *rákṣas*-demons (cf. verse 2 above).

VERSE 6

In *c*, Roth-Whitney emend to *śatáṃ ca śvánvatīnāṃ*. P 2.27.6 omits *ca*. Raghu Vira, however, has [*ca*]. The K manuscript has: *śataṃ sunvatīnām*, 'a hundred female pressers (of Soma)' which, although being a grammatically correct reading, makes little sense. At P 1.89.2 *ab*, we read: *śataṃ jahy apsarasāṃ śataṃ śvanvatīnām* (K: *śatam apsarasāṃ śataṃ sunvatīnāṃ*), "You, [O *bhadrikā*-amulet,] kill the hundred Apsarases, the hundred (females) accompanied by dogs" (cf. Renou, JA, 253: 30). Sāyaṇa, along with the Viśveśvarānanda edition, reads *śaśvanvátīnāṃ*, from *śaśvat-vatī* where the initial 'n' is incorrectly written for 'd' (*dakārasya nakārādeśaḥ*) and glosses it: "diseases beginning with possession and epilepsy which arrive repeatedly for the sake of [causing] pain" (*muhurmuhuḥ pīḍārtham āgantryo grahāpasmārādyā vyādhayaḥ śaśvanvatyaḥ*). This is a rather feeble attempt to justify a bad reading. Roth-Whitney's emendation, therefore, seems to be best; in which case, *śvánvatīnām* could mean 'of those accompanied with dogs.' It receives some support from the fact that at AVŚ 4.37.11 the dog is found in relation to the Gandharvas; and at AVŚ 11.9.15 we read: *śvànvatīr apsaráso*, 'Apsaras accompanied with dogs.' It appears, therefore, that the expression *śvánvatīnām* refers to the Apsarases who bear it as an epithet. Whitney-Lanman's rendering "dog-like ones" is quite wrong here (956; so also Griffith, 294). On Sāyaṇa's mistaken identification of the feminine *durṇā́mnīnāṃ* with the masculine *vyādhi*, 'disease,' see Whitney-

Lanman (956); and on the significance of the pun between the verb *vāraye* (root *vṛ*, 'to ward off,' 'to check'), and *vāra* of *śatávāra*, see verse 1 n above.

Notes to 19.38

Most translators consider AVŚ 19.38 to be a charm involving *gulgulú* or *gúggulu* (bdellium).[23] Sāyaṇa mentions that it and AVŚ 19.39 are found at AthPariś 4.4 where, in the duties of the priest (i.e. *purohitakarmāṇi*), fumigation with *kuṣṭha* and with *gulgulu* is to be offered in the rite of the king's entering into his bed-chamber at night.[24]

VERSE 1

In *a*, Roth-Whitney, based on Sāyaṇa (*rodhaṃ na kurvanti, na pīḍayati*), emend to *ná táṃ yákṣmā ā́rundhate*, "*yákṣmas* do not obstruct him" (see also Whitney-Lanman, 958). In *a*, P 19.24.1 reads *yakṣmā arundhate*. The Viśveśvarānanda edition, following that of Śankar Paṇḍit and all manuscripts of Roth-Whitney, has *ná táṃ yákṣmā árundhate*, "Neither the *yákṣmas*, O Arundhatī, . . . him," which is also found in P. In spite of the accented vocative this reading is supported by Grill (39, 193), Griffith (295) and Bloomfield (40, 675–76). Since Arundhatī figures so predominantly as the goddess *par excellence* of the healing herbs (see AVŚ 19.39.2,3, where *kúṣṭha* is also made efficacious through its association with Arundhatī), it seems quite appropriate for the healer to have invoked her in an incantation which involved the medicinal plant *gulgulú*. (Note: the resinous nature of *gulgulú* brings to mind the sappy *silācī́, lākṣā́*, connected with Arundhatī.) This, then, could lend further support for reading the vocative in *a*. In *c*, Sāyaṇa, Roth-Whitney and some manuscripts have *gugguluóḥ*. Other manuscripts and the P read *gulguloḥ*. It is found at TS 6.2.8.6 as *gúlgulu* (note accent) (cf. also Lanman at Whitney-Lanman, 958). Either reading seems acceptable, with the accent on either the first or last syllable. On the question of the enumeration of the verses in this hymn, see, in particular, Whitney-Lanman, whose suggestion we have followed (958).

VERSE 2 (-3)

In *b*, Roth-Whitney emend to read: *mṛgā́d ṛ́śyā iverate;* in *c*, *guggulu*, and in *d*: *vā́pyási*. P 19.24.2,3 has, in 2*cd*: *viśvañcas takṣmād yakṣmā mṛgā aśvā iverate;* 3*a*: *gulgulu*. 1*cd* is repeated as 2*ab* to make three complete verses in P. The only significant emendation is that which occurs in 2*b*. Sāyaṇa, along with the Viśveśvarānanda edition and P, reads: *mṛgā́ áśvā iverate;*

---

[23] Grill translates it under his section: "Allerlei Übel (Miscellaneous evil)," *Hundert Lieder des Atharva-Veda*, 39, 193; Griffith: "A protective charm," *Hymns of the Atharvaveda*, 2: 295; Bloomfield: "The healing properties of bdellium," *Hymns*, 40, 675, and Whitney-Lanman: "With *gúggulu*: against disease," *Atharvavedasaṃhitā*, Pt. 2, 957.

[24] *purohitakartavye rātrau rājñaḥ śayyāgṛhapraveśanakarmaṇi gulguludhūpaṃ kuṣṭhauṣadhidhūpaṃ ca dadyāt;* cf. also Bloomfield, *Hymns*, 676, and Whitney-Lanman, Pt. 2, 957.

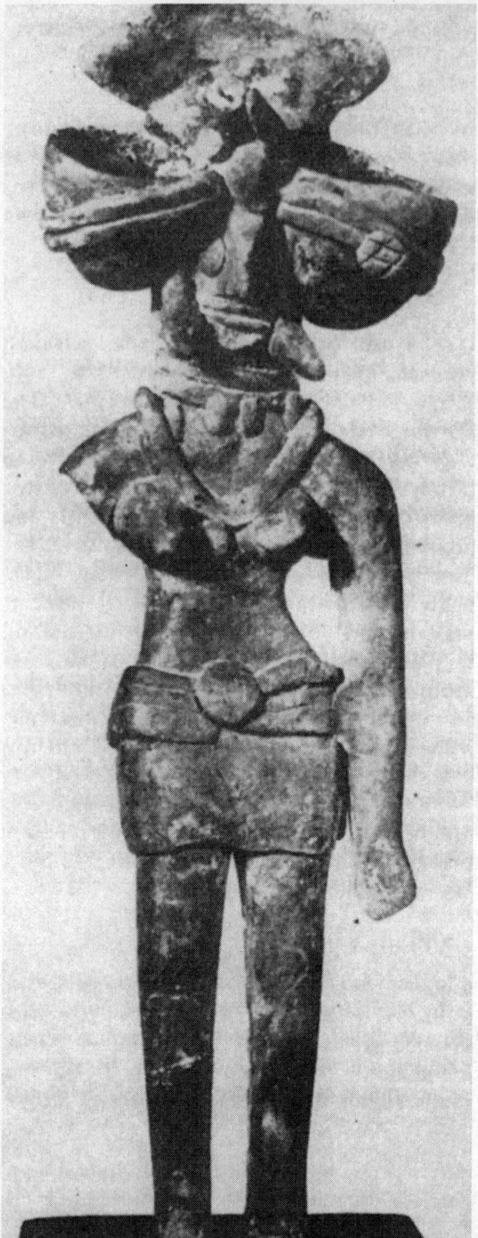

FIG. 5. Earth-Mother Goddess. Terra-cotta. Mohenjo-Dāro. 3rd–2nd millenium B.C.

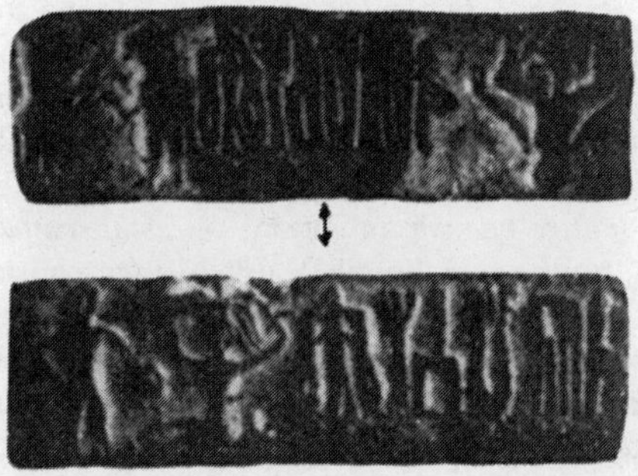

304

FIG. 6. Birth and harvest of plant. Sealing #304. Harappā. 3rd–2nd millennium B.C.

"like wild beasts [or] horses" (so also Grill, 39, 193; Griffith, 295 and Bloomfield, 40, 676) and glosses: "like quick-moving (=*áśvāḥ*) beasts, i.e. like a deer, etc.; or else like beasts, like horses" (*aśvāḥ āśugāmino mr̥gā iva hariṇādaya iva. athavā mr̥gā iva aśvā iva*). Although Roth-Whitney's emendation tends to complete the simile, it does not actually seem warranted. The poet is comparing, as Sāyaṇa implies, the speed of the animals to the quickness by which the *yákṣmas* disperse in the presence of the scent of *gulgulú*. The reading of Sāyaṇa and the Viśveśvarānanda edition may, therefore, be retained. This assumes, of course, that *mr̥gá* had the meaning of 'deer' or, at least, a very quick wild animal. There is, in this verse, a suggestion that *gulgulú* may have been transported by maritime commerce and traded in India (see Filliozat, *La doctrine*, 111; cf. also Zimmer, *Leben*, 28, and Grill, 193). Cf. AVŚ 4.7.6; 5.4.2,8; 8.7.11 where other auspicious plants and plant products were brought from a distance and traded. Note also the well-known practice of the healer stating that he has seized the herbs' two names. This implies that he knows not only their appropriate names, but also their uses.

Notes to 7.76 (80) 3–5

This hymn is a composite charm of which the first two verses are concerned with the *apacíts*; the last (verse 6) is a verse to be recited at the midday Soma-pressing.[25] The middle three verses treat the disease entity *jāyā̃nya*.

VERSE 1 (3)

In *b*, P 19.40.7 has *talīdyam upatiṣṭhati* '[which] comes in contact with the soles of the feet'; in *c*, it reads: *parāstaṃ* (K: *tarās tvaṃ*) *sarvaṃ jāyānyaṃ*,

[25] See notes to AVŚ 7.76 (80).1,2 227, below.

"I have cast away [or less likely: May you subdue (inj. aor. from root *tṝ*)] every *jāyānya*"; and in *d*, it has *kaś ca*. For *a*, Sāyaṇa, reading *prasṛṇāti*, renders: "The disease called *rājayakṣma*, reaching in the bones, i.e. reaching as far as the bones" (*yo rājayakṣmākhyo rogaḥ . . . asthīni . . . prasarati vyāpnoti. asthiparyantaṃ vyāpnotītyarthaḥ*). Sāyaṇa glosses the word *talīdyàm* ('the sole of the foot') as 'being in the vicinity, i.e. the flesh situated near the bones' (*antike bhavaṃ talīdyam . . . asthisamīpagataṃ māṃsam*). Most translators, however, follow Bloomfield who considers it to be 'the sole of the foot' on the following basis: Since the upper (*kakúd*) and the middle (*kīkasa*) parts of the body are represented, *talīdyà* should, therefore, indicate the lower part, and by the fact that Wise (70) defines it as the sole, possibly connected with *talahṛdaya* 'sole of the foot' (AJPh, 11: 329–30; cf. Mayrhofer, Wb, 1: 489). In *c*, *nír hās táṃ* of the Viśveśvarānanda edition is based upon Sāyaṇa who glosses: 'let . . . disappear' (*nirharatu*). Roth-Whitney, however, read *nír āstaṃ*, "I have cast out" (see Whitney-Lanman, Pt. 1, 442). Henry proposes the emendation: *nír āsyaṃ*, "J'ai chassé" (*Le livre* 7, 30; see also *La magie*, 194). Bloomfield has posited yet another reading: *nír āsthaṃ* (from root *as*, 'to throw'), "I have driven out" (*Hymns*, 17, 561–62; cf. also AJPh, 12: 439–40, and Ludwig, *Der Rigveda*, 3: 500). With any of these readings we notice the meaning is basically the same, i.e. the expelling of the demon (cf. also Zimmer, *Leben*, 377 and Filliozat, *La doctrine*, 88). Based on manuscript 'P' of 19.40.7, it appears that *nír āstaṃ* is the correct reading.

VERSE 2 (4)

In *b*, P 19.40.8 has *ya* in place of *sá* and Raghu Vira reads *pauruṣam* [manuscript 'P': *pu(-)ruṣam*] for *pūruṣam*; *cd* are variants of verse (3) 5*cd*, (s.v.) In *d*, Sāyaṇa reads *súkṣitasya* and understands the obscure *ákṣitasya*, in *c*, and *súkṣitasya*, in *d*, to be either from the root *kṣi*, 'to possess,' i.e. "without residing for a long time in the body (*ákṣita*) and residing for a long time [in the body] (*súkṣita*)"; or else from the foot *kṣan*, 'to injure,' with the Vedic addition of 'i,' i.e. the non-injuring, the non-drying of the body (*ákṣita*) and the thorough and complete drying of all the elements residing in the body (*súkṣita*). Thus, both are wasting-diseases (*akṣitasya. kṣi nirvāsagatyoḥ. śarīre cirakālāvasthānarahitasya . . . sukṣitasya cirakālam avasthitasya. yadvā kṣaṇu hiṃsāyām iti dhātuḥ. ikāropajanaś chāndasaḥ. akṣitasya ahiṃsakasya śarīram aśoṣayataḥ sukṣitasya śarīragatasarvadhātūn suṣṭhu niḥśeṣaṃ śoṣayataḥ. . . . ubhayoḥ akṣitasukṣitayoḥ kṣayarogayoḥ . . .*). Ludwig seems to have read the text as Sāyaṇa first suggested (500) and Griffith follows him (365 n). Bloomfield, basing himself on KauśS 31.16–17, its commentaries, and Wise (321), renders: "here is the remedy for sores not caused by cutting, as well as for wounds sharply cut"; the emended *ákṣata* means a 'tumor,' 'boil' and is to be identified with *jāyānya* (18, 562 and

AJPh, 11: 320–22). Both Zimmer (*Leben*, 377) and Henry (30–31, 98) have similar renderings. Bloomfield later changed his mind and considered *jāyā́nya* to be a type of congenital or venereal disease. This, however, is not reflected in his translation, and thus his rendering is ambiguous; unless, perhaps, he has in mind the skin lesions which are commonly associated with advanced stages of syphilis. This, however, may be begging the question. Whitney-Lanman, however, point out quite rightly that the root *kṣan* does not have the primary meaning 'to cut,' but 'to bruise,' thus, calling Bloomfield's interpretation into question (442). Likewise, Filliozat, after Caland (AZ, 101), understands *ákṣita* (or *ákṣata*) to mean 'intact' and thus renders: "Voici le remède des deux, de celui qui est intact et de celui qui est bien crevé" (*La doctrine*, 88 and n 3). Whitney-Lanman, after having examined all these explanations, with the exception of Filliozat and Caland, conclude that *ákṣita* and *súkṣita* are most probably two kinds of *jāyānya*, but quite astutely notice that the two half verses are discordant, and wonder if they even belong together (442). Along these same lines, it should be noted that the P does not have these two *pādas*. With so much difficulty and controversy surrounding this verse, any definite rendering would be futile. We may, however, not go too far astray if we assume that *ákṣita* (*ákṣata*) and *súkṣata* (*súkṣita*) represent two types of *jāyā́nya*. Like the *apacíts* (AVŚ 6.83.1,3), and the *yákṣma* (ṚV 10.97.13), the *jāyā́nya* appears to have the ability to fly; but unlike the *apacíts* it does not make a noise.

VERSE 3 (5)

According to Sāyaṇa, this and the following verse form a separate hymn (7.81). In *cd*, P 19.40.8 (=manuscript 'P' 19.40.9*b*) reads: *kathaṃ ha tatra tvaṃ hanyā yatra kuryām ahaṃ haviḥ*, "How could you harm [him] there where I would make the oblation?" *d* occurs at AVŚ 6.5.3*a*; and at VS 17.52 and TS 4.6.3.1 which have *kurmó* for *kṛṇmó*. Sāyaṇa explains *havír* ('oblation') as "that having the form of melted butter, etc. which is connected with the divinities beginning with Indra who are capable of removing the disease" (*roganirharaṇakṣamendrādidevatāsaṃbandhi ājyādirūpam*). Note the pun on the root *jan*, 'to be born,' and the mythological origin of *jāyā́nya*. This may be alluding to that myth recorded at TS 2.3.5.2, etc. In *cd* we have the use of the rhetorical question. P 19.40.9 (=manuscript 'P': 19.40.10) is an interesting verse, not found in the Śau, which may tentatively be read and translated as follows: *yas* (manuscript 'P': *ya ā*) *saṃprāviśat karoty udaraṃ mahat* (K: *mama*) *yakṣmo yo 'tra jāyate* (K manuscript: *jāyase*) *taṃ jāyānyam anīnaśam*, "We destroy that *jāyānya*, born here [as] *yakṣma*, who has entered completely into [my] abdomen [and] makes it big." We notice a definite connection between *jāyā́nya* and *yákṣma* and the suggestion that *jāyā́nya*, when it entered the abdomen, seems to have been thought to be a type of *yákṣma* causing the belly to swell.

Notes to 2.8

Most translators consider AVŚ 2.8 to be a charm against the disease *kṣetriyá*.[26] A. Weber, however, understands it to be a charm "against crop-damage (gegen Feldschaden)."[27] His basis for this lies in the etymology of the word *kṣetriyá*, which he derives from the word *kṣétra*, 'field,' 'soil,' 'land.' *kṣetriyá*, therefore, means 'related to the land or field.'[28] Sāyaṇa prescribes it "for the cessation of the diseases beginning with skin-disease, consumption and chronic diarrhea, which come from the family"[29] at KauśS 26.41–27.4. At AthPariś 34.7 it is counted in the list of hymns concerned with the destruction of *takmán* (*takmanāśanagaṇa*). Because of the mention of the repetition of the refrain: "Let the *kṣetriyá*-destroying plant [cause] the *kṣetriyá* to disappear," this charm appears to have been originally used to consecrate the plants utilized in the healing rite.

VERSE 1

ab is repeated at AVŚ 6.121.3*ab* and a variant of the entire verse is found at 3.7.4. In *c*, the K manuscript of P 1.99.2 has *sukṣatriyasya muñcatām*, emended by the editors to read as Śau. In *d* it reads: *saṃ granthiṃ* (K manuscript: *saṃgranthya*, Bar., Raghu Vira: *saṃgranthyā*) *hṛdayasya ca*, "and re[lease] the knot of the heart" (cf. Renou: "et re[nouez] le noeud du coeur." He understands *saṃ* [*muñcatām*] to be in opposition to *vi muñcatām*, which does not seem to make sense, JA, 253: 36). P 3.2.4 reads as Śau. In *b*, Sāyaṇa understands *vicṛ́tau* to be the name of two stars in the tail of the constellation Scorpio, and cites TĀ 2.6.1 and TS 4.4.10.2 as support (*etannāmnyau tārake mūlanakṣatram*, see also Whitney-Lanman, 48). Etymologically the word means 'unbinders' which, according to Bloomfield, "enables the word to figure wherever there is a question of the 'fetters' of disease" (288). Thus it could point to a symbolic association. It also suggests the auspicious time, i.e. when these stars are just visible, for the performance of the healing rite. For *pā́śam* ('bond'), Sāyaṇa glosses 'the seed of the disease' (*rogabījaṃ*).

VERSE 2

This verse is wanting in the P. However, P 1.99.1 reads: *apocchantī duḥṣvapnyam apa durhārdam ucchataṃ (K: dussvapnam apa durhādam ucchatām), apoṣṭaṃ sarvaṃ kṣetriyaṃ sarvāś ca yātudhānyaḥ*, "You two (stars), who cause the nightmare to disappear, make the evil-minded one disappear.

---

[26] Ludwig: untitled, *Der Rigveda*, 3: 513; Griffith: "The hymn is a charm against *kṣetriya*, some hereditary disease, perhaps pulmonary consumption," *The Hymns of the Atharvaveda*, 1, 50; Bloomfield: "Charm against *kṣetriya*, hereditary disease," *Hymns*, 13, 186; and Whitney-Lanman: "Against the disease *kṣetriyá*: with a plant," *Atharva-veda-saṃhitā*, Pt. 1, 48.

[27] IS, 13: 149.

[28] Ibid., 149–53.

[29] *kulāgatakuṣṭhakṣayagrahaṇyādirogaśāntaye*; cf. Keśava: *atha kṣetriyavyādhibhaiṣajyam ucyate.*

Disappeared (burned away?) [is] every *kṣetriya* and all the sorceresses" (cf. Renou, JA, 253: 36). In *a*, Sāyaṇa understands *iyáṃ rā̆try* ('this night') to be the night at the time of daybreak (*uṣaḥkālīnā . . . rātriḥ*), which again points to dawn as the time when the rite is to be performed (cf. KauśS 26.42: *apeyam iti vyucchantyām*). He considers the meaning of *abhikṛ́tvarīḥ* ('female demons') in two ways, based on the verb *ápa ucchantu*. In the first instance, he assumes the verb to be transitive and renders: "let the divinities beginning with the Ādityas, who cause the cessation of disease all around, make the mentioned disease (i.e. *kṣetriyá*) go away" (. . . *abhitaḥ rogaśāntiṃ kurvāṇāḥ ādityādidevatā . . . prakṛtaṃ vyādhim apagamayantu*). Secondly, he suggests that the verb may in fact be intransitive and translates: "Let the *piśācīs*, the demons of the diseases beginning with epilepsy, who are disposed to the excision [of the bodily parts], go away" (. . . *kartanaśīlāḥ apasmārādirogakāriṇyaḥ piśācyaḥ . . . apagacchantu*). Based on *pādas cd*, where, according to Sāyaṇa, the only rendering of *ápa ucchatu* is as a transitive (*kṣetriyanāśanī . . . uktaṃ rogam . . . apagamayatu*), it would seem that it would also be transitive in *ab* (cf. Bloomfield, who emends in *b* to *ápa ucchatu* to make both *a* and *b* correspond and thus renders all transitively, 13, 289). According to the P however, it appears that the night and female demons are requested to disappear. Thus, along with Whitney-Lanman (49), *ab* has been rendered intransitively and *cd*, transitively. For night P has nightmare; and female demons are supported by the P reading of *durhārdam* and *yātudhānyaḥ*, suggesting that the *kṣetriyá* was also looked upon as a demon. For the *kṣetriyá*-destroying plant, Sāyaṇa explains: "The herb mentioned in reference to the healing of this or that disease, which is the destroyer of the disease *kṣetriya*" (. . . *kṣetriyavyādher vināśayitrī . . . yā tattadrogabhaiṣajyaprastāvoktā oṣadhir asti . . .*).

VERSE 3

This verse is wanting in the P. In this verse, Sāyaṇa distinguishes three types of plants and plant products in addition to the *kṣetriyá*-destroying plant: 1. a piece of wood from the *arjuna*-tree (*arjunākhyavṛkṣaviśeṣakāṣṭhasya. śakaleneti śeṣaḥ*); 2. a chaff of barley (*yavaḥ prasiddhaḥ. tasya . . . tuṣeṇa . . .*); and 3. the bunches of flowers joined to the sesame-plant (. . . *tilasahitamañjaryā . . .*). These then, according to him, are to be made into an amulet which causes the patient's disease to disappear (. . . *kṛto maṇiḥ . . . tava rogam apocchatu*). Bloomfield, on the other hand, discounts Sāyaṇa's explanation and renders the text philologically, differentiating only two plants and their products: the stalk of the brown and white-sectioned barley, and the sesame-plant's blossom (13, 289; so also Whitney-Lanman, 49, and Griffith, who understands the "white-sections" to refer to "silvery ears," 51). Although one cannot be sure, Bloomfield's interpretation would appear grammatically more correct. Barley is at AVŚ 7.50(52).7 a remedy for hunger and, along with rice, is called a medicine at 8.2.5. In later Indian medicine it also has a medicinal use (see Dutt and King, *Materia Medica*,

270–71). Likewise, sesame has a medical usage in later medicine (ibid., 217–18). In this context, however, it appears that, as Sāyaṇa suggests, they may have been fashioned into an amulet. This is also supported by KauśS 26.43 (see Caland, AZ, 81, and Bloomfield, 287).

VERSE 4

Although the P does not have a parallel to this verse, it does contain a variant at 1.99.3: *namo astu varatrābhyo nama īṣāyugebhyaḥ* (K: . . . *vṛtrahābhyo nama eṣāṃ yugebhyaḥ*), *mṛgāyāraṇye tiṣṭhate kṣetriyāyākaraṃ namaḥ*, "Let there be obeisance to the straps, obeisance to [pairs of] poles and yokes (or, perhaps, "to the demon-slayers and to their ages"?). It stands in the forest for the wild beasts. I have made obeisance to the *kṣetriya*." *pāda c* implies a plant which deer, etc. may eat to cure their diseases (cf. Bh., 29, Renou, JA 253: 36, and Hoffmann, 3, 11: 9). The precise meaning of this verse is obscure. Sāyaṇa explains the first line as follows: "O sick man, for the sake of calming your disease, [let there be] obeisance to the ploughs provided with bulls (or gods; see Whitney-Lanman, 49) and to these limbs of the ploughs, i.e. the poles and yokes" (*he rugṇa . . . tvadrogaśamanāya . . . vṛṣabhayuktasīrebhyo. . . . īṣāś ca yugāni ca tebhyaś ca halāvayavebhyo namaḥ*). He goes on to say that obeisance is made after having effected the worship by the removal of the disease-causing pain; or, even though the ploughs etc. are unconscious, obeisance is made by the intentions of the gods laying claim to them, and cites *Brahmasūtra* 2.1.5 in support of the latter suggestion (*pīḍākararoganivartakatvena pūjyatvam āropya namaskāraḥ kṛtaḥ. yadvā halādīnām acetanatve 'pi tadabhimānidevatābhiprāyeṇa namaskāraḥ* . . .). It appears rather that the obeisance to the ploughs etc., is symbolical. According to the P all these are shown reverence; while in the Śau. only the plough and its parts are given homage. But in the second verse the disease-destroying plant is mentioned, suggesting that the obeisance paid to the ploughs, etc., which presumably were used in the cultivation of the plants such as barley and sesame, was for the purpose of consecration of this plant (*vīrúdh*), destructive of disease. KauśS 27.1 also notices the symbolical use for the plough and prescribes that the patient be placed under it (*namaste lāṅgalebhya iti sīrayogam adhiśiro 'vasiñcati*; see also Caland, AZ, 81, and Bloomfield, 287).

VERSE 5

The Roth-Whitney edition reads, at the end of the first line, *saṃdeśyèbhyo námaḥ kṣétrasya pátaye*. P does not have an exact parallel; but, P 1.99.4 reads: *ākhor idaṃ* (K.: *āṣo hṛdaṃ*) *kṣetrapatyaṃ manoś ca mānavasya ca, manaḥ sarvasya paśyata iha bhūyaḥ syād iti* (K.: *sarvasyāpaśyata iha bhūyamy ādiditi*), "This [is] the lord of the field, [the lord] of the mole, of Manu and of the descendant of Manu. [For it is said:] 'let the mind of everyone, perceiving, be present here(?)' " (cf. Renou, JA, 253: 36–67). In *a*, Sāyaṇa understands the obscure *sanisrasākṣébhyo,* as "empty houses, whose openings of windows, etc. are crumbling completely to pieces (collapsing)"(. . . *atiśayena visraṃsamānāni viśīryamāṇāni akṣāṇi gavākṣādidvārāṇi yeṣāṃ te sanisrasākṣāḥ. śūnyagṛhā ity arthaḥ*); and in *b,* for the difficult *saṃdeśyèbhyaḥ,* he reads *saṃdeśèbhyaḥ* and explains them as "old holes, which are indicated and which are abandoned because of the taking of soil belonging to them" (. . . *saṃdiśyante tyajyante tadgatamṛdādāneneti* . . . *jaradgartāḥ*). It is quite obvious that Sāyaṇa, not knowing the meaning of these words, based his explanation purely on KauśS 27.2–4 (see Caland, AZ, 81–82, and Bloomfield, 287). The word *sanisrasākṣébhyo* is a compound composed of the intensive adjective *sanisrasa,* 'very sunken,' and *ákṣa* (*ákṣi*), 'eye,' i.e. 'to those with sunken eyes' which, as Bloomfield points out, resembles *srastākṣa,* 'with sunken eyes,' at *Suśruta Saṃhitā* 1.115.7 (290). (Note: I have not been able to verify this reference as it is to the volume, page and line of an old Calcutta edition of the text which is inaccessible.) This notion of 'very sunken eyes' may refer to a symptom of the disease or, as Griffith suggests, to the eyes of the farm-laborers who have worked so hard that they can no longer keep their eyes open (51 n). *saṃdeśyà* means 'to be directed together,' but may also have the sense of 'belonging to this place,' 'domestic' (MWSED, s.v.). Bloomfield has noticed that its connection elsewhere is with evils or demons (290). K. Hoffmann has posited the rendering: "zu einer magischen Zuweisung gehörend," but admits that its meaning here is obscure (*Aufsätze,* 1: 300 and note). Since, at AVŚ 3.7.6 (see below), *kṣetriyá* is connected with witchcraft, the notion that they belonged to that evil realm seems probable.

Notes to 3.7

Most translators consider AVŚ 3.7 to be a charm against the disease *kṣetriyá.*[30] Weber, however, defines it further by calling it a hymn for "the banishing of the inherited-evil from a newborn child (Bannung des Erbübels aus e. neugebornen Kinde)."[31] He bases his assertion on two assumptions: 1. *kṣetriyá* is not an inherited sin, but a physical evil, an inborn, inherited germ of disease. 2. The mention of the use of water in verse 5 indicates a removal of the evil by water, which at AVŚ 2.20 is used to wash a newborn child. Or, perhaps, it is a question of brushing the infant by means of the young skin-covered horns of a deer.[32] It is possible that such a rite could have applied to an infant; but there is no justification for specifying it only for a newborn child. Likewise, there is no reference in the charm to a baby. Sāyaṇa prescribes its use "in the healing of the disease, *kṣetriya*"[33] at KauśS

---

[30] Grill: rendered under his section entitled "Krankheit," *Hundert Lieder des Atharva-Veda,* 8, 105; Griffith: "The hymn is a charm to drive away hereditary disease," *Hymns of the Atharvaveda,* 1: 89; Bloomfield: "Charm against *kṣetriya,* hereditary disease," *Hymns,* 15, 336, and Whitney-Lanman: "Against the disease *kṣetriyá,*" *Atharva-veda-saṃhitā,* Pt. 1, 94.

[31] IS, 17: 208.

[32] Ibid., 208–209.

27.29–31. He also mentions its occurrence at *Śāntikalpa* 17.5 and 19.7 in the *Mahāśānti* called *kaumārī.*[34] The first two verses are found at ĀpŚS 13.7.16 and the second again at 10.10.3.[35]

VERSE 1

In *c,* P 3.2.1 has *sukṣetriyaṃ* (K. manuscript: *su kṣettriyam;* Bar., Raghu Vira read as Śau). In *b,* Sāyaṇa explains *bheṣajám* ('medicine') as a disease-removing medicine in the shape of a horn (. . . *roganivartakaṃ śṛṅgarūpam auṣadham asti*). In *c, sá,* according to Sāyaṇa, refers to the deer (*hariṇaḥ*). It could also apply to the healer who may have used a horn in the healing rite (cf. KauśS 27.29). Deriving *viṣāṇā* from the root *sā* plus *vi,* 'to unfasten,' Whitney-Lanman conjecture that it refers to the deciduous horns of certain wild species of deer rather than to the permanent ones of domestic animals (94).

VERSE 2

In *d,* P 3.2.2 has *yat kiñ ca* (K: *yad kiñ cit*). In *ab,* ĀpŚS 13.7.16 reads: *mṛ́gaḥ paḍbhiś;* and in *c: gulphitám,* 'accumulation.' Sāyaṇa reads the difficult *guṣpitáṃ* as ĀpŚS and explains it: 'clumped like the ankle' (*gulphavad grathitaṃ*). Another variant of the word, *guṣṭitáṃ,* occurs at ŚB 3.2.2.20. It is found in connection with a black horn (*kṛṣṇaviṣāṇá*), used for the digging up of a clod of earth and is translated by Eggeling as 'pressed together' (*The Śatapatha-Brāhmaṇa,* 2: 43). The only Ṛgvedic occurrence of *guṣpitá* is found at 8.40.6 and seems to refer to the entanglement of a creeping plant (*vratáter iva guṣpitám;* see Geldner, *Der Rigveda,* 2: 353, and Grassmann, Wb, col. 403). Sāyaṇa here glosses it: 'the projecting branches' (*nigatāṃ śākhām*). It seems, therefore, to have the general sense of snarled or perhaps knotted, as when a vine entangles itself around the limbs of a tree or bush (see Mayrhofer, Wb, 1: 341–42). The reading of *mṛ́gaḥ* (ĀpŚS) for *vṛ́ṣā* is much easier and suggests a class of fleet-footed deer, which the word *háriṇa* later comes to signify. The notion of speed and dexterity, as Bloomfield points out, is implied in the phrase *padbhiś catúrbhiḥ* ('with four feet') (AJPh, 11: 350–46; *Hymns,* 337).

VERSE 3

In *c,* P 3.2.3 has *tena.* The exact meaning of the expression *cátuṣpakṣam iva cchadíḥ* ('like a four-pinioned covering') is rather obscure and has given rise to much discussion: Sāyaṇa suggests that it is either "a remote deer-shaped object situated in the orb of the moon" (*candramaṇḍalasthaṃ viprakṛṣṭaṃ . . . hariṇarūpaṃ vastu . . .*); or else, basing himself most probably

---

[33] *kṣetriyavyādhibhaiṣajye;* Keśava's definition is wanting.

[34] *kaumāryākhyāyāṃ mahāśāntau . . . etat sūktam.*

[35] See Bloomfield, *Hymns,* 337.

on KauśS 27.29, he says it is "a deer's hide appearing in outline [and] which is spread on the ground" (*yadvā . . . paridṛśyamānaṃ . . . bhūmau āstṛtaṃ hāriṇaṃ carma . . .*). He goes on to state that the object or the hide is like "the quadrangular straw-thatch which covers a house" (. . . *catuṣkoṇaṃ. . . . chādyate anena gṛham iti chadistṛṇakaṭaḥ sa iva*). Weber posits that it may refer to a constellation (210) which, according to Whitney-Lanman, might be Aquarius (95). Grill, using the mention of the four feet in verse 2, suggests that it is the deer whose four feet are like posts (*pakṣá?*), with the horns being the roof (*chadís*) (106–107). Griffith, following Grill, renders: "like a roof resting on four walls" (89 and note). Bloomfield states that " 'the roof with four wings (sides)' alludes vaguely to the antlers of the antelope, compared with the roof upon a house" (338). *pakṣá* means literally 'wing,' 'pinion,' but has come to signify also 'side,' 'flank,' etc. (MWSED, s.v.). *chadís* has the sense of 'covering' or 'roof.' At ṚV 10.85.10, it refers to a covering over a cart (*máno asyā́ ána āsīd;* cf. Geldner, *Der Rigveda,* 3: 268, and Grassmann, Wb, col. 461). The idea may, therefore, be one of a covering much like a cart's canopy which has four feathers or pinions as adornment. Or, perhaps, it refers to such a canopy made from a deer's hide, the legs of which, when the whole skin is stretched out as over a cart or wagon, may resemble the four extended wings of two birds in single-file flight (cf. KauśS 27.29, and Caland, AZ, 85). Bloomfield's comparison with the antlers seems forced and in this case may not be warranted.

VERSE 4

See AVŚ 2.8.1 and notes.

VERSE 5

In *cd,* ṚV 10.137.6 has *ā́paḥ sárvasya bheṣajī́s tā́s te kṛṇvantu bheṣajám,* "the waters [are] medicines for every [disease]. [Therefore,] let them make (be) medicine for you." Likewise AVŚ 6.91.3 reads as ṚV in *d.* P 3.2.7 reads as Śau; however, in *d,* P 5.18.9 has *tās tvā kṛṇvantu bheṣajam.* Because of its numerous occurrences it appears that the verse is formulaic and liturgical, recited while the healer consecrates the water to be used in the ritualistic cure (see Grill, 107–108, and Bloomfield, 338; cf. also Weber, 211). Further support for this is obtained from KauśS 27.29, where the patient is given water to sip and is sprinkled with tepid water. Sāyaṇa understands *víśvasya bheṣajī́s* as "another medicine for every disease, i.e. not just a medicine for a certain disease but for all" (*sarvasya rogasya . . . auṣadhāntaravad na kasya cid eva rogasya bheṣajaṃ kintu sarveṣām apīty arthaḥ*).

VERSE 6

a and most of *b* are missing at P 3.2.5 and have been reconstructed by the editors to follow Śau. At the end of *b,* P(K) has *tvābhy ānaśe,* 'has pervaded you. In *c,* P(K) has *tasmin;* and in *d,* P replaces *tvát* with *te.*

Sāyaṇa understands the difficult word *āsutéḥ* ('mixture'), from the passive root of *su* plus *ā*, 'to be wet,' to signify liquefied food and that the *kṣetriyá*-disease has taken possession of the patient because of consumption of bad food (*āsūyate āsicyate ity āsutir dravībhūtam annam. tasmāt ayathopayujyamānād annād yat kṣetriyaṃ kuṣṭhādirūpaṃ vyānase vyāpnot*). Weber, however, renders the phrase *āsutéh kriyámānāyāḥ* as "auf Grund des Zeugungs-Actes" and considers *āsutí* to be "infusio seminis," the cause of the *kṣetriyá* (211). As Bloomfield points out, his interpretation may fit well with the notion of *kṣetriyá* as an inherited disease, but it does not correspond to the general meaning of the root *su* plus *ā*, 'to press out.' He thus suggests the translation "from the prepared (magic) concoction" (15, 338; cf. Grill, 107). A probable interpretation, therefore, might be that the *kṣetriyá* enters and takes possession of its victim by means of a food which has spoiled because of improper cooking (Sāyaṇa), or better perhaps, by a mixture, magically prepared (Bloomfield).

VERSE 7

In *b*, P 3.2.6 has *utoṣasām* and in *cd*, . . . *āmayad apa kṣetriyam akramīt*, "[Every] disease [and] the *kṣetriya* departed. . . ." In *ab*, there appears to be reference to a definite time, when the stars can be seen faintly in the west and the red glow of dawn is beginning to give way to the morning sunlight in the east. It is particularly vivid in plains areas, where the terrain is flat and the entire vault of the sky is exposed. Sāyaṇa, likewise, considers this to be a reference to the early dawn (*uṣasaḥ prārambhe*) or daybreak (*prabhātakāle*) when the ceremony of anointing, etc. begins (*tasmin kriyamāṇena abhiṣekādinā*). The overall sense seems to be that light, here the first light of day, aids in the expulsion of the dark demons, *durbhūtá* and *kṣetriyá* (cf. Weber, 212–13; Grill, 108, and Bloomfield, 338–39). The plural number of *uṣás* suggests that the rite may have taken place over a period of days (cf. Sāyaṇa: *pratidivasam āvṛttyapekṣayā uṣasām iti bahuvacananirdeśaḥ*). As suggested at AVŚ 2.8, it is likely that the ritual began at dawn.

Notes to 4.13

Most translators consider AVŚ 4.13 and its variant ṚV 10.137 to be charms for healing in general.[36] Sāyaṇa prescribes that 4.13 along with other charms be used in two rites for long life (*āyuṣkāma*) at KauśS 58.3–4 and 11. He also mentions its inclusion in the *laghugaṇa*,[37] and its use,

---

[36] Griffith: "A charm to restore a sick man to health," *Hymns of the Atharvaveda*, 1: 148, so also *Hymns of the Rigveda*, 2: 583; Weber: "Gegen miasmatische Krankheit (Massage!?) (Against miasmal disease, with massage)," IS, 18: 48 and Whitney-Lanman: "For healing," *Atharvaveda-saṃhitā*, Pt. 1, 168; to ṚV 10.137, see in particular, Aufrecht, "Ein Heilspruch (A healing charm)," ZDMG, 24 (1870): 204; Lanman: "Exorcism for a sick person," *Sanskrit Reader*, 390; Geldner: "Gegen Krankheit," *Der Rigveda*, 3: 370, and Renou: "À Tous les dieux," EVP, 16: 171.

[37] Cf. also Bloomfield to KauśS 9.4 (*The Kauśika Sūtra*, 28 n 6).

along with AVŚ 2.33 (and 3.11), "in the performance of a healing of a sacrificer who has become ill in the midst of a sacrificial rite"[38] at VaitS 38.1. At AthPariś 34.21, it is included in the *aṅholiṅgagaṇa*.[39] According to Sāyaṇa and the *Sarvānukramaṇī*, ṚV 10.137 is a hymn in *anuṣṭubh* meter, devoted to the Viśvedevas, with each verse ascribed to one of seven great *ṛṣis*, i.e. Bharadvāja, Kaśyapa, Gotama, Atri, Viśvāmitra, Jamadagni and Vasiṣṭha.[40] BD 8.49–50 states that the hymn should be curative of all [diseases] or destructive of *rápas* and that the divinities addressed are as follows: the first verse is to the gods, verses 2–4, to Vāta, verse 5, to the Viśvedevas, and verses 6–7 to the Waters.[41] Finally, *Ṛgvidhāna* 4.9.4–7 specifies its use in a general, healing ritual for one suffering from disease (*roga*) and also mentions specifically indigestion (*ajīrṇānna*).[42]

VERSE 1

This verse is found unaltered at ṚV 10.137.1 and MS 4.14.2. In *b*, P(K) 5.18.1 has *uddharathā*, 'pull out' (O: *uddharatā*); and in *cd*, P reads: *uto manuṣyaṃ taṃ devā daivāḥ* (Raghu Vira: *devāḥ*) *kṛṇutha* (K: *kṛṇuta*) *jīvase*, "and then you divine gods (or, you gods, O gods,) cause that man to live." Geldner (370) and Renou (171) consider that the first line might be a reference to Trita who, according to ṚV 1.105.15 was "dipped into a well" (*kū́pé 'vahitaḥ*). Sāyaṇa to AVŚ, on the other hand, understands it differently: "O gods, make this [man] who is brought near to the realm of Dharma [-rāja, i.e. Yama] cautious, not careless, or else, make him put down, placed down. Carry out thus so that he stays down for a long time" (*he devāḥ imam upanītaṃ dharmaviṣaye avahitam sāvadhānam apramattaṃ kuruta. yadvā avahitam avasthāpitaṃ kuruta. yathāsau cirakālam avatiṣṭhate tathā kurutety arthaḥ*). The meaning is obscure; yet *ávahita* could suggest rather the sense of burial as Sāyaṇa's second explanation seems to insinuate and *únnayathā* would, therefore, imply his unearthing or extracting from the ground (cf. P). In *c*, Sāyaṇa to AVŚ glosses *ā́gaś* as 'transgression, i.e. evil born from neglect of command, etc.' (*aparādhaṃ vihitānanuṣṭhānādijanitaṃ pāpaṃ*). Lanman thus considers the disease to be a punishment for a sin (391). P, as we have seen, makes no reference to transgression, suggesting that the redactor did not consider sin to be a major cause for the individual's malady.

---

[38] *tathā kratumadhye vyādhitasya yajamānasya bhaiṣajakaraṇepi etat sūktam.*

[39] See Whitney-Lanman, Pt. 1, 168.

[40] Anu.: . . . *sapta ṛṣaya ekarcā vaiśvadevam;* Sāyaṇa: . . . *ānuṣṭubhaṃ vaiśvadevaṃ bharadvājakaśyapagotamātriviśvāmitrajamadagnivasiṣṭhā iti krameṇa pratyṛcam ṛṣayaḥ.*

[41] Vs. 49: . . . *uta devāḥ paraṃ tu yat, devānām atra cādyā syād vātadevas tṛcaḥ paraḥ.* Vs. 50: *trāyantāṃ vaiśvadevy ṛk tu séṣas tv abdaivataḥ paraḥ, syād etad viśvabhaiṣajyaṃ rapaso vā vināśanam.* Cf. also Macdonell, *Bṛhat-Devatā*, Pt. 2, 168.

[42] See also Gonda, The *Ṛgvidhānam*, 107–108 and notes. It is interesting to note that in this rite, ghee (*ghṛta*) is a significant element, for it states at vs. 7 that the *sūkta* is to be muttered while anointing the body with ghee (*rogārtasyāpy anenaiva gātram aṅktvā japed idaṃ;* cf. Gonda, ibid.). As we will see at vs. 7 n, the P adds a verse which also mentions ghee which appears to have been utilized in the healing rite, along with water.

VERSE 2

In *cd,* both ṚV 10.137.2 and P 5.18.3 read: *ā́ vātu párānyó;* cf. also TB 2.4.1.7 and TĀ 4.42.1. As Renou points out, *ab* seems to indicate both the wind's source (Sindhu) and its direction towards (here . . . from afar) (171). Sāyaṇa to AVŚ offers this interpretation as one explanation, but then presents another purely conjectural and oversophisticated one which is, nevertheless, interesting from the point of view of the later medical tradition: "Or these two winds, with the nature of *prāṇa* and *apāna,* blowing, (that is to say) moving about in the bodies, from the Sindhu. Here by the word *síndhu,* they mean sweat-ducts from which sweat habitually oozes out. By the word *parāvát,* an area of twelve finger-breadths outside the body is referred to." He continues the analysis in *cd:* "[One] *anyá* is the *prāṇa* or the wind from in front; let it cause your strength to return. [The other] *anyá* is the *apāna* or the wind from behind. What is your evil, let the wind make it, the evil, depart from your presence" (*yadvā imau prāṇāpānātmakau dvau vātau vātaḥ śarīreṣu saṃcarataḥ ā sindhoḥ. atra sindhuśabdena syandanaśīlānisvedāyanāni ucyante. . . . parāvacchabdena śarīrād bāhyadeśo dvādaśāṅgulaparimito vivakṣitaḥ. . . . anyaḥ purovātaḥ prāṇo vā he upanīta . . . tava . . . balam . . . āgamayatu. anyaḥ paścād vātaḥ apānavāyur vā tava yad rapaḥ pāpam asti. . . . tat pāpaṃ . . . tvatsakāśād vigamayatu*). Cf. also Geldner, who understands the winds in the second line to be the same wind (370); Renou, who also sees perhaps a prelude to *prāṇá* of the human body (171); and Weber, who suggests that the wind from in front and that from behind may be the east and west winds or perhaps the winds occurring before and after a thunderstorm (49). Note also the opposition between *dákṣaṃ,* 'dexterity,' or 'skill,' in the sense of possessing the 'full command of the faculties' (cf. Renou, 171, and verse 5, note, below) and *rápas.* The verse implies the reviving of the bodily functions by the restoration of breathing, stimulated perhaps by the ritual fanning of the patient, a practice which takes place over sacred images in temples to this day.

VERSE 3

In *c,* both ṚV 10.137.3 and P 5.18.4 read: *viśvábheṣajo,* which may have been the original and which has been read in this verse. Cf. also TB 2.4.1.7 and TĀ 4.42.1, which also have *viśvábheṣajo.* Sāyaṇa to AVŚ explains *d* as "You move for the protection of all people; or else, you, being like a messenger, i.e. being in the proximity of the sense faculties, move for their nourishment, i.e. you, having permeated the entire body, proceed" (. . . *sarvajagadrakṣaṇāya . . . saṃcarasi. . . . yadvā devānām indriyāṇāṃ dūtaḥ dūtavad āsannavartī san tatpoṣaṇāya īyase. kṛtsnaṃ śarīraṃ vyāpya vartasa ity arthaḥ*).

VERSE 4

In *a,* ṚV 10.137.5 has *ihá* in place of *imáṃ;* and in b: *gaṇáḥ.* In *b,* K 5.18.5 reads: *gaṇaiḥ;* and in *d: agado 'sati,* "[so that he] may be devoid of toxin."

This verse is wanting in O. It is interesting that the redactor of the K has understood *agado* in place of *arapá, agada,* from *gada,* may, as Emmerick suggests, have the sense of 'seizure' ("Indo-Iranian concepts of disease and cure," 14; cf. also ṚV 10.16.6; 97.2; AVŚ 5.4.6–9; 6.95.2 and 18.3.55). In later Indian medicine, however, it refers most often to 'poison.' Sāyaṇa to AVŚ explains *devā́s,* in *a,* as "Indra, etc.; or else (based on AĀ 2.4.2) gods, beginning with Agni, divinities presiding over the sense faculties" and for the *pāda* renders: "Let them protect this man by the gift of clear perception in this or that sense faculty" (. . . *indrādayaḥ. . . . yadvā . . . agnyādyā indriyādhiṣṭhātṛdevatā devāḥ. te tattadindriyapāṭavapradānena imaṃ rakṣantu ity arthaḥ*). In *b,* he understands the troop of Maruts to be "those who are numbered seven among those numbered forty-nine (based on TS 1.8.13.2)–may they protect this (man); or else of those winds, *praṇa, apāna, vyāna* etc., which are established in the body" (*ckonapañcāśatsaṃkhyākānām. . . . saptasaṃkhyākāḥ santi te pi imaṃ . . . saṃrakṣantu. yadvā marutām prāṇāpānavyānādīnāṃ dehe avasthitānāṃ . . .*). This second interpretation is merely in keeping with his attempt to make the charm medically relevant. Aufrecht assumes that the wind is speaking (204). Geldner, however, is perhaps more correct in suggesting that it is the healer addressing the patient (370).

VERSE 5

In *c,* ṚV 10.137.4 and P(K) 5.18.2 read: *te bhadrám ā́bhārṣaṃ* (O: *bhārṣaṃ;* Bar.: *ābharṣaṃ*). In *d,* P(K) has *parā suvāmy anayaṃ te,* "I dispel your adversity"; O has: *parā suvāmy āmayat,* "I dispel what aches," which is the probable reading. For the difficult word *śáṃtātibhir,* Sāyaṇa to AVŚ glosses: '*mantras* which cause pleasure [and] which are beneficial' (*śaṃkaraiḥ sukhakaraiḥ mantraiḥ*); and for *ariṣṭátātibhiḥ:* 'actions which lead to salvation i.e. causing non-injury' (*ariṣṭam ahiṃsā tatkaraiḥ śreyohetubhiḥ karmabhiḥ*); but to ṚV: 'protectings causing non-injury' (*ahiṃsākaraiś ca rakṣaṇaiḥ*). Although the exact meanings for these words are difficult to ascertain, it seems probable that they refer to propitious means brought by the healer; in which case, *śáṃtātibhir* may be understood as beneficial means and *ariṣṭátātibhir,* from *ariṣṭa,* 'unharmed,' as the means to free the patient from his (specific) injury, healthy means, i.e. not merely those which are non-damaging, but also, which are restorative. In *c,* as Whitney-Lanman point out, *ābhāriṣaṃ* is a false reading. The more correct one is *ā́bhārṣaṃ.* In *cd,* as in 2*cd,* there is an opposition between (*dákṣaṃ*) and a disease-entity (*yákṣ-maṃ*) cf. Müller, "Medizin im Ṛg-Veda," 354, 356n).

VERSE 6

This verse is found unaltered at ṚV 10.60.12 and P 5.18.7 (=O verse 5). It appears that the healer is referring to two individual hands: the left, propitious hand, which holds the medicines (cf. ṚV 10.97.11 and *Vendīdād* 3.1, etc., where the priest holds the sacred *baresma* [*barsom*] in his hand, while reciting prayers) and the right, more propitious hand which contains the power to heal by touching and stroking. Sāyaṇa to AVŚ, however, considers there to be only one hand which, because of its possessing all of these qualities, becomes connected with a pleasure-causing touch (*yasmād evaṃguṇaviśiṣṭo madīyo hastaḥ tasmād . . . sukhakarasparśanayukto bhavatu*). This explanation, however, does not fit well with the following verse which distinctly mentions two hands. In place of this verse, ṚV 10.137.6 reads one which occurs at AVŚ 3.7.5 and 6.91.3 and which tends to be formulaic, hinting at the use of water in the healing rite: *ā́pa íd vā́ u bheṣajī́r ā́po amīvacā́tanīḥ, ā́paḥ sárvasya bheṣajī́s tā́s te kṛṇvantu bheṣajám,* "The waters [are] indeed medicinal; the waters [are] *ámīvā*-dispellers; the waters [are] medicines for every [disease]. [Therefore,] let them make (be) medicine for you."

VERSE 7

In *cd,* ṚV 10.137.7 reads: *anāmayitnúbhyāṃ tvā tā́bhyāṃ;* while, P 5.18.8 (=O verse 6) replaces *hástābhyāṃ* with *śaṃbhubhyāṃ,* 'beneficent.' In c, *anāmayitnúbhyāṃ* has the literal meaning 'non-pain-causing' (see J. Narten, St. II, 5/6; 158), which in this context implies 'curative.' In *d,* ṚV has *tvópa spṛśāmasi.* Although this verse seems corrupt, there could be a logical connection between *b* and the rest of the verse. This may occur through an implied simile involving anatomical parts: just as the tongue precedes or is the leader of healing words, so also the fingers of the hand precede the healing touch or stroke. Further, the tongue guides the words to the appropriate place in the same way that the fingers conduct the healing powers to the afflicted spot. Aufrecht (204), and Lanman after him (391), consider that the verse refers to the notion of a spell preceding the act of the laying on of the hands. This interpretation, although possible, does not aim at finding a connection between two seemingly disjointed thoughts. The notion of branch (*śā́khā*) for finger suggests the herbal medicines which, in verse 6, were said to be held in the hand (cf. also Renou, 171). See Lanman on other accounts of the use of hands for healing in the New Testament, ancient Greece, ancient Rome and medieval England (391). P(K) 5.18 has included another verse (6) which seems to indicate that a part of the healing rite involved the use of ghee and the sprinkling of water: *ghṛtena dyāvāpṛthivī ghṛtenāpas samukṣatāḥ, ghṛtena muñcas vainaso yad ā tvā kṛtam ahṛthāḥ* (K manuscript: *āhṛtaḥ*). This verse is wanting in O, suggesting that it may have been a later addition.

Notes to 6.91

Most translators consider AVŚ 6.91, like 4.13, to be a generally remedial charm.[43] Sāyaṇa prescribes its use, along with that of numerous other

[43] Grill includes the charm under his section: "Krankheit," *Hundert Lieder des Atharva-Veda,* 14, 68; Griffith: "A charm against disease," *Hymns of the Atharvaveda,* 1: 295; Bloomfield: "Barley and water as universal remedies," *Hymns,* 40, 507, and Whitney-Lanman: "For remedy from disease," *Atharva-veda-saṃhitā,* Pt. 1, 348.

charms, in a rite 'for the purpose of healing all diseases'[44] at KauśS 28.17–20. It is also counted among the *takmanāśanagaṇa* at AthPariś 32.7.[45]

VERSE 1

For *cd,* P 19.18.7 reads: *sa ghā te tanvo rapaḥ pratīcīnam apa* (Bar.: *upa*) *hvayatām* (cf. *hvayamāsi* at AVŚ 6.90.2), "Indeed, let that [barley] exorcise your bodily *rapas.*" In *a,* Sāyaṇa understands *yávam,* 'barley,' as 'a grain with long awns (or a species of grain plant) suitable for medicine' (. . . *bhaiṣajyāya prayujyamānaṃ . . . dīrghaśūkaṃ dhānyam . . .*). Concerning *yáva,* Bloomfield makes an interesting observation: "The supposed etymology of *yáva,* 'barley', from the root *yu,* 'ward off,' is a fruitful source for the application of barley in charms to cure diseases and ward off demons" (507). It is possible that an amulet of barley was used in the rite as implied at KauśS 28.20 (see Caland, AZ, 91). Cf. also AVŚ 2.8.2, where barley as well as cultivated sesame seem to have been fashioned into an amulet and used against the internal disease-demon *kṣetriyá.* Grill, following Zimmer (*Leben,* 237), renders: four and three yokes of oxen, "wegen des Widerstands des Bodens" (168). The significance of the number of oxen is a mystery. The connection with the ground or cultivated soil, however, is obvious. If the reading is correct, the use of three and four teams of oxen suggests a rather large plough, perhaps with many shares; or, it may be an allusion to many ploughs cultivating the soil at one time [see W. Rau, *Staat und Gesellschaft in alten Indien: nach den Brāhmaṇa-Texten dargestellt* (Wiesbaden: Otto Harrassowitz, 1957), 25]. In either case, it points to a rather high degree of sophistication in agriculture. Since *vyaye,* in *d,* has the sense of 'to wrap' and with *ápa,* 'unwrap,' we are tempted to understand a type of poultice, composed of barley and wrapped in cloth, which, when unwrapped from the affected area, draws the demonic *rápas* out of the body. The P reading (*apa hvayatām*) implies that the *rápas* was thought to be magically removed by means of an amulet of barley. The later ritual tradition supports this view.

VERSE 2

This verse is found at ṚV 10.60.11, which reads in *a: vā̆tó 'va vāti.* It also occurs at P 19.18.8, which reads as Śau, and at P 1.111.1, which has *viṣam* in place of *rápaḥ,* suggesting that *viṣá,* poison, and *rápas* are synonyms (cf. ṚV 7.50.3 below). The notion of it being equated with *gada,* 'poison,' also supports this (see 4.13, verse 4, 127 above). These readings point to the fact that the verse is formulaic. The insertion of the correlative: "[As] . . . [just so]," is supported by Sāyaṇa (*yathā . . . evaṃ*). Since the preceding part of the verse indicates a movement downward, *bhavantu,* in *d,* also implies motion, i.e. 'go' (cf. Grill ". . . abwärts entweich," 14; Bloomfield: "downward . . . shall pass," 41, and Geldner: ". . . soll . . . fahren," *Der*

[44] *sarvarogabhaiṣajyārtham;* cf. Keśava: *atha sarvavyādhibhaiṣajyāny ucyante.*

[45] Cf. Bloomfield, *Hymns,* 507, and Whitney-Lanman, Pt. 1, 348.

Rigveda, 3: 225). The downward movement of *rápas* brings to mind the ground, implied in verse 1.

VERSE 3

This verse is found at ṚV 10.137.6, with the reading, in *c: víśvasya.* It also occurs at AVŚ 3.7.5; at P 3.2.7, which has in *d: tvā muñcantu kṣetriyāt,* "Let [them] release you from *kṣetriya*"; at P 5.18.9 (=O verse 7), which reads, in *d: te* (or, *tvā*) *kṛṇvantu bheṣajam,* "Let [them] make medicine for you"; and at P 19.18.9, which has, in *cd: āpas samudrārthā yatīḥ parā vahantu te rapaḥ,* "Let the waters, going, tending to the sea, carry away [with themselves] your *rapas.*" With such a large number of occurrences of this verse, it is likely that it is formulaic, pointing to the consecration of the water to be used in the healing rite (cf. AVŚ 3.2.7 and notes). P 19.18.9 suggests that the patient may have been ritually placed in a river or swiftly moving water in order to wash away the malady and purify the body. Griffith has referred to an interesting instance of water as a universal healer in Germany: "So Pastor Kneipp, the famous Bavarian water-doctor, maintains that what cannot be cured by water is altogether incurable. Water is the panacea. Hydropathy is the one saving principle which can be applied in every case" (295 n).

Notes to ṚV 7.50

Most translators consider ṚV 7.50 to be a charm against poison.[46] Sāyaṇa, following BD 6.1[47] and the *Sarvānukramaṇī,* describes the charm as a praise of various divinities: the first stanza is to Mitra and Varuṇa; the second to Agni; the third to the Viśvedevas; and the fourth to the river divinities beginning with Gaṅgā. The meter of the first three stanzas is *jagatī;* the fourth is *atijagatī* or *śakvarī.*[48] Sāyaṇa goes on to say that from its character, the hymn is used for the destruction of poison, etc.[49] The charm does not seem to be mentioned in the *Ṛgvidhāna.*[50]

VERSE 1

Sāyaṇa understands the expression "which nests and forms a swelling" (*kulāyáyad viśváyan*) to refer to poison which makes a nest, i.e. abode, and

---

[46] Griffith follows the traditional explanation of Sāyaṇa, *Hymns of the Ṛgveda,* 2: 51; Bolling: "A charm against poison—chiefly that of snakes," ERE, 4: 769; Geldner: "Ein atharvaartiger Zauber gegen Leibsschaden durch Gift u.ä. (An Atharvan-type charm against bodily damage by poison, etc.)," *Der Rigveda,* 2: 227; and Renou: "A divers dieux . . . : type entièrement atharvanique," EVP, 16: 111 (notes only).

[47] *ā māmiti tu sūktena pratyṛcaṃ devatā stutāḥ, mitrāvaruṇāv agniś ca devā nadyas tathaiva ca.*

[48] Anu: *ā māṃ maitrāvaruṇyāgneyī vaiśvadevī nadī stutir jāgatamantyātijagatī śakvarī vā;* Sāyaṇa: *prathamā maitrāvaruṇī dvitīyāgneyī tṛtīyā vaiśvadevī caturthī gaṅgādinadīdevatākā.*

[49] *asya sūktasya pratyṛcaṃ viṣādiharaṇe viniyogo liṅgād avagantavyaḥ.*

[50] Cf. 2.26.2–3 and Gonda, *The Ṛgvidhāna,* 57, and notes.

which increases greatly (*kulāyaṃ sthānam. tatkurvat . . . viśeṣeṇa vardhamānaṃ viṣaṃ . . .*). *viśváyan* has the implication of 'swelling' or 'protuberance' (see Grassmann, Wb, col. 1410). Renou has suggested that there are two separate activities implied in the half-verse: that "qui forme un creux" in opposition to that "qui forme un protubérance" (EVP, 16: 111). The phrase seems rather to refer to one creature which lives, forming a nest (*kulāyáyad*), under the skin, and produces a cutaneous swelling (*viśváyan*). In *c*, *ajakāvá* is difficult. Geldner, following Sāyaṇa, suggests that it may refer to a poisonous insect or to a type of disease (227). The word *tsáruḥ* (creeper) in the last *pāda*, however, seems to indicate that *ajakāvá* is the agent of the infirmity. The meaning would then be: Do not let the evil-looking *ajakāvá*-creature, who creeps along (like a snake, Sāyaṇa), cause injury. Sāyaṇa glosses the verb *dadhe* as an imperative (*dhattām*, i.e. *naśyatu*), which is easier. Cf. also Filliozat, *La doctrine*, 45.

VERSE 2

On *vijā́man*, see AVŚ 6.83, verse 4, note, 226 below, and 7.76(80), verse 2, note, 227 below. For the obscure *vándanaṃ*, in *a*, Sāyaṇa states that it is the name of a poison (. . . *etatsaṃjñakaṃ . . . viṣaṃ*). At ṚV 7.21.5, it occurs in the plural and appears to indicate a class of demons; while at AVŚ 7.113(118).1 and 115(120).2, it designates a type of coarse vine-plant, commonly parasitic (see Mayrhofer, Wb, 3: 142–43). Geldner, following Roth, suggests that it refers to the eruptions on the skin produced by coming in contact with the poisonous plant (227). Because it is described in *b* as covering (*pári déhat*, literally 'may smear around') the two joints of the knee and ankle, the idea of eruption, similar to that caused by the plant of the same name, seems plausible. Cf. also Renou, 111.

VERSE 3

In this verse, the emphasis shifts from an affliction of the leg to poisons and their three sources, two of which are plants, and one is the water of a river. The same refrain that is found in the previous two verses also occurs here, suggesting that the healer is still concerned with a foot problem. Perhaps the healer is mentioning the habitats where such poisonous, crawling creatures were known to reside. We can understand how it may have been considered that the poison originated from those three sources: after walking through damp forests, where the *śalmalí*-tree grows, wading through streams and ponds and brushing against numerous herbs, the symptoms would appear.

VERSE 4

Sāyaṇa explains that the obscure *aśipadā́* means 'not being made of *śipada*, i.e. the name of a kind of disease' and that the equally difficult *aśimidā́* indicates causing no injury; [since] *śími* is one whose action was to kill (i.e. a professional killer)' (. . . *śipadaṃ nāma rogaviśeṣaḥ. tadakurvatyaḥ satyaḥ. . . . śimir vadhakarmā. ahiṃsāpradāḥ . . .*). At AVŚ 4.25.4 and ŚB 7.4.1.27, we find that the feminine *śímidā* occurs as the name of a female demon (cf. Macdonell-Keith, *Vedic Index,* 2: 380, and Geldner, 228). Bolling has suggested that the two words signify 'not causing the disease *śipa* and *śimi*' (769). Franz Specht understands the two words to be connected etymologically because of the common association with evil spirits, stating: "Da diese aber nach altem idg. Volksglauben durch böse Geister hervorgerufen werden, so könnten *aśi-m-adá* und *aśi-p-adá* etymologisch wieder zusammengehören" (KZ, 69: 134). It is impossible to know from these references the exact meaning of these two words. We do, however, have a clue that they may be designations of something evil or demonic. Since the feminine *śímidā* is attested elsewhere, we are inclined to consider that the adjectival form *aśimidā̃* is also feminine; in which case, we could have the male demon and his female counterpart, both of which were thought to pollute the various water sources and help bring about the foot-infirmity.

Notes to 1.22

Most translators consider AVŚ 1.22 to be a charm against yellowness or jaundice.[51] Sāyaṇa prescribes it "for the appeasement of the diseases beginning with *hṛdroga* (chest-pain, angina pectoris?) and *kāmala* (jaundice),"[52] at KauśS 26.14–21. A. Kuhn has pointed to similar healing rites which utilized symbolic color association and birds in ancient Greek, Swedish, Low German, Danish and Dutch legends;[53] and Caland has drawn our attention to those sympathetic rituals practiced among the ancient Romans and the Cherokee Indians of North America.[54]

VERSE 1

In *b,* P 1.28.1 has *hṛddyoto* (K manuscript: *hṛdyoto*); in *cd,* it reads: *yo rohitasya gor varṇas tena tvā pari dadhmasi,* "We surround you with that which is the color of the red bull" (cf. Renou, JA, 252: 430). Sāyaṇa explains that the difficult *hṛddyotó,* being from the causative of the root *dyut,* 'to cause to burn,' 'to inflame,' could mean 'heart-affliction' (*hṛdroga*); or it could be 'the pain born from heart-affliction' (*hṛdayaṃ dyotayati dīpayati*

---

[51] Weber: "Gegen Gelbsucht (Against Jaundice)," IS, 4: 415; A. Kuhn, "Gegen Gelbsucht," "Indische und germanische Segenssprüche," KZ, 13 (1864): 113; Bergaigne-Henry: "Conjuration contre la jaunisse," *Manuel,* 134; Griffith: "The hymn is a charm against Jaundice," *Hymns of the Atharvaveda,* 1: 26; Bloomfield: "Charm against jaundice and related diseases," *Hymns,* 7, 263; and Whitney-Lanman: "Against yellowness (jaundice)," *Atharva-veda-saṃhitā,* Pt. 1, 22.

[52] *hṛdrogakāmalādirogopaśāntaye;* cf. Keśava: *atha hṛdroge kāmale cetyādi bhaiṣajyāny ucyante* and to *sūtra* 21: . . . *apasmāra* (epilepsy) *vismayahṛdrogakāmalakarohiṇakāni bhaiṣajyāni,* cf. Bloomfield, *Hymns,* 264.

[53] KZ, 13: 113–18.

[54] AZ, 75–76 n.

saṃtāpayatīti hṛddyotaḥ hṛdrogaḥ. dyuta dīptau. . . . yadvā hṛdrogajanitaḥ saṃtāpo hṛddyotaḥ. dyuter bhāve ghañ). Filliozat also understands it as "éclat qui est dans le coeur" and discounts the notion that *dyota* is from the root *dyut*, 'to break' (*La doctrine*, 89 and note. Cf. also Bergaigne-Henry, *Manuel*, 134 n). At ṚV 1.50.11 (cf. also TB 3.7.6.22 and ĀpŚS 4.15.1), there is a variant of this verse which tends to support the notion that *hṛddyotá* refers to a symptom characterized by an affliction of the heart or of the inside of the body: "Rising today, O you who have the majesty of Mitra [and] ascending to the highest heaven, destroy my chest-pain, O Sūrya, and [my] yellowness" (*udyánn adyá mitramaha āróhann úttarāṃ dívam, hṛdrogám máma sūrya harimā́ṇaṃ ca nāśaya;* cf. Renou, EVP, 15: 4 and Müller, "Medizin im Ṛg-Veda," 359–60). Meaning an affliction in the region of the heart, it refers to a chest-pain, perhaps angina pectoris. For *harimā́*, Sāyaṇa understands: 'bodily yellowish color born from the disease of jaundice, etc.' (*kāmalādirogajanitaḥ śārīro haridvarṇaḥ*). It is quite likely that, in fact, *harimán* described the bodily condition or disease-symptom which we know as jaundice (see Filliozat, *La doctrine*, 89–90); cf. also Müller, "Medizin im Ṛg-Veda," 359–60, and "Die Gelbsucht der Alt-Inder," *Janus*, 34 (1930): 188–89). Note the sympathetic association between the chest-pain, the yellowness, and the sun, and between the desired, normal and healthy color and the red bull.

VERSE 2

In *cd*, P 1.28.2 reads more effectively: *yathā tvam arapā aso atho* (Raghu Vira omits *atho*) *aharito bhava*, "In order that you be without *rápas*, therefore, be yellowless." The reading implies that when one is without jaundice, he is cured of *rápas*. Sāyaṇa understands *arapā́*, according to *Nirukta* 4.21, to mean 'devoid of evil' (*na vidyate rapaḥ pāpaṃ yasyāsau arapāḥ*). Again the sympathetic color-association is mentioned.

VERSE 3

In *a*, Roth-Whitney read: *yā́ rohiṇīdevatyā̀*, 'who have the red one for divinity.' P 1.28.3 reads: *yā rohiṇīdevatyā* (Bh. *rohiṇīr devapatyā;* Renou, however, casts doubt on it, JA, 252: 430) *gāvo yā rohiṇīr uta, rūpaṃrūpaṃ vayovayas* (K: *rūpaṃ rūpeṇa yo vayas*) *tena tvā pari dadhmasi.* This reading supports the emendation proposed by Roth-Whitney and is followed by us. Bergaigne-Henry also suggest this emendation with the addition of *ṛcas* (135) which, according to Bloomfield, is not necessary (AJPh, 12: 437–38 and *Hymns*, 265). Sāyaṇa, however, reading as *róhiṇīr devatyā̀*, understands it to be the divinely connected red colors which are of types of cows, i.e. those divine ones beginning with *kāmadhenu* ('cow of plenty'), etc., and the earthly ones connected with man (. . . *devatāsu bhavāḥ. . . . devasambandhinyo . . . rohiṇyaḥ lohitavarṇāḥ. . . . uktavarṇā yāḥ kāmadhenvādayo gāvaḥ santi. . . . api ca yāḥ manuṣyasaṃbandhinyo . . . rohiṇyaḥ lohitavarṇā gāvaḥ santi*). Bloomfield follows this interpretation (AJPh, 12: 438; *Hymns*,

7, 265). To whom or to what *róhiṇī,* in *a,* refers is debatable. Bloomfield conjectures that it is "a personification of the red, ascending (*ruh*), ruling sun" (ibid., 265); while Whitney-Lanman suggest that she may be a "red star or lunar asterism" (23; cf. also Renou, JA, 252: 430). In *c,* the exact meaning of *rūpáṃrūpaṃ váyovayas* is vague. Sāyaṇa suggests that the former refers to the full red-brown color in every individual cow, and that the latter is the full youth of every individual (. . . *sarvagovyaktigataṃ kṛtsnam aruṇarūpaṃ tathā . . . sarvavyaktigataṃ kṛtsnaṃ yauvanam*). This interpretation is also implied in Bloomfield's translation (*Hymns,* 7). *váyas,* however, has the sense of 'food' or 'energy' (see Mayrhofer, Wb, 3: 147) and, therefore, may refer to all the nourishing foodstuffs derived from the cow. In this case, both *rūpáṃrūpaṃ* and *váyovayas* could refer to the cows, i.e. in their every shape and in their every nourishment. This receives support from KauśS 26.16–17 where the patient is given cow's milk, in which a piece of bull's skin has been steeped, to drink.

VERSE 4

In *a* and *c,* ṚV 1.50.12 reads *me* in place of *ke;* and in *c,* it has *hāridravéṣu* (cf. also TB. 3.7.6.22 and ĀpŚS. 4.15.1). P 1.28.4 reads as Śau, except Bh. has *prapaṇākāsu* (?) in *b. ropaṇā́kā* is glossed by Sāyaṇa here as a *kāṣṭhaśuka,* perhaps a 'timber-parrot,' i.e. a type of woodpecker (cf. *kāṣṭhakuṭṭa*) or parakeet, and at ṚV 1.50.12 as a thrush (*śārikā*). *hā́ridrava* is glossed by Sāyaṇa here as a yellow-wagtail (*gopītanaka*), at ṚV 8.35.7 as a bird (*pakṣin*), but at ṚV 1.50.12 as a type of tree (*haritāladruma*), presumably where the birds reside. Both are most probably birds which are yellow in color. (Cf., in particular, Bloomfield, *Hymns,* 266; Geldner, *Der Rigveda,* 1: 61, and Müller, "Medizin im Ṛg-Veda," 359–60.)

Notes to 6.14

Most translators agree that AVŚ 6.14 is a charm against *balā́sa.*[55] Sāyaṇa prescribes its use "in a rite for the healing of phlegmatic [diseases]"[56] at KauśS 29.30.

VERSE 1

In *a,* Roth-Whitney read *paruḥsraṃsám,* so also P 19.13.7. In *c,* P 19.13.7 has *niṣkṛdhy,* 'eradicate (cure),' for *nāśaya,* 'destroy.' Sāyaṇa understands the afflictions mentioned in *ab* to be related to *balā́saṃ,* in *c,* which he explains as 'a phlegmatic disease characterized by cough and hard breath-

---

[55] Grohmann renders vs. 1 in his discussion of *balā́sa* in relation to *takmán,* IS, 9: 397; Florenz: "Gegen Balāsa (Against *balāsa*)," "Das sechtse Buch der Atharva-saṃhitā," BB, 12: 265; Bloomfield: "Charm against the disease *balāsa,*" *Hymns,* 8, 463; Whitney-Lanman: "Against the *balā́sa,*" *Atharva-veda-saṃhitā,* Pt. 1, 290. Griffith, following Weber, understands it to be "a charm against consumption," *Hymns of the Atharvaveda,* 1: 252.

[56] *śleṣmabhaiṣajyakarmaṇi;* cf. also Keśava: *ślesmabhaiṣajyam ucyate.*

ing' (. . . *kāsaśvāsātmakaśleṣmarogaḥ* . . .). Likewise, most translators have considered that the first line refers to *balā́sam*, but have rendered *a* along with *b*: 'The internal heart-disease which loosens the bones and joints' (see Grohmann, 397; Florenz, 265; Griffith, 252; Bloomfield, 8, and Whitney-Lanman, 290). Both lines, 1 and 2, seem rather to be describing various residences and afflictions of the internal disease-entity *balā́sa*. Although the subject of the verb is unexpressed, Griffith speculates that it may be a medicinal herb (252 n). On the form of the obscure *aṅgeṣṭhā́(ḥ)*, see Macdonell, *A Vedic Grammar for Students*, #97.2.

VERSE 2

a is found repeated at P 1.90.3*a* in relation to *yákṣma* and *d* is repeated at P 19.2.3*d*. P 19.13.8*ab* reads: *nir balāsaṃ balāsinaḥ kṛṇomi* (manuscript 'P': *kṣiṇomi*) *puṣkaraṃ yathā*, "I eradicate the *balāsa* of the *balāsa*-victim, as [I eradicate] a lotus [from the pond]"; and in *d*, it has *urvārvo yathā*. Sāyaṇa also reads *puṣkarā́m* for *muṣkarā́m* and explains the simile as follows: "As a fully grown lotus in a pool is cut out with its roots, so also do I uproot from the diseased body that disease with its roots" (*mahāhrade prarūḍhaṃ puṣkaraṃ yathā samūlam ucchidyate tathā vyādhitaśarīrāt taṃ rogaṃ samūlam unmūlayāmi* . . .). Bloomfield, understanding *muṣkarā́m* to be "an animal with testicles," offers an interpretative translation of the phrase: "as one gelds a lusty animal" (8, 463–64; cf. also Florenz, who reads *nír akṣṇómi* and renders: "den *balāsa* des *balāsa*kranken verschneide, wie [ich] Hoden tragenden [entmanne]," 266). Cf. Mayrhofer, Wb, 2: 657–58. Since *cd* refers to a plant, however, *puṣkarā́m* may after all be the correct reading. Sāyaṇa equates *urvārú* with *karkaṭī*, a type of gourd. The suggestion here is that the *balā́sa* is some type of external disease which has its origin deep below the surface of the skin.

VERSE 3

P 19.13.9 reads: *nir balāsetaḥ prapata suparṇo vasater iva, adha* (manuscript 'P': *atho*?) [*iṭa*] *iva hāyano 'pa drāhy avīrahan*, "O *balāsa*, fly forth out of here as an eagle from its nest and moreover, O non-destroyer of men, pass away like an annual grass." In *b*, Sāyaṇa reads *śuśukā́ḥ* and understands *āśuṃgā́ḥ* to mean 'quick moving,' glossing the *pāda*: "in the same way that a quick moving deer runs a long way" (. . . *yena prakāreṇa* . . . *āśugāmī śuśukaḥ etatsaṃjño mṛgo dūraṃ dhāvati* . . .). Most translators, basing themselves on Florenz (266), consider *āśuṃgá* to be a foal which runs after the mare (see Griffith, 252, and Bloomfield, 8). T. Chowdhury has suggested that *tā 'śuṅgā́ḥ* may be a corruption for *-ta aśṛṅgā́ḥ*, referring to a "hornless, very young calf (*śiśukó*)" (JBORS, 17: 46–47). *āśuṃgá*, meaning perhaps 'one who moves quickly,' could also refer to a bird (MWSED, 157, col. 3). This seems to be supported by P. We notice also that *yákṣma* is requested to "fly forth" with various birds [ṚV 10.97.13; see also AVŚ 5.30.9 where it is said to have flown forth like a hawk (*yákṣmaḥ śyená iva prā́paptad*

. . .)]. Likewise, cf. AVŚ 6.83.1, where the *apacíts* are requested to fly forth like an eagle from its nest (i.e., perhaps from the bodily hairs). These parallels suggest, therefore, that *āśuṃgá* refers to a bird. In *c*, Sāyaṇa reads *íta*, 'past' (root *i*) for *íṭa* and renders the last line: "and also the past year does not return, thus you, being the non-injurer of our heroes, departing, go the despised path" (. . . *api ca* . . . *gataḥ saṃvatsaro yathā na punarāvartate tathā* . . . *asmadīyānāṃ vīrāṇām ahantā san* . . . *apakramya kutsitāṃ gatiṃ gaccha*).

Notes to 6.127

Most translators consider AVŚ 6.127 to be a charm against a variety of diseases.[57] Sāyaṇa prescribes its use in a rite "for the healing of all diseases beginning with dropsy and erysipelas"[58] at KauśS 26.34, 39. It is also mentioned, along with other hymns, at KauśS 26.33, and is counted among the *takmanāśanagaṇa* at AthPariś 34.7 and among the *gaṇakarmāgaṇa* at AthPariś 34.24.

VERSE 1

For *ab*, P 1.90.1 reads: *asitasya vidradhasya lohitasya vanaspate*, "O tree . . . of the black [and] red *vidradha* (abscess) . . ."; and in *c*, it has *visalpakasyauṣadhe* (K: *vikalpakasyoṣadhe*, Bar.: *-auṣadhe*, cf. Renou, JA, 253: 30). Sāyaṇa explains the four obscure words in *a–c* as follows: *vidradhá* is 'a type of ulcer which usually bursts open' (*vidaraṇaśīlasya vraṇaviśeṣasya*); *balā́sa* is 'that beginning with cough and shortness of breath' (*kāsaśvāsādiḥ*); *lóhita:* 'the red-colored one; i.e. it is the name of a type of erysipelas, or else of a disease characterized by blood-flow' (. . . *lohitavarṇasya. etad visarpakaviśeṣasya nāma. yadvā lohitaṃ rudhiram. rudhirasrāvātmakasya rogasycty arthaḥ*), and *visálpaka*, being derived from the root *sṛp* plus *vi*, 'to creep variously,' is 'the disease erysipelas (*visarpaka*) [which] permeates the inside of the body through the mouth(s) of the tubes' (. . . *vividhaṃ sarpati nāḍīmukhena śarīrasya antarvyāpnotīti visarpakaḥ*). It is likely that *vidradhá* is related to *vidradhī*, 'abscess,' which is defined in detail at CaSūSth. 17.95–100 and SuNiSth. 9.1–38 (cf. AVŚ 9.8.20; see also Filliozat, *La doctrine*, 90 n, 92 n and Mayrhofer, Wb., 3: 210, 794). *lóhita*, as Sāyaṇa suggests, may be a disease characterized by flow of blood; or, it may be a color-designation referring perhaps to the *balā́sa* (see Bloomfield, 531, and Whitney-Lanman, 376). We noticed in P that *vidradhá* (abscess) is described as red and black (cf. the *vātavidradhī* at CaSūSth. 17.99 and SuNiSth. 9.7). In the same way, the Śau. reading could be pointing to the characterization

---

[57] Zimmer renders the charm under his discussion of *balā́sa, Leben*, 386; Griffith: "A charm to banish various diseases," *Hymns of the Atharvaveda*, 1: 315; Bloomfield: "The *cīpudru*-tree as a panacea," *Hymns*, 40, 530; and Whitney-Lanman: "Against various diseases: with a wooden amulet," *Atharva-veda-saṃhitā*, Pt. 1, 376.

[58] *jalodaravisarpādisarvarogabhaiṣajyārthaṃ*. Cf. Keśava to KauśS 26.39: *jalodare bhaiṣajyam ucyate*.

of the *balā́sa* as red in color like the (red and black) *vidradhá.* (Cf. also Karambelkar, *The Atharva-Veda and the Āyur-Veda,* 221–23.) The exact meaning of *visálpaka* is uncertain. Filliozat suggests that it could be erysipelas (Sāyaṇa's *visarpaka*) or a disease "with buds" (*visala* or *bisala,* plus *ya*) (*La doctrine,* 90–91; cf. also Bloomfield, "neuralgia," 40 and Mayrhofer, Wb, 3: 233). *piśitám,* meaning perhaps 'flesh,' has been rendered with Bloomfield: "small bit" (531; see also Whitney-Lanman, 376). The verse appears to be referring to types or stages of cutaneous swellings which the herb *cīpúdru* (verse 2) is able to remove.

VERSE 2

P 1.90.2 reads: *yat te* (K: *ut te*) *balāsa tiṣṭhataḥ kakṣe muṣkāv apākṛtam* (K: *apākṛtau*), *vedāhaṃ tasya* (K: *tasmin*) *bheṣajaṃ cīpadrām* (K: *cīpudrāv*) *abhicakṣaṇam,* "Since your two testicles, O *balāsa,* stand in the armpit because of a defect (or, following K: "Your two defective testicles, O *balāsa,* arise in the armpit"), [therefore,] I know his splendid medicine, *cīpadrā* (or, K: "I know the splendid medicine [is] in this *cīpudri*-herb")" (cf. Renou, JA, 253: 30). Sāyaṇa understands *ab* to refer to two diseases in the form of erysipelas, etc., situated at the base of the arm, and two testicles (or eggs) adjoining the penis (?). (. . . *vikārau visarpakādirūpau* . . . *bāhumūle tiṣṭhataḥ*. . . . *aṇḍau ca* . . . *apakṛṣṭamāśritau* . . .); and for *cīpúdrur,* he reads *cīpadruḥ* (cf. P) and explains it as 'a species of wood having that name' (*cīpadruḥ etatsaṃjño drumaviśeṣaḥ*). *muṣkā́v,* 'two testicles,' seems to be a description of two sack-like swellings or boils located under the arms (see Grohmann, IS, 9: 399; Bloomfield, 531; Filliozat, *La doctrine,* 90 n; and Hoffmann, *Aufsätze,* 1: 93 and note). On the obscure word *cīpúdru,* which is found only here, see Mayrhofer Wb, 1: 392, and F. B. J. Kuiper who, because of the *dru*-ending, suggests that it may be a Proto-Munda loanword ["Two Rigvedic loanwords "in *Sprachgeschichte und Wortbedeutung: Festschrift Albert Debrunner,* ed. G. Redard, (Bern: A. Francke, 1954), 248 n]. *abhicákṣaṇam* has been rendered adjectivally (cf. *vicakṣaṇá*) to *bheṣajáṃ* (medicine). P 1.90 adds a verse (3) which reads: *nirbalāsaṃ balāsino visalpam* (K: *vimalaṃ*) *uta vidradham, paropahatyāṃ te vayaṃ parā yakṣmaṃ suvāmasi,* "We dispel your *yakṣma,* the *balāsa* of the *balāsa*-victim, the *visalpa* (swelling) (or dirt?), the *vidradha* (abscess) [and] the pounding (in the eyes)" (cf. AVŚ 4.13.5; 5.4.10; 6.14.2; 7.5.3,6 and ṚV 10.137.4).

VERSE 3

P 1.90.4 has: *śīrṣarogam aṅgarogaṃ śuktivalgaṃ* (K: *sraktivalgaṃ* ?) *vilohitam, parā te ajñātaṃ* (K manuscript: *jñātaṃ!*) *yakṣmam adharāñcaṃ suvāmasi,* "We dispel downwards your unknown *yakṣma,* head-disease, limb-disease, eye-disease [?, Renou: "vertige (localisé) à l'oreille," JA, 253: 31] and *vilohita*" (cf. AVŚ 9.8.1,2). For *ájñātaṃ yákṣmam,* Sāyana glosses: 'a disease whose nature it not totally known' (. . . *anirjñātasvarūpaṃ* . . . *rogaṃ*). Griffith considers the last line to be a later addition (316 n). *hṛdayāmayám* suggests 'chest-pain,' cf. *hṛdrogá* at ṚV 1.50.11 and *hṛddyotá* at AVŚ 1.22.1. On *vidradhá* see in particular the description of the abscess, *vidradhī,* at CaSūSth. 17.83,90–103 and 106.

Notes to 1.25

Translators and interpreters are in general agreement that AVŚ 1.25 is a charm against the demon *takmán* which is conceived to be severe fever.[59] Sāyaṇa prescribes its use in a rite "for the quieting of the fevers beginning with those recurring daily, of the cold fever, of the continuous fever, and of the remittent fever, etc."[60] at KauśS 26.25. The charm is also reckoned as among the *takmanāśanagaṇa* at AthPariś 34.7.

VERSE 1

In *a,* P 1.32.1 reads as Śau. In *d* K has the more usual form *vṛndhi.* Sāyaṇa, interpreting the verse according to the ritual at KauśS 26.25, explains the obscure *dharmadhṛ́to* 'upholders of the law,' as those who came to bear, i.e. perform [the offering of] oblations and gifts, etc. (=*dharma*) (*dharmaśabdena atra yāgadānādir ucyate. taṃ dhārayanti anutiṣṭhantīti dharmadhṛtaḥ*). Weber (419), Grohmann (403) and Zimmer (*Leben,* 384) consider them to be pious men (Frommen), while Bloomfield, following Ludwig, conceives them to be gods (3, 271). Whitney-Lanman render: "maintainers of duty" (25); Henry: "les grands soutiens de l'ordre divin" (*La magie,* 183) and, similarly, Filliozat: "ceux qui se tiennent à la Norme" (*La doctrine,* 96). The consensus of opinion, therefore, points to mortals who uphold the law. For *saṃvidvā́n,* 'who is all-knowing,' Sāyaṇa glosses: "knowing fully the fire as its own cause" (*samyak svakāraṇam agniṃ jānan*). Others consider it to be an epithet referring to a merciful or complaisant aspect of *takmán* (see, in particular, Weber, 419; Bloomfield, 3, and Whitney-Lanman, 25). It is the only occurrence of the word and, being derived from the root *vid,* 'to know,' has the sense of 'wholly or fully learned,' i.e. 'all-knowing.' In this way, the poet-healer, praising the demon by giving it god-like qualities, desires to win it over by appeasing it. For *takman,* Sāyaṇa glosses: "O one causing a painful life" (*kṛcchrajīvanakārin*) and equates it with fever (*jvara*). As Grohmann first suggested, this verse appears to point to the origin and cause of *takmán* as lightning which, in the form of fire, entered

---

[59] Weber: "Gegen Fieber (Against Fever)," IS, 4: 419; Grohmann also renders the charm in his discussion of *takmán* or fever, "Medicinisches aus dem Atharva-Veda, mit besonderem Bezug auf den Takman," IS, 9: 384–86, 403; Ludwig: "Zauber gegen *takman* (Magic against *takmán*)," *Der Rigveda,* 3: 511; Bergaigne-Henry: "Conjuration contre une fièvre maligne," *Manuel,* 136; cf. also Henry, *La magie,* 182–86; Griffith: "The hymn is a charm against fever," *Hymns of the Atharvaveda,* 1: 29; Bloomfield: "Charm against *takman* (fever)," *Hymns,* 3, 270; Whitney-Lanman: "Against fever (*takmán*)," *Atharva-veda-saṃhitā,* Pt. 1, 25; Müller translates it in his discussion of *takmán,* "Der *Takman* des *Atharvaveda,*" *Artibus Asiae,* 6 (1937): 230–36; and Filliozat renders it under his examination of "Les fièvres," *La doctrine,* 96–97.

[60] *aikāhikādiśītajvarasaṃtatajvaravelājvarādiśāntaye;* cf. Keśava: *atha jvarabhaiṣajyam ucyate,* including, *nityajvare velājvare satatajvare ekāntaritajvare cāturthikajvare ca ṛtujvare ca.*

the waters, i.e. the water-containing clouds, and scorched them. This also implies that the rainy season is the most likely time when *takmán* manifested itself in the form of fever (403–404, see also Griffith, 29–30 note; Bloomfield, 270–71; and Filliozat, who likewise understands it to be *takmán*'s birthplace, *La doctrine,* 96). This agrees with our present-day understanding of the time when the *anopheles* mosquito breeds most abundantly. On the reading of *ā́po* as accusative plural, see Whitney, *Grammar,* #393a and Bloomfield (272) (Sāyaṇa also glosses as *apaḥ*).

VERSE 2

In *ab,* P 1.32.3 (K: 1.32.2) has the clearer reading . . . *yadi vāsi dhūmaḥ śākalyeṣu yadi vā te janitram,* ". . . , or whether you are smoke, or whether your birthplace is among the wood shavings" (cf. Renou, JA, 252: 432). On the basis of this, one could posit that *śākalyeṣú* may be the correct reading for the obscure *śakalyeṣí* (*pada*-text: *śakalya-eṣí*), 'desirous of wood chips' (on possible interpretations of this word, see Weber, 419; Bloomfield, 272, and Whitney-Lanman, 26). In *c,* P reads *huḍur* 'ram' for the problematic *hrū́ḍur;* and in *d,* as verse 1 above. Sāyaṇa reads *rū́ḍhur* which he says is from the root *ruh,* 'to ascend,' i.e. being born of a seed and becoming visible; and it means ascending, i.e. productive in the human body (. . . *rūḍhuḥ rohakaḥ puruṣaśarīre utpādakaḥ. ruha bījajanmani prādurbhāve* [*ca*]). Weber renders it 'cramp' (Krampf) (419–20). Henry has tried to demonstrate its connection with the proto-word **harūdu* which is based on the Assyrian *huraśu* and the Hebrew *harūś,* signifying 'gold.' On the other hand, he suggests that it may be a mysterious or esoteric word which was intelligible only to the initiated and which was the name of a supernatural being who " 'dore' les hommes et à qui l'on attribue en même temps le titre honorifique de 'Dieu du jaune' " (JA, 10: 514; see also *La magie,* 185). R. Müller, whose interpretation is based on that proposed by J. Hertel, offers the translation: 'running' (laufen) or 'flying' (fliegen), presumably from the obscure root *hrūd,* 'to go' ("Der *Takman* des *Atharvaveda,*" 231). For a summary of these and other views, see Mayrhofer, Wb, 3: 617. For want of an exact determination of the word's meaning, it remains in doubt. One may, however, speculate that it could be onomatopoeic. If, in the first verse, the *takmán* was considered to be derived from the lightning, *hrū́ḍur* (or perhaps better, Sāyaṇa's reading, testified in several manuscripts, *rū́ḍhur*) may faintly resemble the sound of the rumblings of thunder which accompanies the lightning. Since the word occurs only in this and the next verse, corroborative evidence is wanting. It is clear that it is a name of *takmán* and that by knowing it and reciting it the healer intends to be able to control the disease.

VERSE 3

In *a,* P 1.32.2 (K: 1.32.3) has . . . *yady abhīśoko* (K: *atīśoko;* K manuscript: *adīśoko;* Bar. *atiśoko,* 'burn excessively'); and in *b: rudrasya prāṇo yadi vāruṇo 'si,* "whether you are Rudra's breath [or] the descendant of Varuṇa" (cf. Renou, JA, 252: 431). Whitney-Lanman propose a slightly different reading: *rudrasya prāṇo yadi vā 'ruṇo 'si,* "whether, you, the golden one, are the breath of Rudra" (26). In light of the Śau. text, *vāruṇo 'si* is more correct, being the equivalent of *váruṇasyā̃si putráḥ* (cf. Renou, JA, 252: 341–42). The breath of Rudra points to the strong winds associated with the thundery storms often connected with the rains. In *d,* P reads as verse 1. Sāyaṇa understands that this verse refers to the cold fever (*śītajvara*) and its origin.

VERSE 4

In *b,* P 1.32.4 reads: *namo rūrāyo kṛṇmo vayaṃ te,* "We make obeisance to that deliriously hot [*takman*]," and in *cd,* . . . *ubhayedyuś caranti* [=*carati*(?), K manuscript: *cahatas,* Bar. *cāgatas* or *cāyatas;* Raghu Vira: *cāgatas*] *tṛtīyakāya* . . . (cf. Renou, JA, 252: 432). As to the kinds of fever, Sāyaṇa, stating that the forms *anyedyúr* and *ubhayadyúr* are irregular, explains that they refer to the fever occurring daily (quotidian) and to [that] recurring every other day, respectively, and that *tṛ́tīyakāya,* being a synecdoche for those appearing every fourth day, etc., signifies the fever recurring every third day (tertian) (. . . *anyedyuḥ ubhayedyuḥ iti śabdau nipātitau. . . . tasmai aikāhikāya dvyāhikāya ca jvarāya . . . tṛtīyadivase āgacchate tryāhikāya jvarāya. cāturthikādīnām api upalakṣaṇam etat*). Filliozat follows this interpretation and presents further support for it from the classical medical texts (*La doctrine,* 97 and note; see also *Magie et médecine,* 101). On the rendering of *rūrā̃ya,* see Mayrhofer, Wb, 3: 71, and Bloomfield, 4. The technique of paying homage to the demon in order to win it over is found in this verse.

Notes to 5.22

Translators agree that AVŚ 5.22 is a charm against the disease-demon, *takmán,*[61] which, Grohmann has suggested, has reached epidemic proportions.[62] The introduction prescribes its use "in a rite for the cure of fever"[63] at KauśS 29.18–19. AthPariś 34.7 counts it as among the list of charms devoted to the destruction of *takmán* (*takmanāśanagaṇa*).

VERSE 1

In *a,* P 13.1.1 reads as Śau; in *b: marutaḥ pūtadakṣāḥ;* in *c,* K: *saṃśiśānā* (O as Śau); and in *d: apa rakṣāṅsy amuyā dhamantu,* "Thus let [them] blow

[61] Ludwig: "Takmanāśanam," *Der Rigveda,* 3: 510; Grill translates it under his section: "Krankheit," *Hundert Lieder des Atharva-Veda,* 12, 154; Griffith: "The hymn is a charm against fever," *Hymns of the Atharvaveda,* 1: 224; Bloomfield: "Charm against *takman* (fever) and related diseases," *Hymns,* 1, 441; Weber: "Gegen des Fieber (Against the fever)," IS, 18: 252; Whitney-Lanman: "Against fever (*takmán*)," *Atharva-veda-saṃhitā,* Pt. 1, 259, cf. also Henry: "La Fièvre," *La magie,* 186.

[62] "Medicinisches aus den Atharva-Veda, mit besonderem Bezug auf den Takman," IS, 9: 412–13; see also Grill, 155.

[63] *jvarabhaiṣajyakarmaṇi;* cf. Keśava: *atha jvarabhaiṣajyam ucyate.*

away the *rakṣas*-demons." On the reading of *marutaḥ* for *varuṇaḥ*, cf. AVŚ 1.25.3 n, where P 1.32.3 reads Rudra in place of Varuṇa. *pūtádakṣāḥ* is difficult; Weber (252) and Whitney-Lanman (259) render it quite literally: "of pure (purified) power (dexterity)"; Henry more liberally: "dont pure est l'habileté liturgique" (*La magie*, 186). Bloomfield presents perhaps the clearest sense: "of tried skill" (1, and 444). Our translation is based on Bloomfield and P. In *d*, *amuyā̄* is understood, with most translators, to imply disgust or contempt (see in particular, Grill, 155; Bloomfield, 444 and Whitney-Lanman, 259).

VERSE 2

In *ab*, P 19.12.12 reads: *janān*, 'people,' for *víśān;* and *kṛṇoty*, for *kṛṇóṣi*. Based on the P reading *janān*, *víśvān* may be understood as 'everybody.' *kṛṇoty* would be preferred in *a*. It does not, however, fit well with the verbs in the second person in *cd*. In *a*, *ayám yó*, literally, 'he who,' has been rendered simply as 'who,' a relative pronoun referring to the subject, *takmann*, in *c*. In *b*, *abhidunván*, 'scorching,' has been taken to modify *agnír*. Weber (252) and Whitney-Lanman (259), conceive it to refer to *takmán*. This also is acceptable. Note the notion of yellowness associated with *takmán* and that of sending the *takmán* downward.

VERSE 3

In *a*, P(K) 13.1.4 has the clearer *pārśvayaḥ*, 'about the flanks'; P(O) reads as Śau. On the meaning of *paruṣáḥ pāruṣeyò*, see Hoffmann, *Aufsätze*, 1: 334, n. 16. In *a*, the implied herb may be *kúṣṭha* (see AVŚ 19.39.10; cf. also Grill, 155, and Bloomfield, 1, 445). *avadhvaṃsá* is obscure. It is derived from the root *dhvaṃs*, plus *ava*, 'to sprinkle,' and suggests a sprinkling of something. Mayrhofer has pointed to a possible, although later, meaning of the word, i.e. 'red sandalwood' (Wb, 1: 57). Since the first line appears to be describing the redness and soreness of joints which accompany a fever (see Müller, "Der *Takman* des *Atharvaveda*," 236–67, and cf. Grohmann, 394), the idea of red dust, resembling the sawdust or chips from red sandalwood, seems to be implied.

VERSE 4

P(O) 13.1.5 reads as Śau. In *b*, P(K) has: *namaḥ kṛtvāya* and in *d: gaccha*. *cd* also occurs at P 5.21.8*cd*. In *c*, *śakambharásya* is difficult. Literally, it means 'of the dung-bearer' and may be the proper name of a demon who personifies abnormal evacuation (see, in particular, Grill, 156; Griffith, 224, and note, and Bloomfield, 1, 445–46). Weber suggests that it may be a mocking name of a people who used dung, but favors rather the notion that it could refer to the city later known as Śākambharī, located in Jaipur state (253–54; see also Law, *Hist. Geog. of Ancient India*, 329). Whitney-Lanman posit that it may refer to the Mahāvṛṣas, "a neighbouring tribe, looked down upon as gatherers of dung for fuel, on account of the lack of wood in their territory" (259). An exact understanding of the word, therefore, is wanting. *mahāvṛṣā̃n* is generally considered to be the name of a tribe whose exact location is debated (see Bloomfield, 446, and Macdonell-Keith, *Vedic Index*, 2: 142–43; cf. Filliozat, who suggests that they may have belonged to the lower Panjab, *La doctrine*, 99).

VERSE 5

For *cd*, P 13.1.7 reads: *yāj* [K: *mahān* (manuscript: *mayā*)] *jātas takman tād* (K: *tad*) *asi bahlikeṣu nyocaraḥ*, "From that which you are born, O *takman*, among the Bahlikas you must reside." The word *nyocaráḥ* is obscure. It is believed to be derived from *ny-ava-cará*, meaning 'belonging to, fit for a place' (see Weber, 254, and Mayrhofer, Wb, 2: 182). With *asi*, it could mean: 'you must reside. . . . The tribal names are as follows: *mū̃javant*, being derived from the name for a mountain, *muñjavant*, may have been the name of a people living in the Himālayas of northern India (see Filliozat, *La doctrine*, 99; cf. Macdonell-Keith, *Vedic Index*, 2, 169–70). *bálhika* (or *báhlika*) is probably the name of a tribe of Bactrians (see Whitney-Lanman, 260, and Filliozat, *La doctrine*, 99).

VERSE 6

P 13.1.8 is as Śau. For the difficult words *vyā̃la*, *ví gada* and *vyàṅga*, see Bloomfield's excellent explanation (447–48) and for *vyā̃la*, see in particular, Mayrhofer, Wb, 3: 270, 796. *ví gada*, according to the *pada*-text, is to be understood as a verb; although it could be a vocative: *vígada* (see Whitney-Lanman, 260). We have rendered it as a verb from the root *gad* plus *vi* 'to speak away,' in the sense of 'not to speak' or 'to keep quiet, silent,' referring to the plea for the demon's thundery noise to stop. *vyàṅga* may be derived from *aṅga* plu *vi*, 'limbless,' 'deformed,' or from the root *añj* plus *vi*, 'to manifest.' Both meanings are rare. The meaning 'deformed' however occurs at AVŚ 7.56(58).4, a healing charm against poisonous snakes. It would be likely, therefore, that it could also fit here, suggesting perhaps, the distorted appearance of a lightning bolt. *yāvaya* is taken to be a causative from the root *yu*, 'to separate,' 'to keep away,' again referring to the plea for the demon's stormy aspects to keep away. The word *niṣṭákvarīm*, 'escaping,' appears to be a play on the word *takmán* (see Whitney-Lanman, 260) and, therefore, may be derived from the root *tak* plus *nis*, 'to run away.' The verse, therefore, appears to be a reference to the lightning (cf. *vájreṇa*, in *d*, and *hetáyas*, in verse 10*c*) and thunder (see next note), which are the obvious manifestations of the beginning of the rains and the rainy season, a time when *takmán* is born (see Grohmann, IS, 9: 404; Bloomfield, 443; cf. AVŚ 1.25.5 n and verse 13 below).

VERSE 7

If we may continue this interpretation, a tentative P 13.1.9 may lend to its support: *giriṃ gaccha girijā asi rautena māyuṣo* [=*mā* – *āyuṣo*?] (O: *girau te mahiṣo) gṛhaḥ dāsīm anv* (O omits) *iccha prapharvyaṃ* (O: *praharvantām*) *tām takman vīva* (K: *nīva*) *dhūnuhi,* "O *takman,* go to the mountains, [for] you are born of the mountain. In the mountain is your radiant power [or, less likely: Do not take away life by (your) resoundings (? *rautena* from root *ru,* 'to roar')]. Seek out the lustful, young slave girl [and] shake her a bit." Here the mountains are stated as being the place where the *takmán* is born and where he must return. Frequently, over mountains one notices thunderclouds forming. Likewise, there is implied an association between the mountain and *mūjavant* (*muñjavant*), the mountain people among whom *takmán*'s home is found (see verse 5). The notion of the resoundings could point to the sound of thunder which would startle and frighten someone young and unsuspecting. On the word *prapharyám,* 'young-lustful,' see Mayrhofer, Wb, 2: 365–66; 3: 763; cf. also Weber, 255.

VERSE 8

In *b* P(O) 13.1.6 has: *oka edhi* (K is corrupted). *cd* is found unaltered at P 13.1.6 *cd* and 13 *cd* (O has *vratāni*? in *c*). Most translators understand *bándhv* to mean 'kinsmen' (see in particular Grohmann, 412; Griffith, 225; Bloomfield, 448–49, and Weber, 255; cf. also Grill, 'young people,' 12, 157). On the basis of P 5.21.2 (not 5.5.1–2!), which states that a portion of a field was transferred to *takmán* in the first half of the earth (*takmann imaṃ te kṣetrabhāgam apabhajan pṛthivyāḥ pūrve ardhe, . . .*), Whitney-Lanman understand *bándhv* to refer to those fields or territories which are connected with *takmán* and render: "thy connection" (260). Although both interpretations could be correct, it appears that, because of the opposition between 'your field (connection)' and 'the others' fields' (*anyakṣetrā̃ṇi* in *d* and *anyakṣetré* in verse 9*a*), Whitney-Lanman's suggestion may have some basis. Since, however, *takmán*'s home is among the *mūjavants* and *mahā-vṛṣás* (verse 5), one naturally assumes that they would be his kinsmen, whose point of identity with *takmán* is with their land or territory from which the rains and *takmán* were considered to have originated. An idea similar to that found in these verses and the previous one occurs at P 5.21.3: *takman parvatā ime himavantas somapṛṣṭhāḥ, vātajūtaṃ bhiṣajaṃ (=bheṣajam?) no akran naśyeto maraṭān abhi,* "O *takman,,* disappear from here [and go] in the direction of the *maraṭas* (?); [for] these Himavant mountains, which bear Soma on their backs, have made for us the wind-driven physician (i.e. medicine)." *ab,* here, suggests the mountain-born *kúṣṭha*-plant which was transported from heaven by a golden sailing ship (i.e. the moon), presumably conceived to be propelled by wind (see AVŚ 5.4.4,5 and 6.95.2). *maraṭa* is perhaps the name of a tribe.

VERSE 9

In *ab,* P 5.21.7 and 13.1.14 have: . . . *na ramate sahasrākṣo 'martyaḥ,* "[If] the thousand-eyed immortal is not satisfied . . ."; P 5.21.7*cd* has *takman sa no mṛlayiṣyati.* P 13.1.3*b* reads as Śau. *b,* but has in *a: takman sārthinaṃ icchasva,* "You, O *takman,* seek out the one attached to the caravan (i.e. the caravan-leader)." On *sārthinam*, cf. *prā̄rthas* in Śau. *c.* The exact meaning of *prā̄rthas* is uncertain. It appears to be derived from *pra-ártha*, 'one having a purpose before him,' in the sense of being eager and prepared for it, i.e. anxious (cf. in particular Whitney-Lanman, 260, and Mayrhofer, Wb, 2: 353). T. Chowdhury, however, suggests that it is a corruption of *prā̄rthya*, 'amendable to supplication' (JBORS, 17: 86–87); in which case, we may render: "[Since] *takmán* has become amendable to supplication (i.e. has understood our request)." This interpretation also fits the context; but, since P 5.21.7 also reads *prārthas*, his suggestion that it is a corruption seems less likely. For a slightly different explanation of this verse, see Bloomfield, 449.

VERSE 10

In *a*, P 13.1.10 has *yas; in d, sa pari*; and in *b*, O has *vā nāśāvīvīyaḥ*. P 5.21.6 presents an interesting variant which may express the idea of this verse more clearly: *yaḥ sākam utpādayasi balāsaṃ kāsam anvṛjam, bhīmās te takman hetayas tābhiḥ sa* (O: *sma*) *pari vṛndhi naḥ*, "[Since] you produce simultaneously *balāsa*, cough [and] *anvṛja*, [therefore,] O *takman*, (always) pass over us with those your dreaded missiles." For *ab*, cf. verse 11, below. For *anvṛjam* Barret suggests *anvṛjum*, 'tending in a straight direction towards' (JAOS, 87: 284) referring perhaps to the thunderbolt-like missiles; and Raghu Vira reads: *anv ṛjum* (?). Both readings are unclear. It is important to note that the missiles (*hetáyas*), which draw us back to the notion of thunderbolts (*vájra*) in verse 6, were thought to be *balā̄sa*, cough and *anvṛja*; while in the Śau., they are shivers and cough. Cough, therefore, is common to both texts and its sound may be sympathetic, resembling that of thunder.

VERSE 11

For *ab*, cf. P 5.21.6 *ab* note 10 above. P 13.1.15 reads quite differently: *ado gaccha mūjavatas tato vā gaḥ parastarām, mā smāto 'bhy ṛṇoḥ punaḥ pra tvā* (O: *abhy nir naḥ punaḥ tat tvā*) *takmann upa bruve*, "I conjure you, O *takman*, go to that place of the Mūjavants; indeed, from there, go further on [and] do not ever leave that place again (or: "do not come to us again from there"; cf. Śau)." This verse resembles Śau. 6, 7 above. In *b*, *udyugā́m* is the only occurrence of the word and may have a meaning similar to that of *udyogá*, 'strenuous and continuous activity'; or, it may mean 'adjoining' and if used to modify *kāsám*, 'cough,' signifies "adjoining cough," i.e. "hiccough," (see Bloomfield, 450, and Whitney-Lanman, 261) or better, "accompanying cough." Weber, however, has suggested a possible explanation that may be more reasonable. He understands *udyugá* to be derived from *ud*, 'free from,' 'without' and *yuga*, i.e. 'unrest,' 'restlessness' (256). More to the point, *yuga*, like *yoga*, could have the sense of 'bodily control'; in which case, *udyugá* would mean 'loss of bodily control,' i.e. the uncontrollable trembling or shaking which often accompanies high fever. P 5.21.6 has *anvṛjam* (*anvṛjum*) which is equally obscure (see verse 10, above).

VERSE 12

ab occurs unchanged at P 13.1.11 which reads *cd: pāmnā bhrātṛvyeṇa naśyeto maraṭān abhi,* "[You, O *takman,*] accompanied with your evil cousin *pāman,* disappear from here [and go] in the direction of those *maraṭas* (?)." Cf. P 5.21.3 (note 8, above) which is a variant of 13.1.11. In *c,* Roth-Whitney read *pāmnā̄* which seems to mean 'with a rash,' 'with mange,' etc. (see, in particular, Filliozat, who considers it not to be a proper medical term, *La doctrine,* 44, 97, and Mayrhofer, Wb, 2: 255–56). The Viśveśvar-ānanda edition, however, has *pāpmā̄,* 'with evil' which, if we consider the parallelism of afflictions between verses 11 and 12, may be equivalent to *udyugá.* It would not be too difficult to understand that uncontrolled shaking or trembling (*udyugá*) was considered to be an evil or misfortune. As we have seen, however, P supports the reading *pāmnā̄* which tends to invalidate such an equation. On the strength of the textual similarity with the P, therefore, the more correct reading seems to be *pāmnā̄.*

VERSE 13

A parallel to this verse occurs at P 1.32.5: *tṛtīyakaṃ vitṛtīyaṃ sadandim uta hāyanam, takmānaṃ viśvaśāradaṃ graiṣmaṃ nāśaya vārṣikam,* "Destroy, [O plant, (perhaps *kúṣṭha,* see verse 3 above)], the *takman* who recurs every third day (tertian), who has the third day free (quartan), who is continual and who lasts the entire year, who recurs every autumn, who arises in the summer [and] in the rainy season" (cf. Renou, JA, 252: 432). There is some controversy surrounding the exact meaning of *vitṛtīyáṃ:* it could signify both the quotidian and the tertian fevers (cf. Filliozat, *La doctrine,* 97, and note; see also Macdonell-Keith, *Vedic Index,* 1: 295); or better, it seems to imply the quartan fever: with the third day free, it should recur on the fourth day.

VERSE 14

In *b,* P 13.1.12 has: *kāśibhyo,* 'to the *kāśis,*' for *áṅgebhyo;* and in *cd: jane* (K: *dhāne;* K manuscript *jāne*) *priyam iva śevadhiṃ takmānaṃ pari dadhmasi,* which may be rendered as follows: "We place the *takman* among the [other] people [or (less likely): in a receptacle] just as if he were a dear treasure." The P reading *kāśibhyo* for *áṅgebhyo* is interesting. Since Aṅga is the region further east of Kāśi (Vārāṇasī, Banaras) and thus further removed from the center of Āryan culture in later Vedic times, there is the suggestion that *kāśibhyo* is the older reading. The exact meaning of Śau. *cd* is not at all clear. Most translators prefer to render *praiṣyán jánam iva śevadhíṃ* as two separate elements: "like a person about to be sent (i.e. a servant, messenger, etc.) [and] like a treasure . . ." (see, in particular, Grill, 13, 158; Grohmann, 412, Weber, 257; Bloomfield, 2, 452, and Henry, *La magie,* 136). Whitney-Lanman, however, translate it as one unit: "like one sending a person to a treasure, . . . ," which implies the emendation of *praiṣyán* to *préṣyan*

(261). Although any interpretation of this line is tentative, it might be possible to read *praiṣyáṃ* as an accusative and render *cd:* ". . . we entrust the *takmán,* as [we entrust with the riches] the man about to be sent to the treasury." The simile, however, is not completely intelligible. The *gandhā́ris* are considered to be people from modern-day Peshawar district in Pakistan; the *áṅgas,* people from present-day North Bengal or Eastern Bihar; and the *magádhas* are people from Bihar (see Filliozat, *La doctrine,* 99, and Macdonell-Keith, *Vedic Index,* 1: 219, 11, and 2: 116–18, respectively).

Notes to 6.20

Translators agree that AVŚ 6.20 is a charm against the disease-demon *takmán.*[64] Sāyaṇa prescribes it for use in a rite to heal bile-fever[65] at KauśS 30.7. It also occurs in the list of hymns for the destruction of *takmán* (*takmanāśanagaṇa*) at AthPariś 34.7.

VERSE 1

P 19.12.10, combining elements of this verse and verse 3 reads: *agnir* (manuscript 'P': *agner*) *iva prasargo 'sya* (manuscript 'P' obscure) *śuṣmiṇa uteva matto vilapann apāyati, tasmai te aruṇāya babhrave tapur maghāya namo 'stu takmane,* "May the discharge, as it were a fire, of this flash (or better: ". . . discharge of this flash, as it were of fire . . .") go away; likewise, [may the discharge] as it were a chattering drunkard, [go away]. Obeisance to *takman,* to that your red [and] brown [color] [and], O glowing one, [your] bounty." Sāyaṇa, based on KauśS 30.7, considers the comparison in *a* as between a forest-fire, which burns both the fresh and dry vegetation and the fever which enters and burns every limb and is provided with a drying force (=*śuṣmíṇa*) (*ārdram anārdraṃ ca sarvaṃ . . . dāvātmakasya . . . kṛtsnam aṅgaṃ dahataḥ śuṣmiṇaḥ śoṣakabalayuktasya . . . jvarasya dāhaḥ . . . kṛtsnam aṅgaṃ vyāpnoti*). In *a,* Florenz translates *śuṣmíṇa* as 'glowing' (glühet) and states that it is a play on the increased blood temperature, giving rise to fever, and that *tápurvadhāya* ('glowing weapon') in *d* extends this pun (275, 76). Whitney-Lanman, on the other hand, suggest the emendation of *śuṣmíṇa* to *śúṣmas* ('vehemence?'), making it the subject of *eti* (295). Rather, the meaning of *śuṣmín* is, as Bloomfield has shown, 'lightning' or 'flashing' (469). Thus, the reading may remain without emendation and points to lightning as the origin of, and the agent for *takmán.* The P also confirms this. In *b, mattó* seems to have the meaning 'drunkard' (from root *mad*) as

---

[64] Grohmann renders the hymn in his discussion of "Medicinisches aus dem Atharva-Veda mit besonderem Bezug auf den Takman," IS, 9: 384–85; Ludwig: "Zauber gegen *takman* (Magical charm against *takman*)," *Der Rigveda,* 3: 511; Zimmer translates the charm under his discussion of *takmán, Leben,* 380; Florenz: "Gegen Fieber (Against fever)," "Das sechste Buch der Atharva-saṃhitā," BB, 12: 273; Griffith: "A charm against fever," *Hymns of the Atharvaveda,* 1: 255; Bloomfield: "Charm against *takman,*" *Hymns of the Atharva-Veda,* 3, 468; and Whitney-Lanman: "Against fever (*takmán*)," *Atharva-veda-saṃhitā,* Pt. 1, 295.

[65] *pittajvarabhaiṣajye;* cf. Keśava: *pittajvarabhaiṣajyam ucyate.*

suggested by Sāyaṇa: "forgetting himself as if intoxicated (or, insane)" (*unmatta iva ātmānaṃ vismṛtya*). Whitney-Lanman, however, suggest the meaning 'from me,' i.e. a quasi-ablative of the pronoun *ma* (295). This explanation would appear to be less likely. In *c*, the emendation of *avratás* to *avratám*, referring to the victim who is always void of virtuous conduct, suggested by Sāyaṇa (*avrataḥ avratam* [*vibhaktivyatyayaḥ*] *sadācārahīnaṃ puruṣam*) and followed by Ludwig (511) and Florenz (276) is, as Bloomfield has demonstrated, not warranted (469). On the meaning of *avratás*, see AVŚ 7.116(121).2 note, 149–50. The entire verse, as supported by the P, seems to be a reference to the association between *takmán* and the lightning and thunder of a rainstorm. The first line, containing two similes, alludes to the origin and to the departure of *takmán*: the lightning flashes and burning arise as it were from Agni (fire) (cf. AVŚ 1.25.1) and the rumbling of the fading thunder resembles the gibberish of a drunkard (cf. AVŚ 5.22.6,7). There is also a suggestion of a sympathetic connection between the babbling of a drunkard and the delirious ravings of a fever-victim. Likewise, in line two, the notion of seeking out another victim and the fiery weapon, i.e. the thunderbolt, point to *takmán*'s connection with lightning (see AVŚ 5.22.6–9, 12).

VERSE 2

In *a*, P 19.12.11 reads: *namo yamāya namo 'stu mṛtyave*, "Let there be obeisance to Yama, to death," and in *cd*: *namaḥ kṣetrasya pataye namo dive namo pṛthivyai namo oṣadhībhyaḥ*, "Obeisance to the lord of the field, to heaven, to earth [and] to the herbs." Note that in *a*, respect is paid to the most dreaded result of *takmán* rather than to *takmán*. In *cd* of both P and Śau, the concern is with venerating the means of bringing about the patient's recovery. Following Sāyaṇa, *tvíṣīmate* in *b* seems to have the sense: 'bright' or 'splendid' (*dīptimate*). Zimmer (380) and Florenz (273) follow Grohmann who renders it as 'impetuous' (385). Both meanings are correct. 'Splendid,' however, seems to fit better in a general attitude of reverence. Rudra, states Sāyaṇa, is the god laying claim to fever (. . . *jvarābhimānī devaḥ*). He goes on to say that there is obeisance to heaven and to earth because they are the mother and father of all living beings and that obeisance to the earth-born grains of rice, etc. (=*óṣadhi*) means that he gains health by worship of the medicinal herb and by a wholesome diet (*dyāvāpṛthivyau hi kṛtsnasya bhūtajātasya mātāpitarau tasmāt tayor namaskāraḥ kṛtaḥ. oṣadhībhyaḥ pṛthivyām utpannābhyo vrīhyādibhyo namo 'stu. auṣadhasevayā pathyakrameṇa ca ārogyam upajāyata ity oṣadhīnāṃ namaskāraḥ*). It is important to notice that in the mind of the poet-healer, *takmán* was a divinity, equal to Rudra and Varuṇa and Yama (in P).

VERSE 3

P 13.1.2 *ab* reads as Śau. *ab*, except *rūro* (O: *ruro*), 'deliriously hot,' replaces *yó*; and in *b*, O has the better reading *kṛṇoti* for *kṛṇoṣi*, which has been adopted as correct in our rendering. P *cd* is the same as P 19.12.10 *cd* (see verse 1 above). In *a*, Sāyaṇa, deriving *abhiśocayiṣṇúr* from the causative of the root *śuc*, 'causing to flame,' plus the prefix *abhi*, 'everywhere, in every limb,' and the suffix *snu* (see Whitney, *Grammar*, #1994c), glosses it as 'burning, i.e. causing heat in all limbs' (*abhitaḥ sarvataḥ kṛtsnam aṅgaṃ sarveṣu aṅgeṣu śocayan śokam utpādayan. śuc śoke . . .*). The prefix *abhi*, when attached to verbs and to their derivatives, can also signify 'to' or 'toward'; in which case, it could refer to the one 'causing flames (to go) toward,' i.e. 'the flame-thrower,' which again suggests a lightning bolt. *pāda b* he explains: "such a bile-fever makes all things completely yellow, i.e. turmeric-colored by means of contaminating the blood" (*īdṛśo . . . pittajvaraḥ . . . viśvāni sarvāṇi . . . haritāni raktadūṣaṇena haridrāvarṇāni . . . karoti*); and in *d*, he glosses *ványāya* as 'to be frequented' (*saṃsevyāya*). It appears, however, to be derived from *vána*, 'forest.' Grohmann offers the translation, 'wild,' yet suggests 'water-born,' presumably thinking of *vána* in the sense of water (385; on *vána* as water, see Turner, IAL, 658, #11277 and 11278). In light of the similarity in form between *ványa* and *grāmyá*, 'tame (of animals),' Grohmann's first interpretation is feasible. Bloomfield, however, proposes that it signifies 'that derived from the forest,' 'forest-born,' understanding wrongly, that it refers to the malaria "which is caused by the decay of the tropically prolific flora" (470). Although his explanation is in error, Bloomfield's translation of the word is possible. Because of its similarity in meaning to *avratás*, 'unruly,' in verse 1, *ványa* might well be rendered as 'wild.' There is implied a color-sympathy between the yellow (jaundice; cf. AVŚ 1.25.2,3; 5.22.2), red and brown color of the fever-victim and the color of the lightning-bolt.

Notes to 7.116 (121)

Translators agree that AVŚ 7.116 (121) is a charm against *takmán* (fever).[66] Sāyaṇa prescribes its ritualistic use "for the purpose of healing all fevers"[67] at KauśS 32.17. At AthPariś 34.7 it is listed as one of the *takmanāśanagaṇa* (charms for the destruction of *takmán*).

VERSE 1

This verse has no parallels in the P. The word *cyávanāya* is an adjective from the root *cyu*, 'to shake' which, as Sāyaṇa points out, may be understood as a verbal noun with a causative sense, i.e., the one causing to shake, (*cyāvayitre . . .*). For *códanāya*, Sāyaṇa and the Viśveśvarānanda edition

[66] Grohmann has translated these two verses in his article "Medicinisches aus dem Atharva-Veda mit besonderem Bezug auf den Takman," IS, 9: 386 and 414 respectively; Zimmer has rendered the charm in his discussion of *takmán*, "Fieber (fever)," *Leben*, 381; Henry: "Contre la fièvre intermittante," *Le livre* VII, 45, 124; Griffith: "A charm against fever," *Hymns of the Atharvaveda*, 1: 384; Bloomfield: "Charm against *takṃan* (fever)," *Hymns*, 4, 565; Whitney-Lanman: "Against intermittent fever," *Atharva-veda-saṃhitā*, Pt. 1: 469; and Filliozat: "Contre la fièvre," *Magie et médecine*, 100–101.

[67] *sarvajvarabhaiṣajyārthaṃ*; cf. Keśava who appears to have also included AVŚ 7.117 (122): *atha jvarabhaiṣajyam ucyate. namo rūrāyeti sūktadvayena.*

read: *nódanāya*. Sāyaṇa glosses it again as a verbal noun with a causative sense: "to the one sending [things] here and there, to the scatterer" (*itastataḥ prerakāya vikṣepayitre*). The vast majority of manuscripts and the Roth-Whitney edition, however, read *códanāya*, and that has been adopted here. In either case, the meaning is essentially the same: it refers to chills produced both from the fever and from the startling effects of thunder (i.e. *takmán* as thunder and lightning). For the difficult compound *pūrvakāmakṛ́tvane*, '[to the *takmán*] who brings about the previous desire [for rain],' Sāyaṇa, deriving the last member, *kṛtvane* from the root *kṛt*, 'to cut,' understands it to mean: 'to the dispeller, i.e. to the one who cuts off previous desires' (*pūrveṣām abhilāṣāṇāṃ kartitre chettre* . . .). Grohmann renders: "der nach altem Triebe thätig ist," and explains: ". . . ich es auf die regelmässige Wiederkehr des Fieberparoxismus beziehe, die im zweiten Verse näher geschildert wird, und wobei der Takman nach einem räthselhaften Naturtriebe zu handeln schien" (386 and n). This interpretation is followed by Zimmer (381), and the translation would be most appealing; the construing of *kā̆ma* as "Trieb" (impulse), however, forces its primary meaning, 'desire,' 'love.' Henry has suggested that the compound could be broken as *pūrva-kāmakṛ́tvan*, i.e. "qui, de temps immémorial, agit à sa guise" (45, 125). Bloomfield, on the basis of ṚV 10.61.6 where *kā̆ma* is found with the root *kṛ* and has overtones of sexual love, hints that *takmán* may be "due to (excessive) sexual intercourse." "This," he says, "finds support in *Suśruta* where 'sexual love,' *kāma* is one of the causes of fever" (569; cf. Grohmann who also points this out, 386 n). He opts, however, for a non-committal rendering: " 'he who in the past fulfilled desires,' " stating, "this may refer to excesses, or to willingness" (569). Whitney-Lanman simply claim that the epithet "is extremely obscure and probably corrupt" (420). If our contention that *takmán* is associated with the thunderstorms is correct, the difficulty with the compound may find some resolution: *pūrvakāma* could refer to the rains which, for these people, would certainly be an object of constant desire, especially during the dry season before the rains arrive; and *kṛtvan* (from the root *kṛ*, 'to do') may be regarded as *takmán* who, in the form of thunder and lightning, brings about, or ushers in, the desired rain. We may add an interesting suggestion by Henry who, because of the imperfect meter, posits a reconstruction of the verse in three *pādas* of *jagatī*:

námo rūrā̆ya cyávanāya dhṛṣṇáve
námo rūrā̆ya códanāya dhṛṣṇáve
námaḥ śītā̆ya pūrvakāmakṛ́tvane.

By a haplology, then, these were fused into the present reading (125). It is a clever suggestion; but, as Bloomfield implies, there is no substantial evidence to support it (568).

VERSE 2

This verse also has no parallel in the P. For *anyedyúr*, Sāyaṇa glosses: 'on the other (or, following) day' (*anyasmin divase*); for *ubhayadyúr*, he reads *ubhayedyáḥ* and glosses: 'on both days' (*ubhayor divasayoḥ*). They appear to refer to the intermittent nature of the *takmán,* i.e. the quotidian or daily fever and the tertian or fever which attacks every other day (the third-day-fever; see AVŚ 1.25.4; cf. also Henry, 125, and Filliozat, *Magie et médecine,* 101). Sāyaṇa understands *avratáḥ* to be 'that fever which has a non-fixed time,' where *vrata* expresses an obligation (*vrataśabdo niyamavācī. aniyatakālaḥ sa jvaraḥ . . .*). Since *avratáḥ* has the general sense of unpredictability, his interpretation is probably correct (see AVŚ 6.20.1; cf. also Filliozat's translation: "qui n'observe pas de règle,. . . ," *Magie et médecine,* 101).

Notes to 5.4

Most interpreters agree that AVŚ 5.4 is a charm against the demon *takmán* and other diseases.[68] Bloomfield and Whitney-Lanman suggest rather that it is actually directed to the plant *kúṣṭha.*[69] In the introduction it states that its ritualistic use is "for the purpose of quieting the diseases beginning with *rājayakṣma* (tuberculosis) and *kuṣṭha* (skin-disease)."[70] The hymn is not mentioned in the KauśS. Dārila to KauśS 26.1, however, includes it among the *takmanāśanagaṇa* (so also AthPariś 34.7); and at KauśS 28.13 he notices that it is one of the *kuṣṭhaliṅga* ('verses having the characteristic word *kúṣṭha*'). This *sūtra* is employed against fever (Dārila) or *rājayakṣma* (consumption), headache, skin-disease and pain in all limbs (Keśava).[71] From the context, it would appear that the charm was originally used to consecrate the *kúṣṭha*-plant, the chief medicine against *takmán.*

The allusions in the first three verses point to a connection between *kúṣṭha* and Soma.[72] This reflects the poet-healer's attitude that the medicinal *kúṣṭha* was a divine plant, equal in importance to Soma, the lord of plants.

VERSE 1

For *a,* P 19.8.15 reads: *yo giriṣu jāyase,* '[you] who are born on the mountains.' *kúṣṭha,* in later Indian medicine, has come to mean a class of skin-diseases in which leprosy occurs, as well as a plant. In the *Atharvaveda,*

---

[68] Grohmann renders vss. 1, 3–6, in his article on *takmán,* "Medicinisches aus dem Atharva-Veda mit besonderem Bezug auf den Takman," IS, 9: 421; Grill includes it under his section "Krankheit." *Hundert Lieder des Atharva-Veda,* 9, 141; Griffith: "The hymn is a charm against fever and other ailments," *Hymns of the Atharvaveda,* 1: 193; and Weber: "Gegen den *takman,* resp. *yakṣma* (Against *takmán,* likewise *yákṣma*)," IS, 18: 178.

[69] Bloomfield: "Prayer to the *kuṣṭha*-plant to destroy *takman* (fever)," *Hymns,* 4, 414; Whitney-Lanman: "To the plant *kúṣṭha:* against *takmán* [fever]," *Atharva-veda-saṃhitā,* Pt. 1, 227.

[70] *rājayakṣmakuṣṭhādirogaśāntyartham.*

[71] See, in particular, Bloomfield, *Hymns,* 415, and Whitney-Lanman, Pt. 1, 227.

[72] On the question of *kúṣṭha*'s relationship to Soma see AVŚ 19.39 notes; Hillebrandt, *Vedische Mythologie,* 1: 244–47; and Grohmann, IS, 9: 423.

however, it refers to the plant *Saussurea lappa* Clarke, which grows in Kashmīr between 8,000 and 12,000 feet in elevation.

VERSE 2

In *a,* P(K) 19.8.14 has *suvarṇasavane girau,* "on the mountain which produces gold"; manuscript 'P' as Śau and in *cd:* . . . *śrutaṃ* (?) *yanti kuṣṭhehi takmanāśana* (K manuscript and manuscript 'P': *takmanāśanaḥ*), "they approach [you], who are well known (?), with riches. [Therefore,] O destroyer of *takman,* O *kuṣṭha,* come [here]." It is virtually certain that *himávatas,* 'from the snowy one' refers to the Himālayas. The suggestion in this verse is that the *kúṣṭha*-plant was famous for its healing properties and that it was an item of trade, demanding a very high price.

VERSE 3

This verse occurs unchanged at AVŚ 6.95.1 and at 19.39.6 *a–c* with the variant in *b: tátaḥ kúṣṭho ajāyata,* "from that place *kúṣṭha* was born" (cf. notes to 19.39.6). Variants are also found at P 7.10.6 *ab,* 19.11.1, which read as 19.39.6 *a–c;* and *a–b* occurs at P 20.51.8 (this verse appears to be wanting in manuscript 'P' at 20.55.8), which has, in *cd, tatra lohitavṛkṣo jātaś śrīguruḥ kṣiptabheṣajaḥ,* "There, was born the red-tree, the Śrīguru (?), the medicine for [wounds from] missiles." The number of similar readings suggests that all or part of the verse may be formulaic. Bloomfield uses *pāda b* to suggest a parallelism between Soma and *kúṣṭha* and also points out that at ṚV 10.135.1 there is mention of a tree in which Yama sits and drinks with the gods (416, see also JAOS, 16: 11). Griffith refers to an interesting Samoan belief which states that the natives' most valuable plants were stolen from heaven by a visitor (194 n). The expression "the appearance of immortality" (*amṛ́tasya cákṣaṇam*) is not at all clear. The same phrase occurs in the Āprī-hymn, ṚV 1.13.5, and is explained by Sāyaṇa as "the appearance of ghee which is identical to ambrosia; or else the appearance of the immortal god, Agni" (*amṛtasamānasya ghṛtasya . . . darśanaṃ . . . yadvā . . . maraṇarahitasya devasya . . . agner darśanaṃ . . .*). Geldner understands it to mean: "auf dem die Götterwelt erscheint!" (*Der Rigveda,* 1: 14) and Renou: "là où (est) le moyen-de-voir l'immortel!" explaining *cákṣaṇa* as "domaine de vue = jusqu'où se laisse voir la gent immortelle" (EVP, 14: 40, 111). K. P. Jog, however, has presented evidence for interpreting *amṛ́ta,* along with Sāyaṇa's second suggestion, as Agni (VIJ 8: 38–47). It appears, therefore, to mean the appearance or manifestation of the divine. In the AVŚ, however, it refers *kúṣṭham* in *d* (cf. verse 4) and, thus, suggests the manifestation of the immortal plant *kúṣṭha* which, by its efficacy, is able to restore life or, to be more exact, to ensure immortality. In the poet's mind, the plant was divine, being called, like the gods, immortal (*amṛ́ta*). Cf. Weber (179), Grill (141), Bloomfield (4) and Whitney-Lanman (227), who understand it to be the manifestation or appearance of the drink of immortality, or of something resembling that drink.

VERSE 4

This verse occurs unaltered at AVŚ 6.95.2. *ab* is found unchanged at AVŚ 19.39.7 and P 7.10.7 which read *cd,* however, as 19.36.6 *cd* (see verse 3 above). These occurrences point to the fact that this verse may also be formulaic, used always in conjunction with verse 3. In *c,* Roth and Whitney have *púṣyam,* 'flower,' *púṣpam,* 'flower.' Either reading is acceptable; the meaning remains unchanged (cf. ṚV 1.191.12). Again, *púṣpam* (*púṣyam*) refers to *kúṣṭham.* It is interesting to note that in later Indian medicine, the flower of the *kúṣṭha*-plant is not mentioned as being used for healing (see Dutt and King, *Materia Medica,* 181–82). This leads one to believe that the literal meaning of 'flower' may not be implied. From the variants at AVŚ 19.39.7 and P 7.10.7, it appears to be rather a metaphorical expression for *amṛ́ta,* or for the divine aspect of the plant, and a deliberate specification of its vegetal nature. The golden boat which sailed about in heaven would most certainly suggest the crescent shape of the moon, which is closely associated with Soma.

VERSE 5

For *ab,* P 19.8.13 reads: *hiraṇmayaḥ* (manuscript 'P': *hiraṇyayaḥ*) *panthā āsīd aritrāṇi hiraṇmayā* (manuscript 'P': *hiraṇyayā*), "Golden was the course [and] golden [were] the oars." In *d,* the verb *nir-ā̄-vahan* implies a transporting of the plant from heaven to the mountain (see verse 1 and cf. Grill, 141, and Bloomfield, 417).

VERSE 6

ab are found at P 1.31.1 with the variant in *b: niṣ kṛdhi.* Bh. has *c* (cf. Renou, JA, 252: 431). For *c,* cf. AVŚ 6.95.3 which reads *d: imáṃ me agadáṃ kṛdhi.* Bloomfield notices that this verse, both in meter (*gāyatrī*) and subject matter, is an interruption of the mythological episode concerning *kúṣṭha.* He does not, however, agree with Grill who, because of these reasons, puts the verse at the end of the hymn (10, 142). In fact, he suggests that it may have been purposely placed here in the original composition (417–18). Such an insertion implies an elaboration of verse 5; whereby, the plant is requested to bring the man as the golden boat (i.e. the moon) of verse 5 brought the *kúṣṭha*-plant. This is further supported by the fact that the verbal prefixes *nir, ā,* are found in both verses. Therefore, as the gods, with the aid of the golden boat brought the *kúṣṭha* from heaven to the mountain, so the herb will bring the sick man from somewhere near death to life.

VERSE 7

Because of the last line, one is led to believe that it is perhaps the patient himself who is speaking. P 19.11.2*cd,* however, reads it more clearly: *sa prāṇāyāpānāya cakṣuṣe 'sya mṛḍa,* "[Therefore] be propitious to his faculty of sight, *prāṇa* and *apāna.*" Note that in place of *vyāná,* diffused-breath' which circulates in all the limbs, P has *apāna*, 'the breath away,' or 'the breath which goes down,' and aids in excretion and childbirth. Both, however, read *prāṇá*, 'in-breath,' or 'breath of the front,' which is in the mouth and maintains the functions of breathing and swallowing (see SuNiSth. 1.11ff; and for a good discussion of the breaths see Filliozat, *La doctrine*, 22–23; 141–52). Bloomfield suggests that *cákṣus*, 'eye,' 'faculty of sight,' does not imply an eye-disease, but the eye with which "to see the sun" and the eye which eventually goes to the sun (418; cf. ṚV 10.16.13 and AB 2.6.13). This interpretation is quite possible; however, since the principal concern of the hymn is with healing, it seems more likely that *cákṣuṣe* implies an affliction of the eyes which is suggested in verse 10 and which occurs in later Indian medicine in association with fever (*jvara*) (see Jolly, *Medicin*, 70–74 passim).

VERSE 8

P 1.31.2 reads as Śau. In *cd*, *nā́māny uttamā́ni* means literally, 'highest names,' which implies the best or perhaps choicest and most healthy looking types or species of plants (cf. Bloomfield, 418, and Whitney-Lanman, 228). The notion that the *kúṣṭha*-plant was a definite article of trade seems to be indicated here (cf. Weber, 180). Cf. also AVŚ 4.7.6 where barter for a healing plant appears to be implied. See AVŚ 19.39.2 where the types of *kúṣṭha* are specified.

VERSE 9

In *a*, P 1.31.3 reads as Śau (K omits *kuṣṭha*). In *cd*, P has: *yataḥ kuṣṭha prajāyase tata ehy ariṣṭatātaye*, "So that [he] may be unharmed, O *kuṣṭha*, come [down] to that place where you are born" (cf. Renou, JA, 252: 431). In *c*, note the association with *yákṣma*.

VERSE 10

In *a*, P 1.31.4 has: *śīrṣahatyām*, 'pounding in the head,' and in *cd*: *kuṣṭho no viśvatas pātu daivaṃ samaha vṛṣṇyam*, "Let *kuṣṭha* protect us on all sides; [for he is,] indeed, divinely potent." (Cf. Renou, JA, 252: 431.) In *a*, *śīrṣā-mayám*, literally 'sickness in the head,' on the basis of P, suggests a throbbing in the head which is a common symptom of high fever. Cf. AVŚ 9.8.1–6 where various types of head-disease are mentioned in association with *takmán*. Note the connection with bodily *rápas*, in *b* (see chapter on *rápas*, 25–28).

Notes to 6.95

Translators agree that AVŚ 6.95 is a charm against disease.[73] Although there is no reference to it in the KauśS, Sāyaṇa counts it as among the *kuṣṭhaliṅga* (charms characterized by the word *kúṣṭha*) mentioned at KauśS

---

[73] Griffith: "A charm to remove disease," *Hymns of the Atharva-veda*, 1: 297; and Whitney-Lanman: "For relief from disease: with *kúṣṭha*," *Atharva-veda-saṃhitā*, Pt. 1, 350.

28.13 and thus prescribes its use in a rite "for the purpose of quieting the diseases beginning with *rājayakṣma* and *kuṣṭha* (skin disease)."[74] He also states that at VaitS 28.20, verse 3 is intended for use in the *agnicayana*-ritual.

The first two verses occur at AVŚ 5.4.3, 4 and the final verse bears a similarity to 5.4.6. Because of its close resemblance to 5.4, one may assume that it represents a shorter version of that charm which somehow found its way into the corpus of the AVŚ.

VERSE 1

See AVŚ 5.4.3.

VERSE 2

See AVŚ 5.4.4.

VERSE 3

a occurs at P 2.32.3*a* in reference to a herb (*oṣadhi*) which in *c* is called the brother of Soma (*somasya bhrātāsi*). *a* and *c*, are also found at P 13.2.6*ac* which reads, in *b: vanaspatīnām* for *himávatām uta*, and in *d: so 'gne garbham eha dhāḥ*, "[Thus] may you, O Agni, impregnate the [egg in the] womb here." *pāda-d* also has a close variant at AVŚ 5.4.6: *tám u me agadáṃ kṛdhi*, "make him indeed without poison." Sāyaṇa, as P 13.2.6 and based on VaitS 28.20, understands this verse to be addressed to Agni who, like an embryo, is situated inside these herbs (*he agne tvam oṣadhīnām . . . tāsāṃ . . . garbhavad antar avasthitaḥ . . . bhavasi*). For *himávatām*, he offers an interesting explanation: 'other trees which are cool to the touch' (. . . *śītasparśavatām anyeṣām api vanaspatīnāṃ* . . .). Both explanations by Sāyaṇa suggest that he had in mind a reading similar to that found at P 13.2.6. Whitney-Lanman point out, quite rightly, that the verse, like the entire hymn, is addressed rather to the *kúṣṭha*-plant (351). The readings from P 2.32.3 and AVŚ 5.4.6 seem to corroborate this viewpoint. The embryo of the Himavant could, therefore, refer to the plant's birthplace (see AVŚ 5.4.1, 8).

Notes to 19.39

Most translators consider AVŚ 19.39 to be a charm against the demonic *takmán* with the *kúṣṭha*-plant.[75] Sāyaṇa mentions its use along with 19.38 at AthPariś 4.4 in a rite which involves the fumigation with the *kuṣṭha*-

---

[74] *rājayakṣmakuṣṭhādirogaśāntyartham*.

[75] Grohmann renders a major part of the charm under his discussion of the two medicinal plants, *jaṅgidá* and *kúṣṭha* which are called upon to heal one affected by *takmán*, IS, 9: 420–22; Ludwig translates it under his discussion of "Gebirge (Mountains)," *Der Rigveda*, 3: 198; Bloomfield: "Prayer to the *kuṣṭha*-plant to destroy *takman* (fever), and other ailments," *Hymns*, 5, 676; Griffith: "A protective charm," *Hymns of the Atharvaveda*, 2: 295; and Whitney-Lanman: "With *kúṣṭha*: against disease," *Atharva-veda-saṃhitā*, Pt. 2, 959.

and *gulgulu*-plants for the king's protection.[76] Like other charms in which the *kúṣṭha*-plant is used for healing (i.e. AVŚ 5.4; 6.95), this one has the primary function of consecrating the plant which was used to ward off and destroy the dreaded *takmán*-fever. It is interesting to note that the plant seems to have been employed as a fumigant. Such a use, however, is not expounded in the text.

VERSE 1

In *c*, P 7.10.1 has the easier reading *nāśayan*, 'destroying.' Cf. AVŚ 5.4.1, 2, 8 where *kúṣṭha* is said to come from the Himavant mountains.

VERSE 2

For *bc*, Roth-Whitney emend: *naghamāró naghāriṣó ná ghāyáṃ púruṣo riṣat* which follows P 7.10.2 and which we follow. In *d*, K has *asmai* for *yásmai;* O reads as Sáu; the Viśveśvarānanda edition follows that of Śankar Pandit. P 1.93.2 has a slightly different version of this verse: *jīvalaṃ naghāriṣaṃ jayatkam aparājitam* (K: *jīvalāṃ naghāriṣāṃ jayata kāmaparājitām!*), *taṃ tvāmṛtasyeśānaṃ* (K: *utāmṛtasyeśāno*) *rājan kuṣṭhā vadāmasi*, "We address you, O *kuṣṭha*, O king, that lord of immortality [who is called] perennial, harmless, conquering [and] invincible" (cf. Renou, JA, 253: 32). The three names, in *ab*, Sāyaṇa explains as follows: *nadyamārá* is killing of the diseases produced by the defilement by water, where *nadī* has the intended meaning, water, i.e. that situated in the rivers; or else, it is the killing of the noise being sounded in a way which is difficult to remove, where *nadyā* is the sounding, *nīya* (. . . *nadyamāraḥ iti ekaṃ nāma. nadyāṃ bhavā nadyāḥ. nadīśabdena nadīsthāni udakāni lakṣyante. udakadoṣodbhavā rogā ity arthaḥ. yadvā nadyā nadanīyāḥ śabdanīyāḥ. atyantaduṣpariharatvena śabdyamānā ity arthaḥ. tān mārayatīti nadyamāraḥ*). *nadyā̆riṣaḥ* (Sāyaṇa: *nadyáriṣaḥ*) is the harming of the previously described *nadyas* (*tathā nadyariṣaḥ. ukto nadyaśabdārthaḥ. tān riṣyatīti nadyariṣaḥ. idaṃ dvitīyaṃ nāma*). The third name is *nadya* alone because, being itself a killer of *nadyas*, it is called *nadya* (*kevalo nadya iti tṛtīyaṃ nāma. nadyānāṃ mārakaḥ svayam api nadya ity ucyate*). He goes on to explain the rest of *c:* "With this being understood, he (the poet-healer) says, 'O herb called *kuṣṭha* (=*nádya*), if there is not the taking of your name, then this diseased man would be harmed.' Hence the uttered name should be understood as the 'protector of the sick' " (*taṃ saṃbodhya brūte—he nadya kuṣṭhākhyauṣadhe tava nāmagrahaṇābhāve ayaṃ vyādhitaḥ puruṣo . . . hiṃsito bhavet. ataḥ vyādhitarakṣaka iti samuditaṃ nāmeti mantavyam*). It is quite clear that Sāyaṇa is merely trying to make the best of a rather bad reading. The text of Viśveśvarānanda Institute is, therefore, totally unacceptable (cf. Bloomfield, 677, and Whitney-Lanman, 959). Roth-

[76] *asya rātrikalpe* (?) *kuṣṭhadhūpapradāne viniyogaḥ pūrvasūktasamaya uktaḥ* (cf. Bloomfield, *Hymns*, 676).

Whitney's emendation, however, is not entirely without basis. It follows P 7.10.2 and at AVŚ 8.7.6 (cf. AVŚ 6.59.3 and 8.2.6*ab*), the names *jīvalā́* (perennial), *naghā́riṣā́* (harmless) and *jīvantí* (life-giving) occur as epithets of the healing plant-goddess Arundhatī (see chapter 21: Simples, 96–102). It seems that Roth-Whitney's emendations are justified. The three names of the *kúṣṭha*-plant may, therefore, be 'non-destroying' (*naghamārá*), 'harmless' (*naghā́riṣa*) and *kúṣṭha* itself, as Bloomfield suggests (5, 677) or 'choicest' (*uttamá*; see AVŚ 6.5.9; cf. also Bloomfield, 677). There also seems to be a direct relationship between the three names and the three times of the day, in *e*, when they are to be recited. In this way, the healer is instructed through the hymn when to pronounce each name.

VERSE 3

For *c*, Roth-Whitney read as 2*c*. P 7.10.3 adds an extra *pāda:* (*c*): *mārṣā nāma te svasā*, "your sister, by name, is *mārṣā* ('respective'; perhaps it is a plant)." The remainder of the P is supplied as at verse 2. Sāyaṇa glosses *jīvalā́* as 'the one causing life,' and *jīvantó*, similarly, as 'causing life' (*jīvayatīti jīvantaḥ. vasanta itivat*; cf. Grohmann, 420).

VERSE 4

a-c are repeated at AVŚ 8.5.11 in reference to an amulet of *sraktyá*. For *d*, Roth-Whitney read as 2*c*. P 7.10.4 reads as Śau; except K has *asmai* in *d*.

VERSE 5

In *a*, Roth-Whitney originally emended to: *trír bhṛ́gubhyo áṅgirobhya;* but later, Whitney-Lanman changed back to the reading: *tríḥ śā́mbubhyo*. In *a*, P 7.10.5 has *triś śāṃbubhyo 'ṅgirebhyas* (Raghu Vira: *triś śā́ṃbhubhyo . . .*); in *d–e* K reads: *sa kuṣṭha* (K manuscript: *kuṣṭho*) *viśvabheṣaja . . . tiṣṭhasi* (O as Śau), and in *f*: *nāśayan*. A slightly different version of this verse is found at P 1.93.1: *tris kuṣṭhāsi vṛtrāj jātas trir divas pari* (K: . . . *vṛtrahā jātas trir ud divas pari*) *jajñiṣe, triḥ somāj jajñiṣe tvaṃ trir ādityebhyas pari*, "Thrice, O *kuṣṭha* you are born from Vṛtra (or: Thrice you, the slayer of Vṛtra, O *kuṣṭha*, are born); thrice, you are born from heaven; thrice, you are born from Soma [and] thrice from the Ādityas" (cf. Renou, JA, 253: 32). Sāyaṇa understands the obscure *śā́mbubhyo áṅgirebhyas* as "the great *ṛṣis* named *Śāmbus* who are the offsprings of the Aṅgirases" (. . . *aṅgirasām apatyabhūtebhyaḥ śāmbubhyaḥ etannāmakebhyo maharṣibhyaḥ* . . .) and explains *trír jātó* as "three times produced for the aid of the three worlds; or else, [it refers to] those characterized by the three *jātis*, i.e. *brāhmaṇa, kṣatriya* and *vaiśya*" (. . . *trayāṇāṃ lokānām upakārāya trir utpāditaḥ. atha vā brāhmaṇakṣatriyavaiśyajātitrayātmanā trir jātaḥ*). The former appears to be more probable. The various origins of *kúṣṭha* point to its divine connection. Note that P 1.93.1 attributes different sources to *kúṣṭha*, avoiding the difficult *śā̃mbubhyo áṅgirebhyas.* For *e,* Sāyaṇa quite rightly explains: "[There is] the title of standing with Soma for the purpose of illuminating its equal strength" (*somena saha avasthānābhidhānaṃ tatsamānavīryatvadyotanārtham*). There is the likelihood that the poet-healer is referring to the habitat of the *kúṣṭha*-plant, i.e., it grew alongside or in the same "plant-community" as the Soma plant (cf. the mutual residence high on the mountains, verse 1, above and Bloomfield, 678).

VERSE 6

Variants of *a–d* are found at AVŚ 5.4.3 and 6.95.1. *e–h* are wanting in the Roth-Whitney edition because they were not found in the manuscripts (see Whitney-Lanman, 960). P 7.10.6*a–d* reads as Śau; and *e–h* are as at verse 5, but supplied. *tátra,* in *c,* and *tátaḥ,* in *d,* seem to refer to the same place, perhaps 'the third heaven from here.' Sāyaṇa considers them to be the *aśvattha*-tree (*aśvatthe . . . aśvatthād,* respectively), and states that because of what CUp 3.1.1 says about the dwelling of *amṛta, āditya* could be meant by the word *aśvattha* (. . . *aśvatthaśabdena āditya ucyate amṛtāvasthānaśravaṇāt,* CUp 3.1.1 . . .). Cf. comments at AVŚ 5.4.3 (6.95.1). Variant versions of this verse occur at P 1.93.3–4:

Verse 3. *antarā dyāvāpṛthivī antarikṣam idaṃ mahat, tatrāmṛtasyeśānaṃ* (K: *tatrāmṛtasyāsiktaṃ;* cf. AVŚ 4.7.1*c*) *kuṣṭhaṃ devā abadhnata,* "This great *antarikṣa* (midspace) [is] between heaven and earth. There the gods attached the *kuṣṭha*-plant, the lord of immortality (or the sprinkling of immortality) [to the earth]" (cf. Renou, JA, 253: 32).

Verse 4. *kuṣṭho 'si devakṛto* (K: *devākṛto*) *himavadbhyo nirābhṛtaḥ* (K: *nirādṛtaḥ*), *tīkṣṇābhir abhribhiḥ khātaḥ* (K: *atribhiḥ vātas*) *sa ca kartārasaṃ* (K: *sa cakarthārasaṃ;* K manuscript: *jagarthārasaṃ*) *viṣam,* "You are *kuṣṭha,* fashioned by the gods [and] brought from the Himavant-mountains, uprooted with sharp mattocks, and the one who makes the poison powerless" (cf. Renou, ibid.).

VERSE 7

Variants of *a–d* are found at AVŚ 5.4.4 and 6.95.2. *e–h* are wanting in the Roth-Whitney edition as at verse 6. In *ab,* P 7.10.7 reads as Śau; *e–h* is as at verse 6. Since these two verses (6–7) always occur together, there is the strong suggestion that they may have been formulaic, and recited whenever the *kúṣṭha*-plant was consecrated.

VERSE 8

In *a,* Roth-Whitney read: *yátra nāvaprabhráṃśanaṃ,* 'where there is no falling downward' (Whitney-Lanman, 961). P 7.10.8 has *yatra nāvaḥ prabhraṃśanaṃ,* 'where the boat descended'; the rest is as in verse 7. Our edition (Viśveśvarānanda) reads: *yátra nā̃vaprabhráṃśanaṃ* (*pada*-text: /ná/ava°/), 'where [there is] no descent.' Sāyaṇa reads it as one word, *nā̃vaprabhráṃśanam*, and considers it to be a place name, glossing: "there is no falling downward of the virtuous ones situated there (i.e. at the place, *nā̃vaprabhraṃśana*) in the heavenly world" (. . . *dyuloke nāvaprabhraṃśanam tatrasthānāṃ sukṛtinām avāṅmukhaprabhraṃśo nāsti*). Most translators understand the word to be the "descent of the ship" which in turn, may refer to the legend of Manu's descent (*manor avasarpaṇam*) at ŚB 1.8.16 and the flood-legend, involving Manu Vaivasvata and the fish, i.e. the place in the Himavants where the boat was moored (*naubandhanam*) at Mbh, Book 3.185.47. (Cf. Grohmann, who is not totally convinced of the connection, 423; Griffith, 298–99 n and Bloomfield, 6, 679–80.) The rendering and understanding of a place where a boat descended is supported by P and has been adopted by us. It probably refers to the descent of the crescent moon ("golden boat") to the top or "summit" (*śírah* in *b*). Such a place could be looked upon as the third heaven, the birthplace of *kúṣṭha* and Soma. The reference to the legend of Manu's descent is forced.

VERSE 9

This verse is very doubtful. In *ab*, Roth-Whitney originally emended to *pū̃rva íkṣvākor yáṃ . . . kusṭhakāmyàḥ*, 'ancestor of *íkṣvāku . . . kuṣṭhakāmyā*' ('those females desirous of *kúṣṭha*?'). Later, Whitney-Lanman, based on Sāyaṇa's reading, *íkṣvākū*(*us?*) and Bloomfield (680), changed the reading to *pū̃rva íkṣvākur yáṃ*. The Viśveśvarānanda edition, following Śankar Pandit, has *íkṣvāko* (*pada*-text: *íkṣvākaḥ*); and in *b*, it reads: *kuṣṭha kāmyàḥ*. Sāyaṇa explains *kāmyàḥ* as 'the son of Kāma' (*kāmaputro*). P(K) 7.10.9 is corrupt; but O has *aikṣvāko* in *a*, *kāsyaḥ* (=Śau?), in *b*, and *sābaso* (=Śau?) . . . *mātsyas*, in *c*. The remainder is as Śau. Roth-Whitney emend: *yáṃ vā̃yaso yáṃ mātsyás*, which is confirmed by O. Sāyaṇa reads: *yáṃ vā váso* [*yaṃ*] *yámā̃syaḥ* and renders: "Since that god, called Vasa whose mouth is like the mouth of Yama, knew [you]" (*yasmād . . . yamasya āsyam iva āsyaṃ yasya sa tādṛsó vasaḥ etannāmā devo veda*). This is obviously a guess. The Viśveśvarānanda edition, again following Pandit who evidently considered that *vasa* was a name, has *yáṃ vā váso* (*pada*-text: *vásaḥ*) *yáṃ ā̃tsyas*. The names mentioned in this verse are extremely obscure and may allow us only to hazard a guess that they could have referred to famous, legendary herbalists: Ikṣvāka, Kāmya, Vasa and Mātsya. Nothing further seems to be known about them.

VERSE 10

In *a*, our text (Viśveśvarānanda) follows Roth-Whitney. P 7.10.10 has *sīrṣālākaṃ* which may be 'pain from inflammation (or poison) in the head' (cf. *alají* at AVŚ 9.8.20). *cd* is the same as AVŚ 5.22.3*cd*. In *a*, Sāyaṇa reads: *sīrṣalókaṃ tṛ́tīyakaṃ* and explains: "O *kuṣṭha*, they speak of your head as heaven (=*loka*), i.e., the third [world] with respect to the earthly world" (*he kuṣṭha . . . bhūlokāpekṣayā tṛtīyaṃ lokaṃ dyusaṃjñakaṃ tava śīrṣa śira āhuḥ*). In *c*, he reads: *viśvadhāvīryam*, glossing: "having [its] efficacy acquired" (*vyāptasāmarthyaṃ*), and makes it refer to *takmā̆naṃ*. His explanations are again simply textual manipulations. On the various types of *takmán*, cf. AVŚ 5.22.13 (also P 1.32.5) and AVŚ 9.8.6 with respect to the relation of *takmán* to the head.

Notes to 6.105

Translators agree that AVŚ 6.105 is a charm against cough (*kā̆sā*).[77] Sȳaṇa prescribes it, along with AVŚ 7.107, for use in a rite "for the purpose of quieting the cough and diseases caused by phlegm, etc."[78] at KauśS 31.27.

VERSE 1

A parallel to this verse can be found at P 19.23.12 at verse 3 below. In *a*, Sāyaṇa glosses *máno manasketáiḥ*: "the *antaḥkaraṇa* with the distant sense objects which are to be known by the *manas* (mind) (and) by the activity of the *buddhi* (intellect)" (. . . *manasā buddhivṛttyā ketyamānair jñāyamānair dūrasthair viśayaiḥ saha* . . . *antaḥkaraṇam*. . .). For the obscure *pravāyyàm*, 'stream' (root *vā* plus *pra*, 'to blow forth'), Sāyaṇa explains: 'the limit to be advanced' (*pragantavyam avadhim* . . .). Bloomfield defines it: 'the course along which the wind blows.' Thus, along with *mánasaḥ*, it could have the meaning 'mind's stream (or course),' or perhaps more colloquially, 'stream of thought.'

VERSE 2

For *cd*, P 19.23.10 (=manuscript 'P': 20.58.4*cd*) has: *evā mūtrasya te dhārā parā patati ketumat* (?), "so also, your flow of urine streams clearly (?) away" (manuscript 'P' 19.23.10 reads as P 20.54.7, below), and P 20.54.7 reads: *evā kāse parā pata sākaṃ vātasya dhrājyā*, "so also, you, O cough, fly forth together with the force of the wind." In both P readings *ad*, are as Śau., suggesting that it may be formulaic. Sāyaṇa glosses *cd*, which includes the difficult word *saṃvátam*, 'contour,' as: "so also, you, O cough, run forth in conformity with the combined-direction (?) of the earth penetrated by the arrow, i.e. go as far as the *pātāla*-region with the speed of the arrow" (. . . *evam he kāse tvaṃ* . . . *bāṇaviddhāyā bhūmyāḥ saṃvatam saṃhatapradeśam* (?) . . . *anulakṣya* . . . *pradhāva. bāṇavegena pātālaparyantaṃ gacchety arthaḥ*). He thus understands distance and speed to be important. *saṃváṭa*, like *pravāyyà* in verse 1, suggests rather the sense of course, path or contour

---

[77] Ludwig: "Kāsā-husten (Kāsā-cough)," *Der Rigveda*, 510; Zimmer: Against "Husten (Cough)," *Leben*, 385; Hillebrandt: "Gegen Husten (Against cough)," *Vedachrestomathie*, 50; Griffith: "A charm against cough," *Hymns of the Atharvaveda*, 1: 302; Bloomfield: "Charm against cough," *Hymns*, 8, 513; and Whitney-Lanman: "To get rid of cough," *Atharva-veda-saṃhitā*, Pt. 1, 357.

[78] *kāsaśleṣmarogādiśāntyarthaṃ*: cf. Keśava: *atha kāse śleṣmapatane ca bhaiṣajyam ucyate*. It is evident that *śleṣman*, given by Sāyaṇa refers to *śleṣmapatane*, 'expectoration,' cited by Keśava.

of the ground along which the arrow flies and the cough is requested to follow.

VERSE 3

Elements of this verse are divided into two separate verses by P. P 19.23.11 reads: *yathā cakṣuś cakṣuṣmataḥ parāpatati ketumat, evā tvaṃ kāse prā* (wanting in manuscript 'P') *pata* (Raghu Vira: [*evā sa parā*] *patat,* 'so may it [?] fly away') *sākaṃ sūryasya raśmibhiḥ,* "As the eye of the seer flies forth clearly, so also, you, O cough, fly forth together with the sun's rays." P 19.23.12 has: *yathā mado manyumatāṃ* (manuscript 'P': *mano manyukety* ?) *parāpatati yojanam* (manuscript 'P': *yotanā*?), *evā kāsā* (Raghu Vira: *evā sa*) *parā patat* (manuscript 'P': *kāse parā pata*) *samudrasyānu vikṣaram,* "As the lust of the passionate ones (or, the intoxication of the spirited ones, i.e., drunkards) streams away a *yojana,* so also may the cough fly away in conformity with the ocean's ebb"; or, following manuscript 'P': "As the mind, marked by order (?), streams away . . . . , so also you, O cough, fly away. . . ." The metaphor in the Śau is somewhat imperfect and unclear; while in the P, it is split, making two separate similes out of the same elements in the Śau. The use of the ocean's ebb, however, seems to fit only marginally in both the Śau and the P. Sāyaṇa renders and explains *cd:* "So also, you, O cough, go forth in conformity with the direction in which the river flows (*vikṣará* is 'pouring forth variously, i.e. a stream'), i.e. having abandoned this man, go quickly like the sun's rays to the end of the ocean" (. . . *evaṃ he kāse tvaṃ . . . udadheḥ vikṣaraṃ vividhaṃ kṣaraṇaṃ pravāho yasmin deśe taṃ deśam . . . anulakṣya . . . pragaccha. imaṃ puruṣaṃ visṛjya samudraparyantaṃ sūryaraśmivat śīghraṃ gacchety arthaḥ*). The word *vikṣarám,* as Sāyaṇa suggests, may be derived from the root *kṣar,* 'to flow,' plus *vi,* i.e. 'pouring out,' 'effluence,' and in relation to *samudrá,* 'ocean,' may have the sense of 'ebb' of the ocean, i.e. the ebb and flow of the tide; cf. Hillebrandt: "Höhe (des Meeres)" (116). Thus, similar to Sāyaṇa, as the sun's rays disappear over the ocean, so also, may the cough flow away and disappear with the outgoing tide. Note the maritime knowledge of tidal flows implied in this verse.

Notes to 9.8

Most translators consider AVŚ 9.8 to be a charm against various diseases.[79] The introduction to the Sanskrit text (by Sāyaṇa?) states that the charm is used "in a rite for the healing of all [diseases] beginning with

[79] Zimmer: The charm is translated in the course of his discussion of *yákṣma* (Auszehrung, Schwindsucht), *Leben,* 378; Henry: "une conjuration . . . contre toutes sortes de maladies," *Les livres VIII et IX,* 105, 141; Griffith: "The hymn is a charm for the cure of various diseases and pains more or less connected, or supposed to be connected, with consumption," *Hymns of the Atharvaveda,* 1: 455; Bloomfield: "Charm to procure immunity from all disases," *Hymns* 45, 600; and Whitney-Lanman: "Against various diseases," *Artharva-veda-saṃhitā,* Pt. 2, 549.

head-disease"[80] at KauśS 32.18–19; and at AVŚ 2.32, Sāyaṇa counts it as among the *aṅholiṅgagaṇa*, 'list of hymns characterized by the word *aṅhas*.'

Although this charm may not be a true composite hymn,[81] as exact parallels are not found elsewhere, nevertheless, from the refrains, we notice conflations which could allow us to interpret its structure as follows:

A. Verses 1–5, an original charm to remove various head-diseases.

B. Verses 6–9 added, which retain the last *pāda* of the refrain, but vary the penultimate *pāda* to include the internal disease-entities: *takmán, yákṣma, balā́sa,* the causes of *yákṣma,* jaundice and Apvā.

C. Verses 10–12, 19–20, a second charm devoted specifically to the expulsion of pain-causing demons by way of the penis and the anus. Verse 10 provides the link to B and begins the new charm which concentrates on the removal of the poisons of the *yákṣmas*.

D. Verses 13–18, a third charm concerned principally with the eradication of the various pain-causing demons through the anus.

E. Verses 21–22 are added to tie the entire charm together.

The link between C and D would be provided, in the redactor's mind, by the word *bíla,* '(anal) orifice,' in verse 11. In other words, he inserted the third charm (verses 13–18) where he did, and not after verses 19 and 20, in order to keep the reference to *bíla* intact. The final redaction, therefore, could have allowed medical incantations, not previously encountered, to be brought together and included in the book of the *Atharvaveda,* which contains some of the work's larger hymns.

VERSE 1

In *a,* P(K) 16.74.1 has *sīrṣaktyaṃ;* manuscript 'P' as Śau; and in *b,* P's *tṛtīyakam,* 'the third,' replaces the obscure *vilohitám.* At AVŚ 12.5.23 a Brāhmaṇa's cow can become headache (*śīrṣaktí*) when it is milked; and at AVŚ 12.2.19, 20, *śīrṣaktí* is said to have been wiped off and settled on to a pillow (*upabárhaṇa*); cf. also AVŚ 1.12.3. SuUtt 20.3 and 6 mention that *karṇaśūla* is one of twenty-eight types of ear-disease and that it is characterized by severe aching in the ear-region and inside the tympanum (verse 6: *samīraṇaḥ śrotragato 'nyathācaraḥ samantataḥ śūlamatīva karṇayoḥ, . . . sa karṇaśūlaḥ kathito durācarah;* cf. also AH Utt 17.12.13 and Wise, 287). The exact meaning of the word *vilohitám* is uncertain. On etymological grounds, i.e. *lóhita,* 'red,' 'blood' plus *vi,* 'without,' 'away,' scholars have suggested various translations: Zimmer (378) and Griffith (455) posit a type of inflammation, perhaps, erysipelas; Henry: "la décomposition du sang," explaining, "il peut s'agir du sang qui se décompose et se transforme en pus?" (105, 142); Bloomfield, suggesting that it may be related to *lóhita,* 'blood-flow' (Sāyaṇa), found at AVŚ 6.127.1 (136, above), renders: "flow

---

[80] *śirorogādisarvabhaiṣajye karmaṇi;* cf. Keśava: *sarvabhaiṣajyam ucyate.*

[81] On composite hymns in the *Atharvaveda,* see Bloomfield, *The Atharva-veda,* 37, 43. P divides the charm rather arbitrarily into two equal hymns: 16.74 and 16.75.

of blood"; and because it is in the head, the flow may be from the nose (45, 600, 657); Whitney-Lanman: "anaemia" (549); and Filliozat merely outlines what has already been said about the word (*La doctrine,* 106). See also J. Narten, St.II., 5/6: 162 n. At AVŚ 12.4.4 it is said to originate from cow-dung. Because the healer is requesting the various head diseases to come out (*bahír*), we are inclined to favor the rendering "outflowing of blood"; and as cow-dung is emitted from an anal orifice, so also, it is implied that the demonic *vilohitá* should be eliminated from an orifice.

VERSE 2

In *b,* P 16.74.2 reads *śuktivalśam,* 'a shell-like branch (of the head),' i.e. 'an ear?' (cf. Barret, AOS, 9: 76, AVŚ 6.127.3 n) and *vilóhitam* (see verse 1). *káṅkūṣebhyaḥ* is obscure, but may refer to the inside of the body (see MWSED, s.v.) or a part of the head (Filliozat, *La doctrine,* 122; Zimmer suggests a part of the ear, 378). The word *ūṣa* can have the meaning 'cavity of the ear' (MWSED, s.v.); in which case, *kárṇa* may refer to the outer ear and *káṅkūṣa* the inner part of the ear. On *visálpakam* (Roth-Whitney: *visályakam*), 'a cutaneous swelling,' see chapter on *balā́sa* (32–33, above) and AVŚ 6.127.1 n. Griffith renders it by "throbbing pain" and comments that it may also be regarded as "the disease that causes throbbing pain or piercing pain in various parts of the body" (455 n). Henry suggests: "la douleur inflammatoire" (106) and Zimmer: "das Reissen" (378). Because of its occurrence with *balā́sa* (swelling) and other words signifying 'abscess,' 'tumor,' etc. at AVŚ 6.127.1 and verse 20 below, we are inclined to consider it also as an 'abscess,' 'pustule,' or 'boil' which is located on the head, perhaps in and around the ear and which causes extreme pain.

VERSE 3

In *b,* P 16.74.4 has *nāsata,* 'from the nose,' for *karṇatá.* In *a,* the phrase *yaśya hetóḥ,* literally, 'because of which,' is difficult to render. Henry's suggestion that *yaśya* refers to the idea of *mantra* in the verb *mantrayāmahe,* rather than to *rogáṃ,* in *c,* seems quite probable (142; cf. also Bloomfield, 45). The idea, therefore, seems to be: because of that charm with which we charm out of you every head-disease. . . .

VERSE 4

In *ab,* P 16.74.3 reads as Śau (Raghu Vira has *kṛṇotu* in *ab*). Deriving the obscure *pramótam* from the root *mū,* 'to bind,' *mūta,* 'bound,' Zimmer conjectures that on the basis of context, it means 'deaf,' which is followed by most translators (see Henry, 106, 142; Griffith, 456; Bloomfield, 45–46, 601); yet, he points out that it may also have the meaning 'dumb,' citing Latin *mūtus* (English, 'mute'; cf. also Sanskrit *mū́ka,* 'mute,' 'dumb') as a possible cognate (378 n). This latter suggestion is adopted by Whitney-Lanman (550) and Filliozat (*La doctrine,* 106). As Henry (142) and Whitney-

Lanman (550) have noticed the word seems to be a corrupted form, yet it is found also in P. Because of the many problems surrounding this word, we can only posit a conjectural meaning of 'deaf' or 'mute' because of the following word *andhám̱*, 'blind.'

VERSE 5

For *ab,* P 16.74.5 reads: *śīrṣarogaṃ aṅgarogaṃ viśvāṅgīnaṃ viśalyakaṃ* (or *visalpakaṃ*), "the disease of the head, the disease of the limbs [and] the *viśalyaka* (*visalpaka*) affecting all the limbs." In *a,* it is clear that *yákṣma* is to be understood: at AVŚ 5.30.8, the healer states that he has exorcised the *yákṣma,* which gives fever to the limbs, from the sick man's limbs (*níravocam ahám̱ yákṣmam áṅgebhyo aṅgajvarám̱ táva*); and at AVŚ 5.30.9, the *yákṣma,* which causes cutting pain in the limbs, fever to the limbs and affliction to heart, is forced by the healer's charm to fly far away like a hawk (*aṅgabhedó aṅgajvaró yáś ca te hṛdayāmayáḥ, yákṣmaḥ śyená iva prā̄paptad vācā̄ sāḍháḥ parastarā̄m;* P 9.13.9 reads: *śīrṣarogam aṅgarogaṃ,* in *a* and *nuttaḥ,* 'driven away,' in *d* and for *a,* cf. P 16.74.5, above); cf. also AVŚ 19.44.2. Filliozat speculates that the compound *aṅgabhedá,* in *a,* denotes, "section des membres," which "peut donc désigner les mutilations spontanées que provoque la lèpre. . ." (*La doctrine,* 90). It would appear rather that *aṅgabhedá* refers to a breaking apart of the limbs or cutting pain in the entire body, brought about by the disease-demon *yákṣma.* Filliozat also suggests that *aṅgajvará* might be a local fever of lymphangitis (ibid.). It is important to note that *-jvara,* 'fever,' in this compound, does not have the same meaning as *takmán;* it simply indicates an intense and localized heat or inflammation. For *yákṣma* and *visálpaka* in association with head-disease, see verses 2 and 3, above.

VERSE 6

For *cd,* P 16.74.6 reads: *takmānaṃ śītaṃ rūraṃ ca taṃ te nirmantrayāmahe,* "We charm out of you that chilly and deliriously hot *takman.*" Cf. AVŚ 5.22.10; see also AVŚ 1.25.4; 5.22.7, 13 and 19.39.10.

VERSE 7

For *anusárpaty,* in *a,* Raghu Vira at P(K) 16.74.7 reads: *anusarpatv,* 'let crawl along' (Bar. as Śau.; K manuscript: *na sarpantv*); for *b,* manuscript P is as Śau (K: *atho ye 'nu gavīnike,* "and who crawls along the two *gavīnikā*"; and for *c: balāsam antaraṅgebhyo,* "the *balāsa* from within the limbs"). On the difficult word *gavīnike,* see AVŚ 1.3.6 n. The doubly accented *antár-áṅgebhyo* is odd. Bloomfield suggests the emendation: *antáraṅgebhyo* (601). If we read the text as it is printed (cf. *pada*-text: /*antáḥ*/*áṅgebhyaḥ*/) the meaning seems to be 'from within the limbs,' rather than, 'from the inner limbs' (cf. Bloomfield, 46, 601; and Whitney-Lanman, 550).

VERSE 8

In *a*, P(K) 16.74.8 has *yat*. Here *balā́sa* has a definite connection to various emotional states.

VERSE 9

P 16.74.9 replaces *b* with *c* of Śau; and in *cd*, reads: *yakṣmaṃ te sarvaṃ aṅgebhyo bahir nirmantrayāmahe*. In this way, the P avoids the troublesome *apvā́*, for which, see 46, above. In *c*, *yakṣmodhā́m*, suggests a producer or causer of *yákṣma*. This is the only occurrence of such a compounded form of *yákṣma*. The only cause of *yákṣma* that the Vedic Indians seem to have noticed was "sin" or "transgression," for which the gods sent the affliction (see chapter on *yákṣma*, 13, above). If this is the meaning which the poet wishes to convey, it is possible that *antár ātmáno* could signify the more metaphysical notion of "self" (cf. Bloomfield, 46). In this way, it could refer to some undesirable psychic state, which encourages *yákṣma* to take up his abode in the body. Note the mention of the emotional states in the previous verse. We may also construe *yakṣmodhā́m* as 'the seat of *yákṣma*' (MWSED, s.v.); in which case, *antár ātmáno* would imply the sense of 'from within the body' (cf. verse 7 n). It should be pointed out, however, that *dhā* (*dha*), from root *dhā*, 'to put,' generally has an active sense, i.e. 'putter,' 'doer,' 'causer,' etc.

VERSE 10

Based on manuscript 'P,' P 16.74.10 reads as Śau (K has [*sa*] *āso balāso bhavan*, 'that ash being *balāsa*'). We can notice a definite pun on *āsó* in *balā́so*. *ā́sa*, 'ash,' in this context, may, as Henry suggests, have the wider sense of "excrement" (142); in which case, the producer of disease is turned into feces and urine and evacuated from the body; or it may refer to the crusty state of the swelling, which the healer requests to become like dry grass and to blow away (see AVŚ 6.14.3; cf. Karambelkar, *The Atharva-Veda and The Āyur-Veda*, 220). In *b*, *āmayát* has been discussed by both Hoffmann (*Aufsätze*, 1: 292) and Narten (St.II, 5/6: 155–56). The two meanings arrived at are: "das Schmerzverursachende" (Hoffmann) and "was weh tut" (Narten). Hoffmann's definition is perhaps best, since Narten's "what aches" implies a part of the body: surely the healer did not desire that to turn into urine; rather it is the agent of the pain, which, in *c*, is indicated by the neuter *viṣám*, 'poison'; elsewhere, the pain is caused by *yákṣma* (P 2.49.1, 2; 50.1, ibid., 156), whose poison is being expelled. The healer then requests the venom-like poison of all *yákṣma*s to become urine and to be discharged from the body.

VERSE 11

P begins a new hymn with this verse. In *a*, P(K) 16.75.1 reads *nir dhāvatu*, which is synonymous with the Śau reading; manuscript 'P' as Śau; and in *b: kahāvalaṃ;* manuscript 'P' as Śau. At AVŚ 1.3.8, there occurs the word *vastibilá,* 'bladder-orifice,' which, Bloomfield suggests, is the probable meaning of *bilaṃ,* in *a* (601). The obscure word *kāhābāhaṃ* appears to be onomatopoeic and, like *bā̄l* at AVŚ 1.3, may be construed as a type of adverb (cf. also Whitney-Lanman, 550). It could also be taken as an accusative, referring to a disease-entity, manifesting this sound, while being directed to stream forth out of the stomach. Since at AVŚ 1.3, urine is released through the *vastibilá* (bladder-orifice) with the sound *bā̄l,* it seems reasonable to assume that the disease-entities, in verses 13–18, would be released through the *bíla* (bodily orifice) i.e. anus, with the sound *kāhābāha,* the rumbling noise in the bowels, or perhaps the noise of passing wind, i.e. flatulence (cf. Mayrhofer, Wb, 1: 206).

VERSE 12

In *a,* between *te* and *klomnáḥ,* P 16.75.2 inserts *pari* which, as noticed by Whitney-Lanman, rectifies the meter (551). For *cd,* P reads as Śau 9*cd,* above.

VERSE 13

In *d,* P 16.75.3 reads *dravanti. arṣaṇī̄ḥ,* from the root *ṛṣ,* 'to thrust,' 'to surge,' with *práti,* 'against,' signifies literally, 'those [pains] who thrust or surge against [the skull (*mūrdhā̄naṃ*)] and therefore, seem to refer to the throbbings or poundings in the head, which accompany a severe headache and which give the sensation that the head is about to split open. The notion of "piercing pain" (Mayrhofer, Wb, 1: 125) does not quite capture the complete significance of the word. This verse appears to begin a series of verses (13–18) by which the healer, although perhaps not in the most systematic manner, works from the head downwards expelling the demons out of the body, through the orifice (*bíla*), i.e. the anus (making the sound, *kāhābāha*!). See also Narten, St.II, 5/6: 158, 163 n.

VERSE 14

Based on manuscript 'P', in *a,* P 16.75.4 has *upasarpanty,* '[who] creep toward' (Raghu Vira as Śau); and in *b,* Henry suggests the emendation, *uttanvánti,* '[qui] distendent' (106, 142).

VERSE 15

P 16.75.5 reads as Śau; but in *b,* K manuscript has *anudakṣanti* '[who] grow along' (Barret mentions that *dakṣanti* may well be emended to *rakṣanti,* AOS, 9: 77).

VERSE 16

In *b,* P 16.75.6 reads: *vakṣaṇābhyaḥ. vakṣáṇāsu,* in the plural, refers to the breast, abdomen or chest (see, Mayrhofer, Wb, 3: 121–22). Literally, the first line would be rendered: "[Let] the pangs, who, moving across, surge forth in your breast." The idea, as suggested by P's reading of *vakṣaṇābhyaḥ*, seems to indicate that the internal pains go across the chest or abdomen.

VERSE 17

Based on manuscript 'P,' P 16.75.7*b* reads: *āntrāṇi* (K has *āntrāti?*) *yopaganti* (K: *yāpayanti*) *ca,* "and who disturb the bowels (or "which cause the bowels to go")." This, as Lanman suggests, may have the same sense as "causing the bowels to move" or "producing diarrhea" does in English (551). Rather than twisting the bowels (Bloomfield, 47), *āntrā́ṇi mohā́yanti ca* has more of the idea of bewildering or confounding the bowels, i.e. those causing irregular evacuations. *pāda a* points to parasitic worms.

VERSE 18

In *a,* P 16.75.8 has *'nusarpanti* '[who] crawl along.'

VERSE 19

In *b,* P 16.75.9 has *saha* which is probably a corruption of *táva.* Manuscript 'P' has *ropaṇāsaḥ.* Zimmer has understood *madáyanti* to mean "paralyze (lähmen)" (379), which is followed by Bloomfield (47, cf. also Henry, 43). Literally, it means 'intoxicate,' which suggests rather the sense of causing the limbs to move irregularly, as a drunken man's legs cause him to stagger. Zimmer (379), Henry (107) and Griffith (457) posit the meaning "colic" for *ropaṇā́s.* Derived from the root *rup,* 'to pain,' it has rather the more general sense of 'those causing pain,' i.e. painers (cf. Bloomfield, 47, and Whitney-Lanman, 551; cf. *ropaṇā́kā,* which, at AVŚ 1.22.4, are yellow birds which carry away the undesired yellowness or jaundice of the patient).

VERSE 20

For *visalpásya,* P 16.75.10 has *viśalyasya* (Raghu Vira: *visalpasya*). For *ab,* manuscript 'P' reads: *visalpakas vidradhas rātīkārās vālakoḥ* (?) *visalpá* is merely a variant form of *visálpaka* in verse 2 above, for which, see chapter on *balā́sa,* 32–33, above. Likewise for *vidradhá,* see chapter on *balā́sa* and AVŚ 6.127.1 n, 136, above. For *vātīkārá,* which is a variant of *vātī́kṛta,* see AVŚ 6.44; 6.109 and the section on "Flesh wounds characterized by bleeding," 75–78, above. In *b, alají* has a close parallel in the later medical texts: *alajī,* which signifies a pustule (*piṭakā*) located on joints, genitals and fleshy parts (AHNiSth 10.25–26; see also CaSūSth 17.83, 88. At SuNiSth 6.17–18, 14.7, and Utt 2.8, two types of *alajī* are indicated: that which is found on the penis and that occurring at the margin of the iris). Whether *alají* in our text has the same meaning as *alajī* in the medical text is difficult to know for sure; but it seems very likely. J. Chowdhury, however, maintains that it is in fact a kind of boil, occurring in any part of the body, which resembles a *vidradhi* (abscess), but smaller (JBORS, 17: 38–39); and similarly

Filliozat states that it is not a disease, but a morbid form known as "phlyctène" (vesicle) (*La doctrine,* 102). Since it is found along with *visalpá* and *vidradhá,* which are types of abscesses or skin-swellings, we also are inclined to consider *alají* as such, perhaps one which is smaller in size. Henry reads *bālajī,* having in mind perhaps a child's disease (107; cf. Bloomfield, 602). Griffith (458) and Bloomfield (47, 602), referring to Wise (296), consider it to be an eye disease.

VERSE 21

After *te,* in *a,* P 16.75.11 has *gulphābhyāṃ,* 'from the ankles,' and *jaṅghābhyāṃ* (wanting in manuscript 'P'), 'from the shanks'; after *jānubhyāṃ, ūrubhyāṃ,* 'from the thighs'; and in *cd,* between *uṣṇíhābhyaḥ* and *śīrṣṇó,* it has *grīvābhyas,* 'from the neck' and *skandhebhyaś,* 'from the shoulders.' On *bhámsasaḥ,* see AVŚ 2.33.5 n, 107, above. In *cd, uṣṇíhābhyaḥ śīrṣṇó rógam* may also be rendered as one unit "the affliction from the head [and] from the nape of the neck."

VERSE 22

In *b,* P 16.75.12 has *viduḥ,* which should be *vidhuḥ;* for the second line, P. 16.75.12 reads: *udyan sūrya ādityo aṅgāni romaṃ nakhāni sarvāṇi sādanāny anīnaśat* [manuscript 'P' has: . . . *ādityo rogam* (?) *anīnaśat,* ". . . the son of Aditi . . . has destroyed the affliction(?)"]. "Arising, the son of Aditi, the sun, has destroyed all the exhaustings(?)—the limbs, hair [and] nails(?)." In *a,* the word *sáṃ,* being unconnected, seems odd. Henry suggests that the verb *anīnaśam* should be supplied and translates: "[J'ai] rajusté" (107, 143). Its primary meaning, 'together,' implies, in this context, a 'healthy' or 'sound' condition of the body; thus it may stand alone. *vidhúḥ* could either be from the root *vidh,* 'to be destitute,' i.e. meaning the moon (see Wackernagel-Debrunner, *Altindische Grammatik,* 2: 476) or from the root *dhū,* 'to shake,' plus *vi,* i.e. 'to agitate,' which suggests the more specific sense of 'flutter' or 'palpitation,' rather than the more general one of 'beat' (see Whitney-Lanman, 552). This, however, implies that the Vedic Indians could distinguish irregular heart beats! At AVŚ 2.32.1, both the rising and the setting sun (*ādityá*) are requested to destroy the worms in cows with their rays; and at AVŚ 1.22.1 (cf. ṚV 1.50.11–12), the sun (*sū́rya*) is asked to remove *hṛddyotá* (*hṛdrogá*) and jaundice. The notion of the rising sun points to the fact that the most auspicious time for the performance of the ritual was early morning (cf. KauśS 32.19).

Notes to ṚV 10.162

Translators generally agree that ṚV 10.162 is a hymn against a demonic disease which destroys the embryo (i.e. miscarriage, abortion).[82] Sāyaṇa,

---

[82] Griffith: "The subject is the prevention of abortion. . . . Stanzas 1, 2 are directed against disease, and 3–6 against evil-spirits which attack women who are about to become mothers," *Hymns of the Ṛgveda,* 2: 615; Hillebrandt: "Gegen Krankheit des Embryo"; "Dämonen aus-

following the *Sarvānukramaṇī,* states that its meter is *anuṣṭubh,* its *ṛṣi*'s name is Rakṣohan, son of Brāhmaṇa; and the *Anukramaṇī* specifically mentions that it is used in the atonement for a miscarriage.[83] BD 8.65–66 states that it is addressed to the *rākṣas*-slaying Agni and that it is known to be used as a prayer-consecration for miscarriage.[84] *Ṛgvidhāna* 4.17–18 prescribes it in a rite to secure the successful birth of a child which otherwise may have been aborted.

VERSE 1

There is some difficulty in rendering *cd* (likewise, *ab* of verse 2). Basically, there is a syllable missing in *c* (*a* of verse 2). The problem may involve the word *ámīvā.* Geldner, following Oldenberg (*Noten,* 2: 361), has construed it as an instrumental, "mit Krankheit" (389–90, he also, however, suggests that it may be in apposition to *durṇā́mā*), thus reading, *ámīvā-ā.* Sāyaṇa merely glosses it as a nominative singular: "that *rākṣasa* which has the form of disease" (*yaḥ rākṣaso amīvā rogarūpaḥ san*). Filliozat, following the suggestion of Hillebrandt (126), renders *durṇā́mā* as adjectival to *ámīvā,* but understands *ámīvā* to be a nominative feminine singular in apposition to *yás:* "étant maladie, ayant un nom sinistre" (107). Renou, agreeing with Filliozat, attempts to explain the form of *ámīvā* by saying: "*ámīvā:* mas. en-*van-* secondairement fait sur *amīva-cā́tana* et *hán*?" (EVP, 16: 174). This suggestion is appealing; but the stem *ámīvan* is not found elsewhere in the Ṛg- or *Atharva-Vedas.* It seems possible to construe both *ámīvā* and *durṇā́mā* in apposition to *yás,* with the missing syllable remaining or perhaps supplied by *ca.* Ultimately, we learn that *yás* relates to *tám̐,* in verse 2*c,* which in turn refers to *kravyā́dam,* 'the flesh-eater' in 2*d.* Sāyaṇa explains *durṇā́mā* as the disease called hemorrhoids (*arśākhyo rogaḥ*). Geldner however suggests: "dessen Name Unglück bringt und nicht in dem Mund genommen wird, weil er ausgesprochen den Dämon ruft, also ominös. Es bezeichnet hier den Dämon, der die Leibesfrucht schädigt" (389–90). Geldner is quite right to consider *durṇā́man* as a demon which damages the embryo. It is, however, a particular type of evil-named one, i.e. it is a flesh-eater who acts like *ámīvā,* entering the domestic abode and causing bodily decay and destruction similar to that of the *káṇva*-demon of AVŚ 2.25 and other evil-named demons who destroy the embryo and cause abortion, mentioned at AVŚ 8.6.

---

treibung (Against the disease of the Embryo; the expulsion of demons)"; *Lieder des Ṛgveda,* 1?6; Geldner: " 'Gegen den Beschädiger der Leibesfrucht.' . . . In Wahrheit ist es eine Beschwörung des den Fötus tötenden Dämons (Against the harmer of the womb. . . . In reality it is an exorcism of the foetus-killing demon)," *Der Rigveda,* 3: 389; Renou: "Contre le démon qui détruit l'embryon," EVP, 16: 174 (notes only); and Filliozat: "Démons et avortement," *La doctrine,* 107.

[83] Anu: *brahmaṇā ṣaḍ brāhmo rakṣohā garbhasaṃsrāve prāyaścittam ānuṣṭubhaṃ hi;* Sāyaṇa: . . . *sūktam ānuṣṭubham. brahmaputra rakṣohā nāmarṣiḥ.*

[84] Vs. 65*cd: rākṣoghnāgneyam ity uktaṃ yat tvetad brahmaṇeti tu.* Vs. 66*ab: sravatām api garbhāṇāṃ dṛṣṭaṃ tad anumantraṇam.*

VERSE 2

ab may be explained as verse 1*cd,* above. In *d,* Sāyaṇa understands *kravyā̆dam* as "that flesh-eater beginning with the *rākṣasa*-demons" (*māṃsāśinaṃ rākṣasādikaṃ*). At AVŚ 8.6.6 the flesh-eater is listed along with other evil-named ones who kill the embryo and who, in turn, are destroyed by the tawny-colored *bajá*-plant (i.e. mustard, Sāyaṇa; or perhaps, both *piṅgá* and *bajá* are meant, cf. AVŚ 8.6.20, 24) (*anujighrā́ṃ pramṛśántaṃ kravyā̆dam utá rerihám, arā̆yāṃ chvakiṣkíṇo bajáḥ piṅgó anīnaśat;* P 16.79.6 same as Śau). Cf. also AVŚ 8.6.23: *yá āmā́ṃ māṃsám adánti páuruṣeyaṃ ca yé kravíḥ, gárbhān khā̆danti keśavā̆s tā̆n itó nāśayāmasi,* "We make perish from here those hairy ones who consume raw meat and human flesh and who eat embryos" [P 16.81.5*cd* reads: . . . *arāyān asyā bhaṃsaso muṣkayor apa hanmasi,* "from her *bhaṃsas* (see, AVŚ 2.33.5 n, 107, above) (and) from (her) two pudenda, we beat away the evil spirits" (cf. AVŚ 3.6.5*cd*)].

VERSE 3

Sāyaṇa considers that in this verse there are three stages of embryonic development culminating in the birth of a child: 1. The flowing (embryo), i.e. the going forth in the form of semen; 2. the embryo which is established there (in the womb); 3. the embryo accustomed to moving about, which arises after three months with all of its limbs intact; and finally, the child born in ten [lunar] months (. . . *patantaṃ retorūpeṇa gacchantaṃ tadanantaraṃ tatra . . . niṣīdantaṃ ca garbhaṃ . . . tato māsatrayādūrdhvaṃ prāptasarvāvayavaṃ . . . sarpaṇaśīlaṃ ca garbhaṃ . . . daśasu māseṣūtpannaṃ . . . śiśuṃ . . .*). Most translators agree with Sāyaṇa's interpretation of the latter phases, but disagree concerning the first stage. The root *pat* generally has the meaning, 'to fly,' 'to jump,' 'to rush on' in the ṚV (see Renou, EVP, 13: 125; 16: 174); in which case, *patáyantaṃ* could imply the sense of the semen which 'flies upwards' or 'leaping,' referring to the passage of the semen via the vagina to the uterus, as Sāyaṇa suggests (see also Hillebrandt, 127, and Geldner, 390). This interpretation may also receive some support from AVŚ 8.6.20 where the notion of the flowing embryo and the fixed embryo appear to be mentioned: "Let the two powerful medicines (*bajá* and *piṅgá,* see verse 24) which are to be worn in the undergarments, protect [and] preserve (P) the embryo which has flown about and which is fixed, so that it may not drop" [*párisṛṣṭaṃ* (P 16.81.1, Sāyaṇa and Whitney-Lanman, Pt. 2, 497 read: *pariśiṣṭam,* 'remained') *dhārayatu* (preferable is P's *dhārayatāṃ*) *yád dhitáṃ mā̆va pādi tát, gárbhaṃ ta ugráu rakṣatāṃ bheṣajáu nīvibhāryàu*]. The root *pat* also has the meaning, 'to fall' i.e. *patáyantaṃ,* 'falling,' which is proposed by Ludwig and R. Müller ("Medizin im Ṛg-Veda," 342). Similarly, Filliozat: "qui est en train de descendre" (*La doctrine,* 107). The exact significance of "falling" or "descending" with respect to the earliest stage of embryonic development is, however, not completely clear. It could suggest, as Filliozat states, the passage of the fetus into the pelvic canal where a prolonged labor could kill it (ibid., 108). It would appear that evidence for stages of embryonic development may, in fact, be present, but only in the most obvious form. The "leaping" and "settled" embryo suggests copulation and impregnation, the embryo which "moves about," the stage when the foetus begins to kick and move, and finally, the birth. In *pāda c,* the death of the newly born infant, suggests a "stillborn" child. References to a "stillborn" baby are found at AVŚ 8.6.18, where there occurs the mention of the demon who causes the embryo to be born dead (*yás . . . gárbhaṃ . . . jātáṃ . . . māráyāti . . .*); and at AVŚ 8.6.26, where the specific mention of a 'stillborn' child (*mā́rtavatsam*) occurs.

VERSE 4

At AVŚ 8.6.8, the flesh-eater (*kravyā́dam,* cf. verse 2 above) is called an excessive licker (*rerihám*). Likewise, at AVŚ 8.6.3, the healer requests the evil-named one not to crawl down between the thighs and states that he is preparing the *bajá*-plant, dispeller of the evil-named one, as medicine (*. . . ūrū́ mā́vo sṛpo 'ntarā́, kṛṇómy asyai bheṣajáṃ bajáṃ durṇāmacā́tanam;* P 16.79.3 as Śau). Finally, at AVŚ 8.6.13, the healer implores Indra to destroy the *rákṣas*-demons who, after putting the excessive mass (of the pregnant woman?) on their shoulders, offer (it), and who spread the women's hips (with a hand-held horn? cf. verse 14) [*yá ātmā́nam atimātrám áṃsa ādhā́ya bíbhrati, strīṇā́ṃ śroṇipratodína índra rákṣāṃsi nāśaya;* for *ab,* P 16.80.5, based on manuscript 'P,' reads as Śau]. Such demons which spread women's hips suggest those who separate their thighs as in *a.* Sāyaṇa also understands this demon to be a *rákṣas.*

VERSE 5

Sāyaṇa states that it is the *rākṣasa*-demon who becomes the form of a brother, of a protector, or of a gallant (*. . . rākṣasaḥ . . . bhrātṛrūpo bhūtvā . . . bhartṛrūpo vā bhūtvā . . . athavā . . . upapatirūpo vā bhūtvā . . .*). We find a very similar verse at AVŚ 8.6.7: *yás tvā svápne nipádyate bhrā́tā bhūtvā́ pitéva ca, bajás tā́nt sahatām itáḥ klībárūpāṃs tirīṭínaḥ,* "He who becomes [like] a brother [or] like a father and lies down with you in sleep—may the *bajá*-plant force hence those who have the form of eunuchs and wear diadems" (in *a,* P 16.79.8 has *yas tvāṃ suptāṃ nipadyate,* "who lies down with you who are asleep"). Cf. also AVŚ 8.6.19, where the tawny colored plant (*piṅgá*) is requested to drive away, as the wind (does) the thundercloud, the Gandharvas who fall to the lot of women, who kill the unsuspecting (new-)born (baby) (cf. verse 3 above), and (who) lie with the woman who has just given birth [*yé amnó jātā́n mārāyanti sū́tikā anuśérate, strī́bhāgān piṅgó gandharvā́n vā́to abhrám ivājatu;* P 16.80.10 has, in *d, abhram iva vāta ajatu* (manuscript 'P': *vāta ivājatu*)]. This verse and its parallel at AVŚ 8.6.7 and at P 16.79.8 shed some light on the sexual ethics of the time: evidently there was a good deal of permissiveness; and even incest does not seem to have been uncommon.

VERSE 6

Sāyaṇa, again, understands this to be a reference to the *rākṣasa*-demons who cause the victim to attain bewilderment by (in) the dream-state and by (in) sleep [. . . *rākṣasādiḥ* . . . *svapnāvasthayā* (°*āyāṃ*) . . . *nidrayā* (°*āyāṃ*) . . . *tvāṃ* . . . *mūḍhatāṃ prāpayya* . . .]. Cf. also AVŚ 8.6.8: *yás tvā svapántīṃ tsárati yás tvā dípsati jā̆gratīm, chāyā̆m iva prá tā̆nt sū̆ryaḥ parikrā̆mann anīnaśat,* "The encircling sun has utterly destroyed, like a shadow, those—[the one] who creeps on to you while asleep [and the one] who desires to injure you while awake." In *ab,* P 16.79.7 reads: *yas tvā*[*ṃ*] *suptāṃ carati* (K: *chinatti*?) *yaś ca* . . . , "who wanders about you who are asleep and who . . . ," and in *c* as Śau. In *a,* Sāyaṇa reads *caránti* for *tsárati. cd* may be understood as "like the encircling sun, a shadow, (so also the *bajá*-plant) has utterly destroyed those . . ." (see Whitney-Lanman, Pt. 2, 495). Note also the presence of the early idea that the sun revolved around the earth, so also Sāyaṇa: *ākāśe paribhraman*. The meaning, 'sleeping' for *svapántīṃ* seems to fit better here than 'dreaming' in the ṚV. Nevertheless, in both places, the demon attacks and causes damage while the victim is asleep (cf. also AVŚ 8.6.7, verse 5 above). See also Renou, EVP, 16: 174.

Notes to 2.4

Most translators consider AVŚ 2.4 to be a charm against various evils or demons, including the disease-demon, *víṣkandha,* with an amulet made from the *jaṅgiḍá*-tree.[85] Sāyaṇa prescribes its use in a rite "for ruining of witchcraft, for protecting oneself and for the removing of impediments"[86] at KauśS 42.23. It would appear from the context that the charm may have originally been recited during the binding of the amulet which was worn to protect one from various demons, including those which could inflict bodily harm.

VERSE 1

In *b,* P 2.11.1 reads as Śau (K: *rákṣamāṇās,* 'protecting ourselves'; note: *ab* is accented in K). *cd* is wanting in K, but Bh. reads according to Śau. In *b,* Sāyaṇa also reads *rákṣamāṇāḥ* and glosses it: 'protecting ourselves, i.e. on account of self-protection' (. . . *ātmānaṃ pālayamānāḥ*. . . . *ātmarakṣaṇād*

---

[85] Weber: "Jaṅgiḍa-Amulett gegen Viṣkandha (Reissen?) [*jaṅgiḍa*-amulet against *viṣkandha* (Rheumatism?)]," IS, 13: 140; Griffith: "The hymn is a charm to win protection and general prosperity," *Hymns of the Atharvaveda,* 1: 45; Bloomfield: "Charm with an amulet derived from the *jaṅgiḍa* tree, against diseases and demons," *Hymns,* 37, 280; Whitney-Lanman: "Against various evils: with a *jaṅgiḍá* amulet," *Atharva-veda-saṃhitā,* Pt. 1, 42; Grohmann translates vss. 3, 4 in his discussion of the plants *jaṅgiḍá* and *kúṣṭha,* "Medicinisches aus dem Atharva-Veda," IS, 9: 417–18.

[86] *kṛtyādūṣaṇārtham, ātmarakṣārtham, vighnaśamanārthaṃ ca;* cf. Keśava, *atha puruṣahave akāryakaraṇena vighnaśamanakarma ucyate* (cf. Bloomfield, *Hymns,* 281) and Dārila: "for the driving away of *piśāca*-demons" (*piśācacātanam*).

dhetor ity arthaḥ). In *c*, he, along with the *pada*-text, reads *viskandhadūṣaṇaṃ* and explains it as the one who wards off the obstruction (i.e. trouble) characterized by an impediment to going caused by the demons beginning with the *rakṣas* and *piśāca* or [the trouble] having the form of the drying up of the body (=*vískandha*) (*viskandhaḥ rakṣaḥpiśācādikṛtagatipratibandhātmakaḥ śarīraśoṣaṇarūpo vā vighnaḥ tasya nivārakam*); and in *d*, he defines *jaṅgiḍáṃ* simply as a type of tree well known in Vārāṇasī' (. . . *vṛkṣaviśeṣo vārāṇasyāṃ prasiddhaḥ*). *jaṅgiḍá* appears to be a plant which is indigenous to India (cf. Bloomfield, 280–81, and Grohmann, IS, 9: 417–19). The word *maṇím* in *c* denotes any small perforated object strung on a thread and worn on a part of the body (cf. Mayrhofer, Wb, 2: 556–57), but in the context with *jaṅgiḍá*, suggests 'amulet,' implying perhaps that it was composed of the precious plant and worn around the neck. Caland, based on Dārila's commentary to KauśS 8.15, 26.43 and 43.23, speculates that the plant may have been the *arjuna*-plant (AZ, 15, 81; cf. also Karambelkar, *The Atharva-Veda and the Āyur-Veda*, 301). Griffith draws the amusing analogy with the moly-plant (garlic?) which Hermes gave to Ulysses (45 n).

VERSE 2

P 2.11.2*ab* reads as Śau (it is wanting in K). *cd* is also found at P 7.7.1 in reference to an amulet fashioned from *darbha*-grass. P(K) *cd* is as Śau; O has *sa* for *maṇíḥ*, in *e*. For the obscure words in *ab*, Sāyaṇa defines as follows: *jambhá* is either the enemy such as sorceress, etc.; or else, it is the name of a kind of tooth, i.e. the chewing caused by a kind of demonic tooth (. . . *hiṃsakāt kṛtyādeḥ. yadvā jambha iti dantaviśeṣasya ākhyā. rākṣasadantaviśeṣakṛtāt khādanād ity arthaḥ*); *viśará* is the dissolution of the body (*śarīraviśaraṇāt*); and *abhiśócana* is the pain caused by sorceresses (*kṛtyākṛtāc chokāt*). Although these names appear to be demonic in character, they may, as Sāyaṇa suggests, also imply abnormal bodily states caused by them: references to *jambhá* point to its meaning as 'convulsion,' 'teething,' 'lock-jaw,' or as Caland, following Sāyaṇa, suggests, "ein Rakṣasa . . . der die Mundsperre . . . verursacht" (AZ, 103 n); *viśará* reflects the sense of 'tearing or contorting pain'; and *abhiśócana*, 'a burning or scorching pain.' The latter two are derived purely on etymological grounds (see, in particular, Filliozat, *La doctrine*, 106–107; cf. also Weber, 142; Bloomfield, 283–84; and Whitney-Lanman, 42).

VERSE 3

ab occurs at AVŚ 1.16.3 which has *idáṃ* in place of *ayáṃ* in *a* and *b* and which reads in *cd*: *anéna víśvā sasahe yā́ jā́nāni piśācyā́ḥ*, "with that [lead-amulet (*sísa*), see verse 2], I have overpowered all the types of *piśācī́*-demon" (P 1.10.2 has *jātāni* in *d*). In *b*, P 2.11.3 (verse 2, Barret) reads: *ayaṃ rakṣo 'pa* (Raghu Vira: *rakṣān apa*) *bādhate*, "It expels the *rakṣas*-demon"; and in *d*, K has *jaṅgiṇaḥ*, which Barret explains may be a peculiarity of K (JAOS, 30: 199). Bh., however, reads as Śau; K has *jaṅgiṇa* throughout. In *c, viśvábheṣajo* may also, as Sāyaṇa points out, mean that in which there is all (i.e. complete) medicine. The meaning is that it is entirely medicinal in character (. . . *viśvaṃ kṛtsnaṃ bheṣajaṃ yasmin. sakalauṣadhātmaka ity arthaḥ*).

VERSE 4

P 2.11.4 reads as Śau. In *b,* Sāyaṇa explains *mayobhúvā* as that which becomes pleasure (*maya iti sukhanāma. tad bhavaty asmād iti mayobhūḥ*); thus, 'pleasurable' or 'delightful'; and in *c,* he states that *rákṣāṃsi* is a synecdoche for the demons beginning with the *bhūtas, pretas* and *piśācas* (*rakṣaḥśabdopalakṣitān bhūtapretapiśācādīn*).

VERSE 5

In *ab,* P 2.11.5 has *śaṇaś* (K: *khanaś*) *ca tvā jaṅgiḍaś ca viṣkandhād adhi* (K: *abhi*) *muñcatām,* "Let both the hemp[-cord] [or K: uprooting one (?)] and the *jaṅgiḍa*[-amulet] release you from *viṣkandha*"; *cd* is as Śau. We, with Sāyaṇa, understand *śaṇáś* to refer to the cord used to bind the amulet (. . . *prasiddhaḥ maṇibandhanasūtraprakṛtibhūtaḥ;* cf. KauśS 42.23: . . . *mantrokta bandhāti,* and Weber, 142; Bloomfield, 284 and Whitney-Lanman, 42). In *d,* he defines *kṛṣyā́* as agriculture, i.e. the type of occupation of husbandmen (*kṛṣiḥ karṣakavyāpāraviśeṣaḥ*) and *rásebhyaḥ* as a wood consisting of the essence of herbs (*oṣadhisārabhūtakāṣṭhebhyaḥ*). *kṛṣyā́ . . . rásebhyaḥ,* meaning literally, 'the saps of agriculture,' suggests rather the sense of best parts of products of the ploughed land, i.e. 'the essences of cultivation.' There is some disagreement concerning the origin of the hemp and the *jaṅgiḍá.* Weber assumes that the hemp was wild-growing, i.e. in the forest, and the *jaṅgiḍá* was cultivated in the field (142). Bloomfield, on the other hand, supposes the opposite: "The hemp, of course, comes from the sap of the furrow; *jaṅgiḍá* the tree, from the forest" (284). We have no way of knowing for sure which interpretation is correct; however, hemp commonly grows in the wild and such an important plant as *jaṅgiḍá* may well have been cultivated. The parallelism in the verse would tend also to support this supposition.

VERSE 6

This verse is repeated at AVŚ 19.34.4. In *ab,* however, it has the slight variant: *kṛtyādū́ṣaṇa evā́yám átho arātidū́ṣaṇaḥ.* P 11.3.4 follows 19.34.4, but has *kṛtyādūṣaṇa vā ayam,* in *a. pāda d,* as Bloomfield points out, may be formulaic (284). Since this verse is not found at P 2.11, Whitney-Lanman imply that it may have been added, spoiling the book's normal five verses in each hymn (43). Sāyaṇa explains the import of the verse as describing the efficacy of the indicated result accompanied by the praising of the amulet (*maṇeḥ praśaṃsāpūrvakam abhilaṣitaphalasādhanatvaṃ pradarśyate . . .*).

Notes to 3.9

Most translators consider AVŚ 3.9 to be a charm against *víṣkandha* and other evils or demons.[87] Sāyaṇa prescribes its use "in a rite for the removing of impediments"[88] at KauśS 43.1–2. Like AVŚ 2.4, this charm appears from the context to have originally been recited during the ritualistic binding and consecration of the amulets which include, as verse 6 implies, the *víṣkandha*-ruining, *jaṅgiḍá*-amulet.

VERSE 1

Two parallels to this verse occur at P 3.7.2 and 2.64.3. In *a*, P(K) 3.7.2 has: *karṣabhasya viṣabhasya* (Bh. as Śau); and in *d*, Bh. reads, along with K manuscript, *tathāpi kṛṇutā punaḥ*, "so also you must produce again." Bar. and Raghu Vira emend to read as Śau. P 2.64.3*a*, however, has *kaśyapasya pratisaro dyauṣ*, "[There is] the cord of Kaśyapa; heaven . . ."; and in *d*, it reads *tathāpi* (K: *tathābhi*) *kṛṇutā punaḥ*, "so also you must produce it again." The two words *karśáphasya* and *viśaphásya* are rather obscure. Sāyaṇa explains them as follows: *karśápha* is that having hoofs (?) or a small-hoofed one, i.e. a wild beast beginning with a tiger (*karaśaphasya kṛśaśaphasya vā śvāpadasya vyāghrādeḥ* . . .), and *viśaphá* is that devoid of hoofs, i.e. black snakes, etc., which rival man or one whose hoofs are manifested, i.e. fierce cattle, buffaloes, etc. (*vigataśaphasya spardhamānapuruṣakālasarpādeḥ vispaṣṭaśaphasya vā krūragomahiṣādeḥ* . . .). These explanations are merely guesswork based on fanciful etymologies. Weber, on the other hand, understands the words to be derived from the root *kṛś*, 'to be lean,' and *viś*, 'to enter,' plus the suffix *(a)pha* = *(a)bha* (see Whitney, *Grammar*, #1199 and Wackernagel-Debrunner, 2:745 and 746f.) and translates: "of the emaciating one" and "of the piercing one," respectively (215). This derivation of the two words receives some support from P(K) 3.7.2. The roots involved, however, are *kṛṣ*, 'to dig' and *viṣ*, 'to subdue,' suggesting that *karṣabha* might mean 'an animal which digs' and *viṣabha*, 'an animal which subdues' (i.e. a poisonous animal). Since, however, the P(K) reading of this verse is open to question, this interpretation receives only limited support. The PW defines the two terms as goblins or diseases (cf. also Mayrhofer, Wb, 1: 176). Whitney-Lanman suggest, although hesitatingly, that they appear from the context to be "two varieties of *víṣkandha*" (so also, Karambelkar, *The Atharva-Veda and the Āyur-Veda*, 272). P 2.64.3*a*, however, implies the *kaśyapa* is an amulet which is bound to the patient by means of a *pratisara*, 'cord' or 'string' (cf. also Kaśyapa as the author of a medicinal

---

87 Weber: "Spruch gegen Viṣkandham (Charm against *viṣkandha*)," IS, 17: 215; Griffith: "The hymn is a charm against Viṣkandha or Rheumatism," *Hymns of the Atharvaveda*, 1: 91; Bloomfield: "Against *viṣkandha* and *kābava* (hostile demons)," *Hymns*, 67, 339; and Whitney-Lanman: "Against *víṣkandha* and other evils," *Atharva-veda-saṃhitā*, Pt. 1, 98.

88 *vighnaśamanakarmaṇi*; cf. Keśava: *punar vighnaśamanam ucyate* and Dārila: *piśācanāśanam*, 'for the destruction of the *piśāca*-demons.'

hymn at AVŚ 2.33.7). By analogy, therefore, *karśápha* and *viśapha* may also be types of amulets which were divinely given and must be divinely removed (or, if we read *api*, along with P, in *d:* they must repeatedly be prepared). It follows that they would have been auspicious because elsewhere we find that medicinal herbs are said to have had heaven as their father and earth as their mother (see AVŚ 8.7.2 and 3.23.6; cf. also Bloomfield, 339–40). It seems possible, therefore, given the context of the entire hymn, that *karśápha* and *viśaphá* were auspicious elements, perhaps vegetal amulets. We may, also, propose on the basis of P 3.7.2 and 2.64.3 the reading of *api* (or *abhi*) in *d*. In this way, the verse may be understood as consecrating two vegetal amulets by imposing on them divine parentage and by requesting the gods, who once produced them, to do the same again now for the purpose of the rite.

VERSE 2

In *a,* P 3.7.3 has: *aśleṣmāṇo;* and in *c,* K has *kṣiṇomi,* 'I destroy.' In *a,* Sāyaṇa also reads *aśleṣmā̃ṇo* and, basing himself on KauśS 43.1, 2, explains it as "people unaffected by hindrances, i.e. void of the attainment of the effects desired [by the hindrances]; or else, gods with divine bodies devoid of [material] bodies defiled by the three *doṣas* ('humors') characterized by phlegm and who bear (=*adhārayan*) the amulet made from the *aralu*-tree and the staff, etc. for the purpose of calming the hindrances" (. . . *aśliṣṭāḥ vighnair abhimatakāryasaṃprāptiśūnyā janāḥ. . . . yadvā śleṣmopalakṣitatridoṣadūṣitaśarīrarahitāḥ divyadehā devāḥ. . . . vighnaśamanāya araluvṛkṣavikāramaṇiṃ daṇḍādikaṃ ca dhṛtavantaḥ*). Weber renders the word "without nooses" (*a—śreṣmā̃no*) and explains that the injured one is covered firmly and laced around with bonds (verses 3, 4) of hemp (AVŚ 2.4.5). Continuing, he states: ". . . dadurch wird die Krankheit gebunden, ihrer mascula virtus beraubt, gerade wie die Castration der Ochsen durch Abbinden, Abschnüren den Hoden herbeigeführt wird . . ." (216). This suggestion receives some support from Griffith (92) and Whitney-Lanman (98). Bloomfield offers another purely conjectural translation: "Without fastening they (the protecting plants) held fast . . ." (67, 340). Karambelkar renders: "Without fastenings they held it" and offers a completely different interpretation: he assumes without question that the word *víṣkandham* (in *c*) is formed from *vi* + *skandha* and that *skandha* in the first instance means "shoulder (the joint with muscles)" and secondarily "all the joints with their muscles." In this way, the fastenings would be the muscles and the phrase *aśreṣmā̃ṇo adhārayan* would mean: "the joints were hanging loose without support from the muscles." The treatment for such a condition, therefore, involved the tying of the joints with the amulet of *jaṅgiḍá* or *aralu* in the same way that the bull's testicles, which are about to be castrated, are tied. In support of his interpretation, he quotes from vaguely related passages in the *Suśruta-* and *Caraka-Saṃhitās*, all but one of which he has identified (*The Atharva-Veda and The Āyur-Veda,* 272–74). The principal meaning of *aśreṣmā̃no*, as we gather from the P and Sāyaṇa, is 'without bonds,' 'without fasteners.' From the context, it would appear that the charm was recited while the healer bound an amulet which had the power to destroy various demons. For this reason, it is unlikely that the "fasteners" referred either to people, gods, bands of hemp, or unsupported joints. They may, however, refer to vegetal amulets which Manu had once, in the distant past, bound without the use of thread. On Manu's possible connection with an Atharvavedic rite, compare ṚV 1.80.16.

VERSE 3

In *b,* P 3.7.4 has: *yadá badhnati;* and in *c,* K manuscript has *sravasyaṃ* (Raghu Vira: *sravasyuṃ,* 'swift'); Bh. *śravasyaṃ.* For the obscure *khṛ́galaṃ,* Sāyaṇa, on the strength of ṚV 2.39.4 where the word has the meaning, 'armor,' glosses it as "protection for the body" (*tanutrāṇam*). Weber conceives it to be related to *kharju* (root *kharj*), 'itching,' 'scratching,' 'biting'; and thus it is a brush for scratching (217). Bloomfield accepts the explanation of Sāyana, and, on the authority of KauśS 43.1, where an amulet from the wood of the *aralu*-tree is tied to the possessed one by means of a reddish brown thread, understands it to mean a "talisman" (67, 339–40). On the same basis, T. Chowdhury further equates it with *daṇḍa* and defines it as 'stick' (JBORS, 17: 67). Cf. also Kuiper, who derives it from a proto-Munda word **ya-ḍa* plus the prefix **ker* and defines it as 'stock' (Mayrhofer, Wb, 1: 310–11). Because it was bound on to the red thread, and because of the mention of this practice at KauśS 43.1, one would tend to favor the interpretation of an amulet, perhaps in the form of a stick or stock. In *c,* Sāyaṇa, like P(Bh), reads *śravasyáṃ* for the difficult *śravasyúṃ* and understands it to be a food (?) (*śrava ity annanāma. bālarūpam annam arhati . . .*). Weber assumes it to refer to a greedy demon who is eager for glory (216–17). On the strength of the P(K) reading *sravasyaṃ* (*sravasyuṃ*), from root *sru,* 'to flow,' *sravasyuṃ* has been rendered as 'flowing' or perhaps 'fleeting,' which brings to mind the notion of an apparition (cf. verse 4, and Whitney-Lanman, 98). On the general fiery sense of *śúṣmam,* see Bloomfield, ZDMG, 48: 574. *kā̃bavám* is also obscure. Sāyaṇa explains it as "a hindrance related to the *kabu,* which is a ferocious animal with a spotted color" (*kabuḥ karburavarṇaḥ krūraḥ prāṇī. tatsaṃbandhī vighnaḥ kā̃bavaḥ*). Weber suggests that it may be onomatopoeic for groaning (217). Mayrhofer states that it might be the "name of a certain evil spirit" and that the connections with the Slavic words meaning protecting-spirit are hardly correct (Wb, 1: 199). Although its exact meaning is unknown, it would appear from the context to be an inauspicious name or a demon whom, like *víṣkandha,* the healer, by the use of the bound wooden amulet, hoped to make devoid of harmful power. In *d, bandhúraḥ* is troublesome. Sāyaṇa explains it either as "that amulet [of *aralu*-wood] bound by us; or else, he reads *bandhúrā̃ḥ,* i.e. the amulet, staff, etc. being carried by us" (*asmā̃bhir api bandhaḥ sa maṇiḥ. . . . yadvā̃ bandhuraḥ. . . . bandhurā̃ḥ as-*

mābhir dhāryamāṇāḥ maṇidaṇḍādayaḥ . . .). Weber reads *bandhúrāḥ* and conceives it as "bonds," perhaps referring to the Ṛgvedic meaning 'strap,' or 'strap-material.' He, thus, offers the interpretation that a brush for scratching was given to the sick man partially to alleviate his pains; and partially, the suffering parts were laced firmly around with ties (217). Bloomfield speculates "fastenings" (67 and 341) and Whitney-Lanman translate: "binder," quoting Sāyaṇa (98). It would appear that it refers to an amulet or amulets, as Sāyaṇa suggests, which are fastened on to the thread and on to the victim, as opposed to those, in verse 2, which are "devoid of fasteners."

VERSE 4

In *a,* P(K) 3.7.5 has *sravasyavaś* (K manuscript: *sravasyo;* Bar: *sravasyāś*); Bh.: *śravasyo.* Sāyaṇa here explains *śravasyavaś* as "people seeking food or honor by the conquest of the enemy" (*he janāḥ. . . . śravaḥ annaṃ yaśo vā. tat śatrujayena ātmana icchantaḥ*). On *bándhurā,* see previous note. Karambelkar argues that *kapír* is the name of a plant, either *kapivalli* or *kapiśāka* and renders *cd:* "the tying is the effective check of *kābavá* as *kapi* (a plant?) is that of the dog's bite" (*The Atharva-Veda and the Āyur-Veda,* 274 and notes). It seems, rather, to mean 'monkey' whose noises and commotion ward off dogs as the bound amulet does the *kābavá*-demon.

VERSE 5

P(K) 3.7.6, although quite corrupted, has been emended to read *ab* as Śau (following the Roth-Whitney edition). Bh., however, has: . . . *bhantsyāmi dūṣayitvā kābavam,* ". . . , having ruined *kābava,* I will bind. . . ." In *c,* Bar. and Raghu Vira have suggested: *uttarāvanto rathā,* 'victorious chariots'; Bh. reads as Śau. In *a,* the Roth-Whitney edition has *bhartsyā̃mi,* 'I will revile.' Sāyaṇa reads *bhatsyā̃mi* and glosses "I bind" (*badhnāmi;* i.e. root *bandh*) or "I burn" (*dīpayāmi;* i.e. from root *bhand,* 'to be bright'?). This reading is followed by the Viśveśvarānanda edition. Whitney-Lanman, however, suggest the emendation, *bhantsyā̃mi,* 'I will bind,' which we have accepted. In *c,* Sāyaṇa reads *údāśávo* as one word, glossing: "fast horses, i.e. like chariots yoked with horses, looking up ready to go" (*āśuraśvaḥ. gamanonmukhair vegavadbhiḥ aśvair yuktā rathā iva . . .*); and in *d,* he reads *cariṣyatha,* glossing "go as one pleases" (*yatheṣṭaṃ saṃcarata*). He understands *d* to mean: "you people being separated from the curses, i.e. the abuses caused by the hindrances made by others (i.e. your enemies), go as you please" (. . . *he janā yūyaṃ . . . śapathaiḥ parakṛtair vighnanimittair ākrośaiḥ. viyuktāḥ santa iti seṣaḥ. . . . yatheṣṭaṃ saṃcarata*). It might be better, however, to render *śapáthebhiḥ,* like the previous translators, as an instrumental of accompaniment, i.e. "along with the curses" (see in particular Weber, 217, Bloomfield, 67, and Whitney-Lanman, 99). The plural subject of *sariṣyatha* may be the 101 *víṣkandhas* mentioned in verse 6*a.* In fact, it would make better sense if we reversed 5*ab* and 6*ab* and then reversed the order of the half-verses in 6, making it verse 5. In this way, we would render for verse 5: "Of these [amulets], the [gods] originally selected you, the *víṣkandha*-ruining amulet. Indeed, for the sake of ruining, I will bind you [O, amulet and] I will ruin the *kābavá*"; verse 6: "[Likewise,] together with the curses, you, the hundred and one *víṣkandhas*, scattered over the earth, will go forth like speedy chariots." One suspects this to be the meaning of the last two verses.

VERSE 6

In *cd,* P 3.7.1 reads *teṣāṃ ca* (Bh: *teṣān tu*) *sarveṣām idam asti* (Bh: *astu*) *viṣkandhadūṣaṇam,* "and of all those [amulets], this one is *viṣkandha*-ruining"; or following Bh: "Indeed, of all those [amulets], let this one be *viṣkandha*-ruining." For *cd,* Sāyaṇa renders: "For the cessation of the hindrances (=*téṣāṃ*), the gods previously drew you, O amulet, out (reading: *újjahruḥ*). Hence, I bear this amulet fashioned from the *aralu*-tree" (*teṣāṃ vighnānāṃ nivṛttaye he maṇe tvām . . . pūrvam ujjahruḥ devā uddhṛtavantaḥ. ataḥ . . . imam araluvṛkṣavikāraṃ maṇim. aham api dhārayāmīti vākyaśeṣaḥ*). Similarly Bloomfield: "for these . . . they brought out thee, the amulet, that destroys *viṣkandha*" (67; cf. also Weber, 218 and Griffith, 92). Although this is a forced sense of the genitive, the interpretation is possible. One would suppose rather that *téṣāṃ* refers to various amulets (see verses 1, 2, 3) as implied by the P and Whitney-Lanman (99), of which the gods (verse 1) originally selected the *víṣkandha*-ruining one which, on the basis of AVŚ 2.4.1, was the amulet fashioned from the *jaṅgiḍá*-plant. On the inauspicious number 101, see, in particular, Kuhn, KZ, 13: 128ff. and Griffith, 92 n.

Notes to 19.34

Most translators consider AVŚ 19.34 to be a charm for protection and against diseases with the *jaṅgiḍá*-amulet.[89] Sāyaṇa mentions that it, along with AVŚ 19.35, is found at *Śāntikalpa* 17.4 and 19.6 in the *mahāśānti,* 'great consecration,' called 'wind,' where an amulet made from the wood of the *jaṅgiḍá*-plant is employed.[90]

Although the charm does not expressly so state, it is clear from AVŚ 2.4 that the *jaṅgiḍá* mentioned here is an amulet fashioned from the parts of the so-called *jaṅgiḍá*-tree. Like AVŚ 2.4 the principal function of the amulet appears to have been protection from evil forces and from the effects of witchcraft as well as destruction of disease.

---

[89] Bloomfield: "Charm with an amulet derived from the *jaṅgiḍa*-tree, against disease and demons," *Hymns* 38, 669; Griffith: "A protective charm addressed to the panacea called *jaṅgiḍa,*" *Hymns of the Atharvaveda,* 2: 291 and Whitney-Lanman: "With a *jaṅgidá*-amulet: for protection, etc.," *Atharva-veda-saṃhitā,* Pt. 2, 950. Parts also rendered by Grohmann, IS, 9: 417–18.

[90] *vihitāyāṃ vāyavyākhyāyāṃ mahāśāntau jaṅgiḍavṛkṣanirmitaṃ maṇiṃ badhnīyāt.*

VERSE 1

Based on verse 6 below, Roth and Whitney suggest that *a* should be emended to *áṅgirā asi jaṅgiḍa,* "You are an Aṅgiran, O *jaṅgiḍá* . . ."; and at the end of *b,* they emend to *jaṅgiḍa* (vocative). This reading is followed by Grohmann (417), Griffith (291) and Bloomfield (38, 670–71). Later, however, Whitney-Lanman withdrew the suggested emendations and read *ab* as we do: *jaṅgiḍó 'si jaṅgiḍó rákṣitā 'si jaṅgiḍáḥ.* In *a,* P 11.3.1 reads as Śau. Sāyaṇa reads the second *jaṅgiḍá,* in *a,* as a vocative: *jaṅgiḍa.* The translation would certainly be easier if both in *a* and *b* vocatives are read. For the sake of emphasis, however, the nominative seems to have been preferred (cf. AVŚ 4.12.1 and Whitney-Lanman, 951). Sāyaṇa explains that the *jaṅgiḍá* is the name of a certain type of herb well-known in the north (*jaṅgiḍo nāma kaścid oṣadhiviśeṣaḥ, sa ca uttaradeśe prasiddhaḥ*) and considers it to have been used as an amulet (*he jaṅgiḍa maṇe* . . . and again . . . *jaṅgiḍo jaṅgiḍākhyo maṇi*). See also AVŚ 2.4.1, 2, 4, 6 where it is called an amulet (*maṇí*). Its protective or prophylactic aspect is also mentioned at AVŚ 2.4.1–3, 5. That is, in fact, the dominant quality of the amulet. In *c, divpā̃c* and *cátuṣpād* are accusative adjectives, governing *sárvaṃ* in *d,* and may be rendered: "our whole [property consisting of] bipeds [and] quadrupeds" (cf. Sāyaṇa: . . . *yad* . . . *pādadvayopetaṃ manuṣyādilakṣaṇam asti tathā* . . . *pādacatuṣṭayopetaṃ gomahiṣādilakṣaṇam asti*).

VERSE 2

In *a,* Roth-Whitney originally suggested the emendation: *akṣakṛtyā̃s,* 'the sorceries with dice,' which was followed by Griffith (292). Later, Whitney-Lanman changed the emendation to *kṛtyā̃s,* 'the witchcrafts' (951) which is based on Bloomfield's suggestion and reading (38, 671). P(K) 11.3.2 has *yāḥ kṛcchrās,* "the causers of pain, who . . . ," which is also possible; but O has: *mā* (=*yā*?) *gṛtsyas.* We read: *yā̃ gṛtsyas,* "the clever ones, who . . . ," which Sāyaṇa glosses: "witches who are accustomed to greed" (. . . *gardhanaśīlā yāḥ* . . . *kṛtyāḥ* . . .). In *c,* Roth-Whitney, based on Sāyaṇa (i.e. *hatavīryān svavyāpāre kuṇṭhitaśaktīn,* "powerless ones who have a dulled ability in their own function"), emended to *sárvān vínaṣṭatejaso 'rasā̃m,* which is followed by Griffith (292) and Bloomfield (38, 672). P has *sarvān vinaktu tejaso* (O: *vinaktatejaso*) which is our reading. *vinaktu,* from the root *vic,* 'to shift,' 'to separate,' has the sense of separation from, as grain from the chaff (MWSED, s.v.). Cf. Whitney-Lanman's long note on these various readings (951–52). In *b,* Sāyaṇa understands *kṛtyā* in the compound *kṛtyākṛtáś* to be "an effigy, etc. fashioned with clay and wood, etc." (*kṛtyā nāma mṛddārvādinā nirmitaputtalyādi*). Since *pādas a* and *c* are rather doubtful, the entire verse is questionable. Our translation implies that the healer is requesting the *jaṅgiḍá*-amulet to remove from the sorcerers their effectual power, thereby, making them powerless. The clever ones may have been types of wizards who, like the practitioners of witchcraft, were skilled in "black magic."

VERSE 3

In *b,* Roth-Whitney read: *visrásaḥ* (accent on the second syllable). In *a,* P(K) 11.3.3 has *nāḍam* which may mean, 'a hollow stalk' (=*nāla,* related to *nāḍī,* 'tube'); and in *d: sādhaya,* 'cause to succeed'; 'subdue'; O has *viśasaḥ,* in *b,* and *jaṅgiḍāmātīm iṣuva uteva sādhaya,* in *cd.* The P reading of *nāḍam* suggests a type of ritualistic instrument used for making sounds. *pādas a* and *b* are rather obscure. We have rendered them by borrowing the subject and verb from verse 2*d.* Sāyaṇa does so for *a;* but in *b,* he understands *arasāḥ saptá vísrasaḥ* as nominative feminine plurals. It is easier to construe them as accusative feminine plurals in agreement with the accusatives in *a.* Sāyaṇa considers the "seven debilities" (*saptá vísrasaḥ*) to be "seven sorcery-produced slackenings, i.e. discharges [from] within the seven skull-situated-openings having the form of the two nostrils, the two eye-sockets, the two ear-cavities and the mouth-cavity" (. . . *saptasaṃkhyākā visraṃsanāḥmūrdhaniṣṭheṣu nāsārandhradvayacakṣurgolakadvayaśrotracchidradvayamukhakuhararūpeṣu saptasu cchidreṣu abhicaratā utpāditāḥ sapta niṣyandā* . . .). Bloomfield, on etymological grounds, suggests that they refer to "seven debilitating (charms)" (38, 672); and Griffith, rendering: "seven decays," conjectures that they are the "gradual stages of increasing debility as old age comes on" (292 and n). It is difficult to know to what exactly the deceitful sound and the seven debilities refer. The artificially produced, deceitful sound may suggest the noises produced by an instrument other than the human voice, as P seems to imply, which were employed in the witchcraft rite. The seven debilities or declines (root *sraṅs,* 'to fall' plus *vi,* 'away') could also refer to the ritual practices of sorcerers; what they exactly signify, however, has been lost in obscurity. In *c, ámatim,* 'indigence,' from the root *am,* like *ámīvā,* seems to reflect the sense of disease, i.e. a demonically caused malady, perhaps the illness associated with malnutrition and poverty (see chapter on *ámīvā,* 49–53, above).

VERSE 4

In *ab,* P(K) 11.3.4 has *vā ayaṃ atho 'rātidūṣaṇaḥ,* "This . . . [witchcraft-ruining] or else enemy-ruining . . ."; O, however, is as Śau. Cf. also AVŚ 2.4.6. Again it seems clear that the word "amulet" (*maṇí*) is implied by *jaṅgiḍá.*

VERSE 5

In *c,* Roth-Whitney read: *sāsahé.* P 11.3.5 is the same as Śau. Sāyaṇa defines *víṣkandha* as a great wind-type disease causing the dislocation of the shoulders (. . . *viśliṣṭaskandham evaṃ nāmānaṃ vātaviśeṣaṃ mahārogam* . . .). *sáṃskandha,* being the only occurrence of the word, appears to be the opposite of *víṣkandha,* as Sāyaṇa implies: "The disease by which the shoulder becomes curved [or] closed" (*yena rogeṇa skandhaḥ saṃnataḥ saṃlagno bhavati sa rogaḥ saṃskandhaḥ;* cf. also Whitney-Lanman, 952, and

Mayrhofer, Wb, 3: 506). Zimmer simply suggests that it is the contracting of the shoulders (*Leben,* 391) and Griffith states that *víṣkandha* and *sáṃskandha* are "apparently different forms of acute rheumatic pains in the shoulders and neck" (292 n). Filliozat considers that their precise meanings are uncertain (*La doctrine,* 106–107). In *cd,* Sāyaṇa reads *saha* for *sāsáha* and construes it with *ójasā:* "[Its] greatness [=*ojáḥ*] together with the disease's power destroys the great disease characterized by wind" (*taṃ mahārogaṃ vātalakṣaṇam ojaḥ mahimā ojasā saha rogasya sāmarthyena saha nāśayati*). In other words, Sāyaṇa suggests a sympathetic healing; whereby the power of the amulet together with the disease's own power brings about the destruction of the malady. While it is unlikely that *saha* should be read for *sāsáha,* it is possible that *sāsáha . . . ója ójasā* could mean the conquering of the power by its own power; or *ójasā* may, like *mahimā* in *a,* refer to the power, energy or force which the *jaṅgiḍá* possesses. *ojás* may also be the power or energy of the disease entities *víṣkandha* and *sáṃskandha* (cf. Bloomfield, 38) and any, perhaps evil, force (cf. Griffith, 292, and Whitney-Lanman, 952). Since the *jaṅgiḍá* was considered to be an amulet which protects one from evil, we are inclined to regard *ojás* as a power possessed by hostile sorcerers and that one of the functions of the amulet was to turn the evil back on itself, thereby causing its own destruction. In this way, it illustrates a type of sympathetic or associative magic found in the context of the healing ritual.

VERSE 6

For *trís,* P(K) 11.3.6 has *niṣ*(?); O: *tṛṣṭrā* (=*triṣṭrā*?). We have condensed *cd* for the sake of a better translation. Literally it would be rendered: "The ancient Brāhmaṇas knew him indeed as you the Aṅgiras." Sāyaṇa understands *áṅgirā* as the name of a great *ṛṣi;* or else, it is *aṅgāras*, the name of a people (. . . *aṅgiraākhyo maharṣiḥ. yadvā aṅgirā aṅgārāḥ*). Bloomfield states that it seems to be a trumped pun on the word *jaṅgiḍá* (673). It could refer to the well-known Aṅgiras from whom the use of the amulet was derived. It would, therefore, have borne their name. Note the mythological reference to its divine origin and to its auspiciousness deriving from its having been known for a long time in the tradition of the Brāhmaṇas. Since the *jaṅgiḍá* is "fixed in the earth," it would appear to have been a tree or woody plant, from which an amulet was fashioned.

VERSE 7

For *taranti,* 'surpass,' P(K) 11.3.7 has *caranti,* 'pervade'; O: *tarantu,* 'Let . . . [not] surpass.' In *c,* Sāyaṇa reads *jaṅgiḍáḥ* as a vocative (*he jaṅgiḍa* . . .), which is easier; and in *d,* the *pada*-text resolves *páripāṇaḥ* as *paripānaḥ* which, from the root *pā,* 'to drink,' could mean 'beverage.' Sāyaṇa, however, reads as *páripāṇaḥ* and glosses: "one who protects all around" (*paritaḥ pātā* . . .). In *d, sumaṅgálaḥ* has the literal meaning: 'having good luck' or 'very auspicious.' In this context, however, it may be better to render it as "bringer of success," "bestower of good fortune," etc. The old herbs, mentioned in *a*, may help to elucidate the mythology of verse 6; or, they could merely refer to herbs which have been kept for a long time and thus have become withered and dry, in contrast to those which are new and fresh; or better, they may point to the developing stage of ancient Indian materia medica, when new medical substances were being discovered.

VERSE 8

This verse is hopelessly corrupted. For *a*, Roth-Whitney emend: *átho yadā́ samábhavo,* "and when you . . . arose." This is followed by Griffith (293) and Bloomfield (673). P 11.3.8 has *aśva yo padāni* (O: *aśvo padān*) *bhagavo jaṅgiḍāmitavīrya* (O: °*yaḥ*). In *c*, Roth-Whitney emend to *ugrāgratá,* ". . . O Powerful one, at first . . . ." Again, this is followed by Griffith and Bloomfield. P offers a plausible alternative to *cd: purā te ugrāya sata upendro vīryaṃ dadhau* (O: *vīryān dadau,* 'added strengths'), "to you, being previously powerful, Indra adds strength" (cf. Whitney-Lanman, 953). In *a, upadāna* is the only occurrence of the word. Sāyaṇa explains it as a vocative from the root *dā* plus *upa, ā,* " 'to be acquired,' i.e. you who are appropriated in the functions beginning with the removal of witchcraft" (*he upadāna upādīyate svīkriyate kṛtyānirharaṇādivyāpāreṣv iti upadānaḥ. tasya saṃbodhanam*). This explanation is purely conjectural and offers no real solution to the meaning of the word. For *pādas cd,* he suggests: "[O *jaṅgiḍá*], Indra, having recognized that beings having raised strength will eat you (=*purā́ grasta*), has given [you] strength unsurpassed by others, so that the powerful ones do not eat you" (. . . *he jaṅgiḍa . . . tvām . . . udgūrṇabalāḥ prāṇinaḥ purā graste bhakṣayiṣyantīti vijñāya indraḥ yathā tvām ugrā na bhakṣayanti tathā . . . parairanabhibhāvyaṃ sāmarthyam . . . prādāt*). Here again, Sāyaṇa is merely playing with the text, for *grasta(e)* is a singular middle, not a plural; yet *ugrā́* is understood by the *pada*-text as *ugrā́ḥ,* nominative or accusative feminine plural. If we read *ugrā́* as a nominative feminine singular and as the subject of *grasta,* which is to be understood in the past sense because of *purā́,* we may render tentatively as above. It is uncertain, however, to what the "powerful female" refers; perhaps she should be thought of as a female demon (cf. Bloomfield, 673). Since *ugrá* is used to describe *jaṅgiḍá* in the previous verse and Indra in the next verse (cf. Sāyaṇa there), we would expect it to have one or the other function here; but it is feminine. The verse is quite impossible; and any rendering is purely speculative. Our translation is based on the Viśveśvarānanda edition and has tried to incorporate the notions suggested in P's reading of *cd.*

VERSE 9

For *cd,* P(K) 11.3.9 reads: *amīvās sarvā rakṣāṃsi jahi raksāṇsy oṣadhe,* "O herb, kill the *amīvā*s [and] all the *rakṣas*-demons"; O has *tāmāvaḥ* (=*amīvāḥ*?), in *c,* and the remainder is as Śau. The repetition of *rakṣāṃsi* in K is merely a mistake or it serves as an intensifier. AVŚ 4.19.8*cd* (a hymn against enemies with a plant) reads very similarly to *ab: índras te vīrudhāṃ pata ugrá ojmā́nam ā́ dadhat,* "May powerful Indra grant energy to you, O lord of the plants." The idea of verse 8 seems to be carried over to verse 9*ab* and is also found elsewhere in the AVŚ. Sāyaṇa understands *vanaspate* to refer to *jaṅgiḍá* and reads *ugrá* as a vocative to agree with *vanaspate (jaṅgiḍá).* This keeps the continuity of the hymn, but does not follow the grammar of the verse (cf. notes to previous verse).

VERSE 10

In *a,* P 11.3.10 is as Śau (K has *āśarīraṃ*); and in *d,* it reads: *arasaṃ.* Sāyaṇa conceives *ā́śarīkaṃ* to be the name of a disease which is completely injurious (*sarvato hiṃsakam etannāmānaṃ rogaṃ . . .*) and *víśarīkaṃ* to be the name [of a disease] which is selectively injurious (. . . *viseṣeṇa hiṃsakam etannāmānaṃ . . .*). Both words, being derived from the root *śṛ,* 'to crush,' suggest a disease or pain which wrenches the body. *ā́śarīkaṃ* could, therefore, be a pain which causes the body to constrict; and *víśarīkaṃ,* a pain which seems to twist the body apart. At AVŚ 2.4.2, there occurs the word *viśará* which may have the sense of 'tearing or contorting pain' (cf. Filliozat *La doctrine,* 106). *pṛṣṭyāmayám,* literally, 'pain in the ribs [or sides],' may indicate more generally, as Filliozat suggests, "backache" (mal des reins) or "lumbago" (ibid., 101). It is clearly a symptom of disease (see Narten St.II, 5/6: 162). Sāyaṇa simply states that it is the name of a disease which extends to all limbs (. . . *sarvāṅgavyāpinam etannāmānaṃ ca rogaṃ*). Cf. AVŚ 1.25.4; 5.22.7, 11, 13 and 9.8.6.

Notes to 19.35

Most translators consider AVŚ 19.35, like 19.34, to be a charm for protection, especially from diseases, with the *jaṅgiḍá*-amulet.[91] Sāyaṇa mentions that is to be used along with 19.34 in the rite for the binding of the *jaṅgiḍa*-amulet at *Śāntikalpa* 17.4 and 19.6.[92]

This charm, like 19.34, is riddled with obscurities. It is, however, apparent that it was recited while the healer ritually tied the plant-amulet on to the victim of disease and of misfortune for the purpose of protecting him from further mishap. In fact, it appears to be essentially a shorter and a more condensed version of 19.34.

---

[91] Grohmann translates the charm in the course of his discussion of the two medicinal plants *jaṅgiḍá* and *kúṣṭha,* which are called upon to heal one suffering from *takmán*'s attacks, IS, 9: 418–19; Zimmer translates the charm under his discussion of the healing plant (Heilpflanze), *jaṅgiḍa, Leben,* 65; Bloomfield: "Charm with an amulet from the *jaṅgiḍa*-tree, against disease and demons," *Hymns,* 39, 674; Griffith: "A protective charm addressed to the magical *jaṅgiḍa,*" *Hymns of the Atharvaveda,* 2: 293; and Whitney-Lanman: "With a *jaṅgiḍá*-amulet: for protection, etc.," *Atharva-veda-saṃhitā,* Pt. 2, 953.

[92] *tasya jaṅgiḍamaṇibandhane pūrvasūktena saha ukto viniyogaḥ.*

VERSE 1

P 11.4.1 reads as Śau. In *ab,* Sāyaṇa renders: "previously the *ṛṣis*, uttering the name of the god, gave the amulet called *jaṅgiḍa* to men desiring protection for [their] superior strength" (*pūrve ṛṣayaḥ . . . devasya nāma . . . uccārayanto . . . jaṅgiḍākhyaṃ maṇim atiśayitavīryatvāya rakṣākāmebhyaḥ puruṣebhyo . . . dattavantaḥ*). In *cd,* he reads *viṣkandhabheṣajam* and glosses "the medicine for the great disease called *viṣkandha*" (*viṣkandhākhyasya mahārogasya auṣadhaṃ . . .*). Our translation follows on these general lines, reading, however, *viṣkandhadūṣaṇam,* in *d,* which goes with *bheṣajám* in *c.* Here as at AVŚ 19.34, the amulet fashioned from the *jaṅgiḍá*-plant is meant. At AVŚ 2.4.1 and 3.9.6, the *jaṅgiḍá*-amulet is called *víṣkandha*-ruining; at AVŚ 2.4.3, it is mentioned as being the medicine for all diseases; at AVŚ 2.4.4, the gods are said to have given it; and at AVŚ 19.34.6, they are stated as having created the *jaṅgiḍá*-plant.

VERSE 2

P 11.4.2 reads as Śau. At AVŚ 19.34.6, ancient Brāhmaṇas are said to have known *jaṅgiḍá* as "Aṅgiras"; at AVŚ 2.4.6 and 19.34.4, *jaṅgiḍá* is called enemy-ruining; and at AVŚ 19.34.7, it bears the epithet of protector.

VERSE 3

In *a,* Whitney-Lanman suggest the emendation: *durhā́rdaṃ ghorácakṣuṣam,* "The enemy of terrible aspect" (956; originally, Roth-Whitney read: *durhā́rdas tvā́ṃ ghorā́ṃ cákṣuḥ . . .*). In *b,* they read: *ā́gatam* for *ā́gamam;* and at the end of *d,* they emend to *jaṅgiḍa* (vocative) (also in Roth-Whitney's edition). P(K) 11.4.3*a* has *durhārdaṃ ghoracakṣuṣam* (O: *durhārdasaṃghoracakṣuṃ,* which looks like Śau); and in *b, āgatam* which is also read by Sāyaṇa. Both the reading of K and that of Sāyaṇa serve as the basis of Whitney-Lanman's suggested emendations. Sāyaṇa posits that *a* means: "the excessively ferocious eye of the evil-hearted enemy" (. . . *duṣṭahṛdayasya śatroḥ . . . atyantakrūraṃ cakṣuḥ*). It is likely that in our text *sáṃghoraṃ cákṣuḥ* refers to 'evil-eye' (see Grohmann, 419; Zimmer, 65; Bloomfield, 39, and Griffith, 293; cf. also Gonda, *Eye and Gaze,* 73). It may also, however, imply, along with Whitney-Lanman, the more general idea of horrible, dreadful or terrifying aspect or appearance of the evil-hearted one (i.e. the enemy). One is tempted to make *cákṣuḥ* the single object of the first line and to translate: "I have approached the evil-causing, dreadful eye of the enemy." The plural *tā́ṃs,* 'them,' in *c,* which refers to *ab,* however, suggests that there is more than one element in the first line. It might be better, therefore, to read *durhā́rdaḥ,* in *a* as a genitive singular and *ā́gamam,* in *b,* as a noun meaning, 'approaching,' governed by *pāpakṛ́tvānam,* i.e. "the very terrible eye of the enemy [and] the approaching [of that] which has done evil." In this way, there are two elements in *ab.* Zimmer (65) and Griffith (293) isolate three elements in the first line: the enemies, the evil-eye and the approaching sinner; Grohmann (149) and Whitney-Lanman, two: the enemy's dreadful glance or aspect and the evil doer; and Bloomfield notices two elements, but reads *ā̄gamam* as a first person singular aorist: "the evil eye of the hostile-minded (and) the evil doer I have approached" (39, 674). No reading is entirely satisfactory and a definitive translation is wanting. In *c*, Sāyaṇa, along with the *pada*-text, reads *pratibodhéna* and explains: "by your repugnant mind, or else by revealing the crime committed by them" (. . . *pratikūlayā tava buddhyā. yadvā tatkṛtāparādhodghāṭanena* . . .). At AVŚ 6.20.2, 4, 6, a thousand-eyed (*sahasrākṣá*), divine herb is used to discover types of evildoers (see also Gonda, *Eye and Gaze*, 72–73).

VERSE 4

P 11.4.4 reads as Śau. In *c*, Sāyaṇa understands *bhūtā̄t* to be the past time, i.e the living beings belonging to the past (*atītāt kālāt. bhūtasaṃbandhinaḥ prāṇijātād ity arthaḥ*), so also Zimmer (65) and Bloomfield (39). Grohmann (419), Griffith (293) and Whitney-Lanman (954) consider it to be the present time. This is possible; but, since the healer is asking for complete protection now from all abodes and plants, it would be logical for him to request it also from all times, the past, the future and the present; the last does not need to be expressed because he is, at the moment, making the request.

VERSE 5

This verse is difficult. For *ab*, Roth-Whitney emend: *yé kṛ́tvano devákṛtā yá utó mártyebhyaḥ*, "[Those] sorcerers who are divinely formed and also [those] who [are formed] by mortals." Most translators have followed this reading (see Grohmann, 419; Zimmer, 65; Bloomfield, 39, 674–75; Griffith 293 and Whitney-Lanman, 954). P 11.4.5*ab* reads: *ya ṛṣṇavo devakṛtā ya uto bibhṛte 'nyaḥ*. In *a*, Barret suggests the possible emendation: *he kṛṣṇā̄vo* "[Those] dark (i.e. sinister) ones who." We have, hesitatingly, followed the P-supported Viśveśvarānanda edition which has *yá ṛṣṇávo*, in *a*, and *vavṛté 'nyáḥ*, in *b*. Sāyaṇa understands the obscure *ṛṣṇávo* as from the root *ṛṣ*, 'to move,' and glosses: "movers, i.e. men who are injurers" (. . . *gantāro hiṃsakāḥ puruṣāḥ santi*); and in *b*, he reads: *yé utó vavarté 'nyé*, and renders: "and also oppressors urged by men, etc., who have remained" (. . . *api ca* . . . *manuṣyādipreritā bādhakā* . . . *vavṛtire* . . .). Although Sāyaṇa's explanation of *ṛṣṇávo* is rather fanciful, we can notice perhaps a contrast between those who move about (*ṛṣṇávo*, root *ṛṣ*) and those who have remained (*vavṛtá*, root *vṛt*). The exact meaning of the first line, however, is vague. The *ṛṣṇús* and the others who have remained may refer to individual practitioners of evil, as suggested by Sāyaṇa; or, they may be particular practices or effects of the sorcerers, or even, disease entities, demons and misfortunes which come and go. Since one is said to be "divinely made," we would tend to favor the latter two possibilities.

Cf. AVŚ 2.4.3, where the *jaṅgiḍá* is called the medicine for all diseases and is requested to protect one from distress (*áṃhas*). Because of the uncertain readings in *ab*, any translation is conjectural.

Notes to 6.111

Translators agree that AVŚ 6.111 is a charm against insanity.[93] Sāyaṇa considers it to be among the *mātṛnāmagaṇa* ("list of charms having the name mother")[94] and prescribes its use in a rite "for the quieting of pain from the Gandharvas, from the Rākṣas-demons, from the Apsarases or from *bhūtagraha* ('demonic seizure'?), etc."[95] at KauśS 26.29–32. It is also found at SVB 2.2.2 in the same context.[96]

VERSE 1

In *b*, P 5.17.6 reads *yo vibaddho grāhyā lālapīti*, "who, bound by seizure (*grāhī*) babbles senselessly" (O: *yā vibho grāhā lālapīti*?); and in *cd: ato 'dhi te* (Bar.: *atho 'dhi te*) *kṛṇavad bhāgadheyam* (O: *athatodi te kṛṇuva* or *kṛṇava*?) *anunmadito* (Bar: *anunmudito*, 'unexulting'?) *agado yathāsat*, "Therefore, he shall make an offering to you, so that he may become healthy [and] sane." Similarly, Sāyaṇa understands *b* as: "This man, who is tied by the bonds having an evil form [and who is one] having his progress restrained, cries forth very much (or loudly)" (*yo 'yam puruṣo . . . pāparūpaiḥ pāśair baddhaḥ san . . . suṣṭhu niyamitaḥ niruddhaprasaraḥ san . . . bhṛśaṃ pralapati*; cf. also Bloomfield, 520). The phrase also implies that the madman was tied and secured as if by a type of primitive straight-jacket. For *cd*, he renders: "Because of this, O Agni, let this man make your part of the offering excessive, so that he may become sane, i.e. free from the confounding of the *buddhi* (intellect) caused by seizure by Gandharvas and Apsarases" (. . . *asmād dhetoḥ he agne . . . tava . . . havirbhāgam . . . adhikaṃ karotu ayaṃ puruṣaḥ. . . . yathā yena prakāreṇa asau . . . unmādarahitaḥ gandharvāpsarograhajanitabuddhiskhālityarahitaḥ . . . bhavet*). In *d*, Sāyaṇa also reads *yáthā* in place of *yadā́* (cf. *pāda d* of verses 2, 4). *yáthā* is, therefore, a possible alternative reading. It implies, however, that the victim must present a gift in order to secure a better mental condition, though he is hardly well enough to do that (cf. P 5.17.7*cd*, where, in fact, the healer is said to make the offering). By reading *yadā́*, however, it is understood that he

---

[93] Ludwig: "Wansinn (Madness)," *Der Rigveda*, 3: 512; Zimmer: "Wahnsinn (Madness)," *Leben*, 393; Hillebrandt: "Gegen Wahnsinn," *Vedachrestomathie*, 50; Grill: "Irrsinn (Insanity)," *Hundert Lieder des Atharva-Veda*, 21, 170; Griffith: "A charm to cure insanity," *Hymns of the Atharvaveda*, 1: 306; Bloomfield: "Charm against mania," *Hymns*, 32, 518; and Whitney-Lanman: "For relief from insanity," *Atharva-veda-saṃhitā*, Pt. 1, 361.

[94] Cf. AthPariś 34.4; KauśS 8.24; Bloomfield, *Hymns*, 518–19; and Whitney-Lanman, Pt. 1, 361.

[95] *gandharvarākṣasāpsarobhūtagrahādipīdāśāntaye*; cf. Keśava: *gandharvarākṣase āpsarase bhūtagrahādiṣu bhaiṣajyāny ucyante.*

[96] See Caland, *AZ*, 78 n.

presents the offering to Agni in gratitude for rescuing him from the grip of insanity.

VERSE 2

For *b,* P 5.17.7 has: *yat te tan mana uddhṛtam,* "If your mind has been separated [from your body]"; and for *cd* it reads: *juhomi vidvāṃs te havir yathānumadito* (Bar.: *yathānumudito*) *bhavaḥ,* "[For] I, being skilled, sacrifice the offering to you, so that you may become sane." Sāyaṇa reads *údyatam,* 'raised,' in *b,* and renders it: "if your mind has risen up because of the seizure-disease" (. . . *tvadīyaṃ manas yadi udyatam grahavikāreṇa udbhrāntaṃ vartate*). The tradition, therefore, implies that insanity was characteristically understood as the mind leaving the body. At AVŚ 8.1.7, in a prayer for the continuation of life, the mind is requested not to depart [to the region of Yama (commentary)] and not to be lost (*mā́ te mánas tátra gān mā́ tiró bhūn* . . .). Cf. P 5.17.8, at n. 4 below. In *cd,* P continues the notion of sacrifice mentioned in verse 1; and for this reason, it may be a more correct reading. Śau, however, implies that more a healing than a sacrificial ritual was performed.

VERSE 3

P 5.17.1 reads: *devainasād unmaditaṃ kṣetriyāc chapathād uta, muñcantu tasmāt tva* [*ṃ*] *devā unmattaṃ rakṣasas pari,* "Therefore, let the gods release you, insane because of a sin against the gods, because of an imprecation and because of *kṣetriya,* and demented because of the *rakṣas*-demons." For the difficult *devainasā́d,* Sāyaṇa glosses: "a sin committed by the gods" (*devakṛtam enaḥ*) and renders *a:* "[him] possessed of insanity, i.e. the confounding of the *citta* because of that violation, i.e. evil committed by the gods" ([*tasmāt*] *devakṛtāt pāpād upaghātād* . . . *unmādaṃ cittaskhalanaṃ prāpitaṃ* . . .). Bloomfield (likewise, Grill, 21) also gives strong evidence for the interpretation of a sin committed by the gods (526). Others tend to favor the notion that there was an infringement against the divinities (see, in particular, Zimmer, 393; Griffith, 306 and Whitney-Lanman, 361). Both renderings are possible. Against the *pada*-text and Sāyaṇa, however, the compound could be read *deva-ainasá,* where *ainasá* is equivalent to *énas;* in which case, it would imply, like Bloomfield, the gods' action against the victim who has infringed their taboos and sacred norms. In *ab, únmaditam* and *únmattaṃ* are practically synonymous. *únmaditam,* literally, 'made demented,' however, implies that the victim has brought the condition on himself because he has offended the gods; while *únmattam,* 'demented,' suggests the demons, i.e. *rákṣas,* caused it. In *d,* the preferable reading is *yáthā* for *yadā́* (see Bloomfield, 526, and Whitney-Lanman, 361). As we have seen, P avoids the entire issue by presenting a completely different reading. Sāyaṇa merely refers to his previous comments where he has understood *yáthā* for *yadā́.*

VERSE 4

P 5.17.8 reads: *punas tvā dur* (O: *tvād*?) *apsarasaḥ punar vātaḥ punar diśaḥ, punar yamaḥ punar yamasya* (O: *punar yamaḥ asya*) *dūtās te tvā muñcantv aṅhasaḥ, jīvātave na martave atho ariṣṭatātaye,* "Let the Apsarases return you; let the wind [and] the directions re[turn you]; let Yama [and] Yama's (his) messengers re[turn you; and] let them release you from distress, to live and not to die, so [you] may not be harmed." In *a,* Sāyaṇa understands the *apsarásaḥ* to be a synecdoche for *gandharvas*, etc., citing TS 3.4.8.4 as support, (*etad gandharvādīnām api upalakṣaṇam*) and as those "causing insanity to him who is seized by insanity" (*he unmādagṛhīta puruṣa . . . tvām. . . . unmādakāriṇyo 'psarasaḥ . . .*). At AVŚ 2.2.5, they are called noisy, dusky, dice-loving, mind-confusing(!) and the wives of the Gandharvas. See also Bloomfield, 520–21. The verb *púnas . . . dur* (root *dā*, 'to give'), as Bloomfield suggests, has the sense of "to give back again," "to return" (ibid.). This fits well with the notion that madness was considered to be characterized by the mind leaving the body; and in order to become sane, it must be returned.

Notes to 2.31

Translators agree that AVŚ 2.31 is a charm against worms (*krími*).[97] Sāyaṇa prescribes it for use in a rite against "disease [caused by] various [types] of worms which have entered the body"[98] at KauśS 27.14–20.

VERSE 1

P 2.15.1 reads as Śau. In *a,* "Indra's great stone-slab" (*índrasya . . . mahī́ dṛṣát*) appears to be, as Bloomfield suggests, an allusion to his thunderbolt (*vájra*) (315; cf. also Grill, 98, and Griffith, 71 n), as opposed to the ordinary stone-slab (*dṛṣádā,* Sāyaṇa: *peṣaṇī,* 'grind-stone'), in *d.* Sāyaṇa understands *khálvāṁ,* in *d,* to refer to 'chick-peas' (*caṇakān*), similarly, Keśava to KauśS 27.14, i.e. *kṛṣṇacaṇakān* ('black chick-peas').

VERSE 2

In *a,* seen and unseen (*dṛṣṭám adṛ́ṣṭam*) appear to be designations of poisonous vermin (see, in particular, Grill, 99, and Bloomfield, 315). In *ab,* P(K) 2.15.2 reads *adruham atho kurīram adruham,* "I have injured . . . and

---

[97]Kuhn renders it under his discussion of "Segen gegen Würmer (Charms against worms)," KZ, 13 (1864): 137; Weber: "Gegen Würmer," IS 13: 199; Ludwig translates the charm in the course of his discussion of Indra's battle with the life-threatening demons, *Der Rigveda,* 3: 323; Grill: "Würmer," *Hundert Lieder des Atharva-Veda,* 6, 98; Griffith: "The hymn is a charm against all sorts of worms," *Hymns of the Atharvaveda,* 71; Bloomfield: "Charm against worms," *Hymns,* 22, 313; and Whitney-Lanman: "Against worms," *Atharva-veda-saṃhitā,* Pt. 1, 73.

[98] *śarīragatavividhakrimirogeṣu;* cf. Keśava: *aruṣīudaragaṇḍulakabhaiṣyāny ucyante,* "for the healing [of one suffering from] red worms and *gaṇḍulaka*-worms in the stomach (?)."

I have injured the *kurīra*"; Bh. as Śau.; and in *c*, P has *chalūlān*. In *b*, Sāyaṇa also reads *kurī́ram* for the difficult *kurū́rum* and explains it as "a net, i.e. a multitude of worms inwardly situated" (. . . *jālam. tadvad antaravasthitaṃ krimikulam*. . . .). Sāyaṇa's K-supported reading and explanation suggests maggots or larvae which are sometimes found inside living beings and are connected especially with open wounds. An equally valid reading is *kurūrum* which, from the context, points to the name of a species of worm (see Macdonell-Keith, *Vedic Index*, 1: 170; cf. also AVŚ 9.2.22). In *d*, Sāyaṇa defines the obscure word *algáṇḍūn* as the name of types of worm (*etan nāmnaḥ krimiviśeṣān* . . .); but in verse 3 he glosses it as "worms which corrupt the blood and the flesh" (*śoṇitamāṃsadūṣakān jantūn*). For *śalúnān* he reads *śalgā́n* and explains that it refers to worms with that name (*etan nāmnaś ca*). They appear, therefore, to be names of types of *krími* (cf. Whitney-Lanman, 73, and A. Sharma, *Beit. z. Ved. Lex.*, 46).

VERSE 3

In *cd*, P 2.15.3 has *sṛṣṭān asṛṣṭān ni kirāmi* (Bh. as Śau), "I overcome the produced [and] unproduced." In *ab*, Sāyaṇa, basing himself on KauśS 27.14-20, explains *mahatā́ vadhéna* as "the act of subduing of the *hanana*-worms, beginning with the charm and the herbs" (. . . *hananasādhanena mantrauṣadhādinā* . . .) and *dūnā́ ádūnā* as "those which are burned and unburned all around by the herbs, etc., prepared by me" (. . . *matkṛtauṣadhādinā paritaptāḥ* . . . *aparitaptāśca ye santi* . . .). Bloomfield, following Grill (99) suggests that the great weapon (*mahatā́ vadhéna*) is in fact the charm (*vácas*) which is called *vájra* ('thunderbolt') at AVŚ 6.134, 135, and that it could be the fire from this symbolic bolt which is called upon to burn the worms mentioned in *b*. It seems possible that the burned and unburned may allude to the ritual act of burning the vermin with a symbolic *vájra* in the form perhaps of a caustic medicine or a flame. Through the efficacy of the charm being recited and by the ritual burning (cf. KauśS 27.14.16: *pratapati* and AVŚ 5.23 13), the healer endeavors to destroy the *algáṇḍu*-worms. After the burning any remaining worms (cf. Sāyaṇa: *prāg ahatān krimiviśeṣān*, "types of worms previously not destroyed") are defeated by the recitation of the charm.

VERSE 4

In *b*, Roth-Whitney read *krímim*. In *ab*, P 2.15.4 has *anvāntryaṃ* (Bh.: *anvāntriyaṃ*) *śīrṣṇyam* (Bh. as Śau) *atho pārṣṭeyaṃ* (K manuscript: *pārśvayaṃ*, being in the region of the side') *krimīn* (Bh: *krimim*). For *pā́rṣṭeyaṃ*, Sāyaṇa reads *pā́rṣṇeyaṃ* and glosses: "a worm arising from heel" (*pārṣṇibhavaṃ krimim*), suggesting perhaps a type of maggot which occurs from a fly-blown wound. In *b*, Sāyaṇa also reads *krímīn*, which is followed by the Viśveśvarānanda edition. This reading implies that *krímīn* refers to all the types of worms mentioned in *ab*, as *krímīn*, in *cd*, does for those in *c*. Because of this parallel occurrence, we have also read *krimīn*, in *b;* yet *krímim* does not alter the meaning. The two words *avaskavám̐* and *vyadhvarám̐* are rather obscure. Sāyaṇa derives the first from the root *sku*, plus *ava* in the sense of to flow downward and defines it as that having the nature of going downward; i.e. having entered inside [the body], it remains [there] (. . . *avāggamanasvabhāvam. antarantaḥ praviśya vartamānam ity arthah. skuñ āpravaṇe. asmād avapūrvāt pacādyac*); and he explains the second as either that which has entered into various paths, i.e. having made different holes, it goes there; or else, *dhvara* means injury, and it thus signifies: he, who is called *dhvara*, is not injured by various drugs, etc. (. . . *vividhamārgopetam. nānādvārāṇi kṛtvā tatra gacchantam ity arthaḥ. . . . yadvā dhvaro hiṃsā. vividhair auṣadhādibhir api na vidyate dhvaro yasya sa tathoktaḥ*). Weber derives *avaskavám* from the root *sku* in the sense of 'to cover' and renders: "he who uncovers, peels off (der da abdeckt, abschält?)" (201; cf. also Bloomfield, 316, and Whitney-Lanman, 74). For *vyadhvarám̐*, Weber points to unaspirated alternative readings *vyadvará*, at AVŚ 6.50.3 and SB 7.4.1.27, and *vyádvarī* (note accent), at AVŚ 3.28.2, which are derived from the root *ad*, 'to eat,' and thus assumes *vyadvarám̐* to be the correct reading here, meaning 'that which gnaws' (201; cf. Zimmer, *Leben*, 393). Bloomfield (316) and Whitney-Lanman (74), however, derived it from the root *vyadh*, 'to pierce,' i.e. that which bores. Cf. also A. Sharma, *Beit. z. Ved. Lex.*, 260–61. We can see that with the widely differing views on the etymological meaning of these two words a definitive statement about them is problematic. From the context, however, it is evident that they refer to types of *krími* or worms.

VERSE 5

P 2.15.5 reads: *ye krimayaḥ parvateṣu ye vaneṣu ya oṣadhīṣu paśuṣv apsv antaḥ, ye asmākaṃ tanvaḥ* (Bh.: *tanvaṃ*) *sthāma cakrur* (Bh.: *cakrira*) *indras tān hantu mahatā vadhena*, "Let Indra, with [his] great weapon, kill those worms which are in the mountains, in the forests, in the plants, in the domestic animals, in the waters [and] those which make our bodies (body) [as their] seats." Concluding the charm with a petition to Indra, P preserves the continuity of the hymn. In *c*, Sāyaṇa reads *té* and, *tanvàḥ*.

Notes to 5.23

Most translators consider AVŚ 5.23 to be a charm against worms, perhaps those specifically found in children.[99] In the introduction the hymn is said to be used "in a rite for healing of [one afflicted with] worms"[100] at KauśS 29.20–26.

---

[99] Kuhn translates it under his discussion of "Segen gegen Würmer (Charms against worms)," KZ, 13 (1864): 139; Ludwig: "Würmertod (For death to worms)," *Der Rigveda*, 3: 501; Bergaigne-Henry: "Conjuration contre les vers parasitaires," *Manuel*, 148; cf. also Henry, *La magie*, 188; Griffith: "Charm for the destruction of parasitic worms," *Hymns of the Atharvaveda*, 1: 226; Bloomfield: "Charm against worms in children," *Hymns*, 23, 452; Weber: "Gegen Würmer in Kindern, etc. (Against worms in children, etc.)," IS, 18: 257; Whitney-Lanman: "Against worms," *Atharva-veda-saṃhitā*, Pt. 1, 261.

[100] *kṛmibhaiṣajyakarmaṇi*; cf. Keśava: *atha kṛmibhaiṣajyam ucyate*.

VERSE 1

a-c are found again at AVŚ 6.94.3. For the difficult words *óte, ótā* and *ótau,* P(K) 7.2.1 reads respectively: *oṣate, okatā* and *okato.* Barret, however, after emending to the Śau reading, suggests that the correct reading may in fact be *oṣṭe, oṣṭā* and *oṣṭau,* all of which are derived from the root *vas* plus *ā,* 'to shine hitherward,' 'to abide here,' i.e. those abiding here (JAOS, 40: 148). O has *okte, oktā* and *oktau,* 'invoked,' 'called' (*ā* plus root *vac*). At the end of *d,* P has *imaṃ.* Some translators derive *óte,* etc., from the root *u* plus *ā,* i.e. 'called, invoked' (see in particular Kuhn, 140, Bloomfield, 453–54; Griffith, 226; and Bergaigne-Henry, 206). Others, however, basing themselves most likely on Sāyaṇa to AVŚ 6.94.3, who derives it from the root *vā* plus *ā* and glosses: "mutually extended or connected through confrontation" (*ābhimukhyena saṃtate parasparaṃ saṃbaddhe vā*), understand it to be from the root *vā* (*uta*) plus *ā,* 'to weave in,' in the sense of "brought in for my aid" (Whitney-Lanman, 262) or "spell-bound" (Weber, 258–59; cf. also Bloomfield, 453–54). Either interpretation may be correct and fits well into the context of the verse. Based on the reading from the Orissa manuscripts, however, we are inclined to favor the interpretation of the root *u* (or *vac*) plus *ā* and to translate the three words as "has (have) been invoked."

VERSE 2

In *b,* P 7.2.2 has *krimiṃ,* corresponding to *krímiṃ* in verses 1 and 3; and in *d,* O has *'nena vacasā mama.* The sense seems to be that once the way has been made safe by the destruction of the evil entities, Indra, the king (cf. Bloomfield, 454) and the possessor of the fiery thunderbolt, can approach and (continuing the idea of verse 1) aid in the removal of the worms from the afflicted child. The means for the eradication of the vermin may, therefore, have included their scorching or burning (cf. verse 13 below and AVŚ 2.31.3).

VERSE 3

In *b,* P(K) 7.2.3 has *nāsau* (stem: *nās*); O reads, in *a, yo 'kṣau* and as Śau in *b.*

VERSE 4

In *a,* P 7.2.4 reads: *virūpau dvau sarūpau* (K manuscript: *surūpau*) *dvau;* and, in *d,* O has *gṛdhrās.* The precise meaning of *d* is difficult. Bloomfield (454) and Whitney-Lanman (262), on the strength of Sāyaṇa's gloss (at AVŚ 8.6.2): *cakravāka* ('*cakra*-bird'), translate the onomatopoeic *kókaś,* as 'cuckoo' (cf. also Henry, 189). Others, however, on the basis of ṚV 7.104.22, have understood it to refer to the wolf (see, in particular, Mayrhofer, Wb, 1: 268; 3: 682). The meaning of wolf may be appropriate because, as Weber notices, along with vulture (*gṛ́dhraḥ*), it suggests the worms' voraciousness (258). On the other hand, the poet-healer may be desiring to make a comparison between two birds, a vulture and a cuckoo. Neither explanation is wholly satisfactory. Because of the worm's parasitic nature, however, we would tend to favor Weber's suggestion.

VERSE 5

In *a*, P(K) 7.2.5 reads *śitivakṣā*, 'white-chest'; O, however, is as Śau. In this and the previous verse we have descriptions of worms which could hardly be applied to what we know them to be today. One can only speculate that the Vedic Indian conceived of various types of parasitic fauna in terms of worms which inhabited the body and fed on it.

VERSE 6

ab is found unchanged at ṚV 1.191.8*ab;* and for the same two *pādas*, P 7.2.7*ab* reads: *ud asau sūryo agād viśvadṛṣṭo adṛṣṭahā*, "that yonder sun has risen, seeing all, destroyer of the unseen." In this verse, as AVŚ 2.31.2, the description of seen and unseen applies particularly to vermin. The notion of the unseen or invisible worms which are destroyed by the rising sun suggests species of nocturnal vermin; and by logical extension, the seen or visible worms could be diurnal vermin which the sun can also destroy. The idea that fire or heat was ritually used to eradicate these parasitic pests is also suggested in this verse. A similar notion is found at AVŚ 2.32.1: "Let both the rising and setting sun destroy with [its] beams of light those worms which are in the cow" (*udyánn ādityáḥ krímīn hantu nimrócan hantu raśmíbhiḥ, yé antáḥ krímayo gávi*). Cf. also verse 13 below, ṚV 1.191.9 and AVŚ 6.52.1 and Henry's comments to ṚV 1.191.12 at MSL, 9: 242–43.

VERSE 7

For *ab*, P(K) 7.2.8 reads: *yavāṣāsaḥ* (O and Raghu Vira as Śau) *kaṣkaṣāso dhukṣāmaś* (K manuscript: *dhukṣāmaś*, O: *dhḷkṣanāsaḥ*?, Bar: *dhuṅkṣāsaś*) *ca parivṛkṇavaḥ* (O: *sípavitnavaḥ*); and in *d*, it has *ca uta*. *yavāṣāsaḥ*, being perhaps an older variant of *yévāṣāsaḥ*, is found at KS 30.1 and appears to be the name of a noxious insect (see Bloomfield, 155, and Mayrhofer, Wb, 3: 11, 783). Pisani has suggested a more exact meaning of the word based on etymology: It could be derived from *yava* plus *aśa* (root *aś* 'to eat') where *ṣ* and *ś* are interchanged, indicating an 'eater of grain,' i.e. a grasshopper, etc. (*Paideia*, 20: 328). For the *káṣkaṣāsa* (*o*), Weber has suggested that it may be a reduplicated form from the root *kaṣ*, 'to scrape' (259). Mayrhofer, however, mentions that this is unlikely (Wb, 1: 191). Cf., however, *maṣmaṣākaram* in verse 8. If we conceive it to be a variant of *kákṣāṣa*, where the *ṣ* and *k* are transposed through metathesis, we may, on analogy with *yávāṣa*, consider it to be composed of *kákṣa(ā)*, 'underparts' plus *aṣa(aśa)*, i.e. 'the vermin who eats the underparts.' Śau's *ejatkāḥ* may be from root *ej*, 'to stir,' 'to move,' i.e. *ejat* plus *ká* (cf. *avat-ká* at AVŚ 2.3.1 and *éjati* in connection with *krími* at AVŚ 12.1.46), meaning 'the stirring ones' (see

Mayrhofer, Wb, 1: 126; cf. Whitney-Lanman, 262, and Bloomfield, 455). P's *dhukṣāmaś* (*dhū°, dhḷ°*) may be worms which somehow are related to "agitating-ground." Barret's suggestion of *dhuṅkṣāsaś* occurs at VS 24.31 and refers to a kind of bird, which does not fit into the context of parasitic vermin. For Śau's *śipavitnukā́ḥ,* Weber suggests that it may actually be *śipayitnu(kā́),* from the root *śíp,* 'to be sharp, pointed,' meaning: 'the sharp-drilling ones' (259; cf. also Mayrhofer, Wb, 3: 337). K's *parivṛkṇavaḥ* points to a similar meaning, i.e. from root *vraśc,* plus *pari,* 'the ones which cut round.' O's variant of Śau, however, suggests a corruption in K. An interesting verse which contains two of the above names along with three other equally obscure ones occurs at P 19.29.4: *kaṣkaṣā[ḥ]kaṣkaṣāḥ piṣṭā yevāṣāyevāṣāḥ piṣṭāḥ, gaveṣayantaḥ svayuktāḥ pāśavā dṛṣṭā adṛṣṭāḥ,* "Each and every *kaṣkaṣa* has been crushed; each and every *yevāṣa* has been crushed. [Likewise,] the *gaveṣayants* ('the cow-seeking ones'), the *svayuktas* ('the self-adhering ones'), the *pāśavas* ('the ones belonging to animals') [as well as] the visible and the invisible ones [have been crushed]." Manuscript 'P' has difficult readings but overall seems to follow K manuscript. We notice further *kaṣkaṣa* and *yevāṣa* (*yavāṣa*) seem always to occur together, suggesting perhaps parasites of the same genus (cf. verse 8, below).

VERSE 8

d is found at AVŚ 2.31.1*d.* P(K) 7.2.9 reads differently: *hato yavāṣo hataś ca pavir hatas sagaṇavāṃ* (K manuscript, Raghu Vira: *ṣaṃgaṇavāṃ*) *uta, hatā viśvā arātayo anena vacasā mama* (cf. verse 2*cd* above), "The *yavāṣa* has been destroyed; the *pavi* ('pointed one') has been destroyed; so also, the ones of similar type [have been destroyed]; [in fact,] all the enemies have been destroyed with this my spell." This verse appears to be wanting in O. In *b,* the word *nadanimā́* appears to be derived from the root *nad,* 'to sound' and to mean 'buzzing' or 'humming ones' (see Weber, 259; Bloomfield, 455; and Whitney-Lanman, 263). In this verse, the poet-healer seems to be describing the noxious vermin which are characterized by their ability to make a "buzzing" or "humming" noise. The *yévāṣa* may also be included among such insects; and, therefore, also perhaps the *kaṣkaṣa* (see verse 7 n, above).

VERSE 9

b-d are found at AVŚ 2.32.2*b–d.* 2*a,* however, reads: *viśvárūpaṃ catura-kṣáṃ,* "with various forms and four eyes." In *ab,* P 7.2.6 has the easier reading: *yo dviśīrṣaś* (O: *dviśīrṣā*) *caturakṣaḥ krimis sāraṅgo arjunaḥ,* "the spotted [and] whitish worm with two heads [and] four eyes"; and for *ápi,* it reads *apa.* Our rendering implies the nominatives in *ab.* Sāyaṇa to AVŚ 2.32.2, however, contrives an explanation for reading accusatives in *ab:* He suggests that they should be the objects of *śṛṇā́mi,* in *c,* i.e. "I crush the spotted [and] whitish worm . . . [and] I cut off his ribs and head." It is clear from the variants to *a* that poets or redactors (?) were confused about the exact description of the worm. It is difficult to conceive of any worm, insect or vermin, visible to the naked eye, which would fit into any of the characterizations presented in the above three readings. Cf. Weber (202) and Bloomfield, (318), who hazard a guess that the one with four eyes (AVŚ 2.32.2: *caturakṣáṃ*) may refer rather to the spots in (or over) eyes.

VERSE 10

This verse is found unaltered at AVŚ 2.32.3. In *a,* P 2.14.5, in keeping with the singular in the previous verse, reads: *tvā krime;* and in *d: sarve te krimayo hatāḥ,* "all those worms have been destroyed." Bergaigne and Henry notice that the names are those of mythical sages and composers of powerful charms who were called upon to increase the efficacy of the exorcism (*Manuel,* 149 n; cf. *La magie,* 189 ṇ. See also Ludwig, 3: 137, and Weber, IS, 18: 114–17). In fact, they tend to reflect the Purāṇic tradition. This is another example of a verse in which the name of the charm being recited is given in the charm itself (cf. AVŚ 2.33.7 where Kaśyapa's spell is named).

VERSE 11

This verse is found unchanged at AVŚ 2.32.4. P 2.14.2 reads: *yo dviśīrṣā caturakṣaḥ* (Bh.: *visvarūpaś caturakṣaḥ*) *krimis sāraṅgo arjunaḥ, hato hatabhrātā krimir hatamātā hatasvasā,* "The spotted and whitish [or, the variegated (and) four-eyed] worm with two heads and four eyes, whose brother, mother and sister have been destroyed, has [also] been destroyed" (cf. verse 9 above). On the derivation of the word *sthapátir* and its meaning, see in particular Bloomfield, *Hymns,* 319–20; Wilhelm Rau, *Staat und Gesellschaft,* 114; and R. C. Hazra, "The word *sthapati,*—its derivation and meanings," *Our Heritage* (1974), 397–423.

VERSE 12

This verse occurs at AVŚ 2.32.5. P 2.14.3*cd* reads as Śau's *ab;* but P's *ab* is the same as verse 11*ab* (=AVŚ 2.32.4*ab*). In *a,* Sāyaṇa to AVŚ 2.32.5 glosses *veśáso* as "principal homes" (*mukhyagṛhā . . .*), and in *b, páriveśasaḥ* as "adjacent homes" (*samīpagṛhāś*). *veśás,* being derived from *víś,* 'house,' suggests rather the meaning 'subject' (cf. *váiṣya*); and *páriveśas,* being the one around him, might be his "dependent" (cf. also Rau on *veśa, Staat und Gesellschaft,* 49).

VERSE 13

P(K) 7.2.10 reads as Śau. This verse appears to be wanting in O. The reference to grinding brings to mind the stone-slab mentioned in verse 8 and at AVŚ 2.31.1. We notice that fire is specifically mentioned. Its use in the ritual, as we have seen, seems quite likely. The verse is referred to at KauśS 29.24. AVŚ 2.32 concludes with a different verse (6): *prá te śṛṇāmi śṛ́ṅge yā́bhyāṃ vitudāyási, bhinádmi te kuṣúmbhaṃ yás te viṣadhā́-*

naḥ, "I break off your two horns with which you pierce [and] I split your sac which is your poison-receptacle." In this verse *kuṣúmbham* is difficult. Our rendering is based on P 2.14.4, where *kumbham,* 'sac,' is read. Cf. also Sāyaṇa who reads *ṣukámbham* and glosses: "a kind of limb" (*avayavaviśeṣam*), Bloomfield, *Hymns,* 320, and Mayrhofer, Wb, 1: 246. Likewise, the translation of *viṣadhā̃naḥ* is based on P's reading: *yasmin te nihitaṃ viṣaṃ,* "[The sac] in which your poison is kept."

Notes to 1.3

Most translators consider AVŚ 1.3 to be a charm against urine-retention and/or constipation.[101] Sāyaṇa prescribes it for one suffering from the confinement of feces and urine[102] at KauśS 25.10–19. Concerning the number of verses in this hymn, Whitney-Lanman remark: "It is easy to reduce this hymn to the substance of four verses, the norm of the book, by striking out verses 2–5, as plainly secondary variations of verse 1, and combining verses 7–8 (as in Ppp.) into one verse, with omission of the sense-disturbing refrain."[103]

VERSE 1

P has no parallel. The expression *bā̃l íti* occurs at AVŚ 18.2.22 referring to the sprinkling of rain water: . . . *varṣéṇokṣantu bā̃l íti.* At TS 3.3.10.1–2 we read: *ví te bhinadmi takarī̃ṃ ví yóniṃ ví gavīnyàu, ví mātáraṃ ca putráṃ ca ví gárbhaṃ ca jarā̃yu ca, bahís te astu bā̃l íti,* "I breach your *takarí* (pudenda?), womb, *gavīnī̃* (see verse 6 below), the mother, the son, the embryo and the placenta; let it be out of you, [sounding like] '*bā̃l.*' " Cf. also JB 3.360: *tasmād āpo 'sṛjyanta balbalbal ity etayā vācā,* "from there, the waters are released with the sound: 'balbalbal' " (see Hoffmann, *Aufsätze,* 2: 519–21; cf. also 1: 43 n. 1). These references point to the fact that *bā̃l íti* is an onomatopoeic expression, in this case, for the discharge of urine. Sāyaṇa also understands *bā̃l* to be an onomatopoeic word for the evacuating urine which is brought about by its recitation in the *mantra;* yet he also suggests that "*bā̃l*" could stand for *bala* in the sense of "animating" and *íti* may mean "cause." Thus, he would render: "for the sake of life, let the urine of the one afflicted by disease be out" (*niṣecanaprakāram āha—. . . tava śarīrāntarniruddhaṃ mūtraṃ. . . . anukaraṇasabdoyam. . . . anena prakāreṇa*

[101] Weber: "Gegen Urinzwang (Against urine-retention)," IS, 4: 395; Bergaigne-Henry: "Conjuration contre la rétention d'urine," *Manuel,* 130; Griffith: "This hymn is a charm against acute diarrhoea or dysentery," *Hymns of the Atharvaveda,* 1: 3; Bloomfield: "Charm against constipation and retention of urine," *Hymns,* 10, 235; and Whitney-Lanman: "Against obstruction of urine: with a reed," *Atharva-veda-saṃhitā,* Pt. 1, 3.

[102] *mūtrapurīṣanirodhe;* cf. Keśava: *atiduḥkhamūtre duḥkhapurīṣakaraṇe ca śamanabhaiṣajyāny ucyante.*

[103] *Atharva-veda-saṃhitā,* Pt. 1, 4.

śabdaṃ kurvat . . . bāhyapradeśe bhavatu. mantrasāmarthyād vividhaṃ śabdaṃ kurvat tvarayā śarīrāt nirgacchatu ity arthaḥ yadvā bāl. bala prāṇe. . . . itir hetau. asya rogārtasya jīvanahetoḥ mūtraṃ bahir astv iti). His second explanation is also found at TS 3.3.10.1–2. Parjanya seems to have a connection here because he is the god of rain which is represented by *śatávṛṣṇya*. The rain as we have seen also makes the desirable sound *bāl*. The mention of the other gods in verses 2–5 appears to be, as Bloomfield (236–37) and Lanman (Pt. 1, cliv) suggest, mere secondary and mechanical repetitions. Sāyaṇa, however, conjures explanations based on TS 1.7.10.1, 2; 2.4.10.2; *Nirukta* 10.3, 11.5; TB 2.2.10.4 and TU 2.8 for their inclusion in the charm (see Bloomfield, 236–37) and understands the malady from which the patient is suffering to be 'the disease beginning with urine retention' (*he mūtranirodhādivyādhigrasta . . .*).

VERSES 2–5

P has no parallels. See previous note (end).

VERSE 6

P has no parallel. In *b*, Roth-Whitney read *sáṃsrutam*, 'has flowed together' for the difficult *sáṃśritam*. Weber suggests the emendation of *sáṃsrutam*, 'united' (396). In *b*, Sayaṇa reads *sáṃśritam* (as does our Viśveśvarānanda-edition) and glosses, "remained fixed, i.e. because of the power of the disease, at the proper time [of discharging], it was withheld" (. . . *samavasthitaṃ rogaváśād yathākālaṃ . . . niruddham abhūt . . .*). This reading and interpretation is also followed by Bloomfield (10,237). Sāyaṇa glosses the obscure *gavīnyór* as "two tubes of urine situated in the two lateral parts of the trunk, which allow access to the bladder for the urine that has come out of the bowels (?)" (*āntrebhyo vinirgatasya mūtrasya mūtrāśayaprāptisādhane pārśvadvayasthe nāḍyau . . .*). Based on this explanation Bloomfield suggests that it may refer to the urethra and ureter (10,237) and Filliozat, the two ureters (*La doctrine*, 123). Such interpretations imply a fairly advanced anatomical knowledge which the Vedic Indians indeed possessed; but a major difficulty lies with a more precise identification of the internal parts. Weber (396) and Whitney-Lanman (4) offer the more conservative translation of "groins," which is, however, unsatisfactory. A form of the word *gavīnike* (dual) occurs at AVŚ 1.11.5 along with, among other things, the urethra (*méhana*), female genital tract (*yóni*) and placenta (*jarāyu*) and at AVŚ 9.8.7 in the dual. As we have seen *gavīnī* also is found at TS 3.3.10.1–2 in a similar relationship to that found at AVŚ 1.11.5. It always occurs in the dual, is associated with the genitalia and, from this verse, is the place where urine was thought to be held. This information, however, does not allow us to determine the exact identity of the *gavīnī*; but, "ureters" seems probable (cf. also Mayrhofer, Wb, 1: 331).

VERSE 7

For a parallel in the P see next verse. For *a*, Sāyaṇa, based on KauśS 26.16 and Keśava, renders: "O one affected with the urine-disease, for the sake of urine-discharge I open, with a metal probe, your urine tube by which the urine discharges . . ." (*he mūtravyādhipīḍita . . . tava. . . . mihyāti siñcati aneneti mehanam mūtranālaḥ. . . . lohaśalākayā mūtranirgamanārthaṃ vidārayāmi* . . .); here Sāyaṇa suggests the use of a metal catheter (cf. Whitney-Lanman, 4). Cf. also AVŚ 1.11.5 (see previous verse) and TS 3.3.10.1–2 (see verse 1).

VERSE 8

P 19.20.12–14 and 20.40.2–3 are interesting variants to this and the previous verse. P 19.20.12 reads: *yathāśvāso yathā dhūraṃ yuktā vahanti sādhuyā, evā mūtra pra bhidyasva vi vaster ā saṃ sṛja*, "Just as horses yoked to the front of a chariot draw [it] on a straight course, so also you, O urine, are to be breached (?) [and] you must pour out from the bladder." P 20.40.2 has *cd* as P 19.20.12 but in *ab*, reads: *parā patanty āśavo 'śvā adho dhuraṃ* (K: *'śvasādo dūraṃ*) *yathā*, "Just as fast horses fly (i.e. speed) away from under the front of the chariot. . . ." P 19.20.13 has: *viṣitaṃ te vastibilaṃ samudrasyodadher iva, pra te bhinadmi mehanaṃ vartraṃ veśantyā yathā* (manuscript 'P': *iva*), "Released is your bladder-orifice as [the orifice] of a water-holding ocean. I breach your urethra as the dike of a lake [is breached]." P 20.40.3 reads as P 19.20.13. Note the combination of Śau verses 7, 8 into one P verse. P 19.20.14 reads: *yās samudrād uccaranti vīcīr api śuṣmikāḥ, pramehaṇasya* [manuscript 'P': (*tā*?) *mehaṇasya*] *tā vidur ubhayor mehanasya ca*, "Of both the urine-promoting [amulet] and urethra, they know those roaring waves which issue forth from the ocean (?)" (cf. KauśS 25.10). In this series of verses from the P, like those of the Śau, including verse 9, the emphasis is on the free-flowing of urine after the penis has been breached or opened. With *pramehaṇa*, verse 14 brings to mind KauśS 25.10. On *vastibilám*, 'bladder-orifice,' cf. AVŚ 9.8.11, etc., 164–65 above.

VERSE 9

Cf. P 19.20.12 and 20.40.2 in verse 8, above. Sāyaṇa understands *parā́patad* in the present sense as "departs with unobstructed speed, i.e. goes quickly aiming at its mark" (. . . *parāpatati aniruddhavegā śīghraṃ lakṣyoddeśaṃ gacchati*). This rendering has been followed by Bloomfield (11).

Notes to 4.12

Translators generally agree that AVŚ 4.12 is a charm for the curing of bodily injuries.[104] Sāyaṇa prescribes its use in a rite "for the ceasing of a

[104] Ludwig: "[Against] Knochenbruch (Broken bone)," *Der Rigveda*, 3: 508; Hillebrandt: "Beinsegen (charm for a broken leg)," *Vedachrestomathie*, 48; Grill: translates in his section entitled, "Durchfall und Wundkrankheit (Diarrhoea and Wound-fever)," *Hundert Lieder*, 18,

blood-flow born from an injury by a sword, etc. and for the quieting of the fracture of a bone, etc."[105] at KauśS 28.5–6. According to Dārila, it is to be employed, along with AVŚ 5.5, at KauśS 28.14 in a healing rite against wounds, in which the use of lac (*lākṣā*) is also mentioned.[106]

VERSE 1

P 4.15.4 reads: *rohiṇī saṃ rohiṇy asy asthnaḥ śīrṇasya rohiṇī, rohiṇyām ahni jātāsi rohiṇy asy oṣadhe,* "You, the *rohiṇī,* are like *rohiṇī,* the healer of the broken bone. You, O herb, are *rohiṇī* and you are born on the *rohiṇī*-day(?)." Sāyaṇa reads *rohiṇi* in *a,* and glosses it as a vocative: "O red-colored *lākṣā* (lac)" (*lohitavarṇe lākṣe*). This interpretation suggests a symbolic association between the dark red color of lac and the blood issuing from the wound caused by a broken bone (see AVŚ 5.5; and cf. Bloomfield, 386–87; Weber, 46–7; and Whitney-Lanman, 166–67). In the ṚV and later however, *róhiṇī* is generally considered to be a cow or a *nakṣatra* ('star') (see Macdonell-Keith, *Vedic Index,* 2: 228, and 1: 418). *a* has been rendered to give emphasis to the *róhiṇī.* One may speculate that this was the intent of the poet-healer as a similar construction occurs with *jaṅgiḍá* at AVŚ 19.35.1 (cf. Bloomfield, 385). Whitney-Lanman, however, being tempted to read one *róhaṇī* as a vocative and being influenced by P(K), suggest that the true reading may have been: *róhaṇy asi rohiṇi,* "thou art a grower, O Red one" (167). The word *róhaṇī,* being derived from the root *ruh,* 'to grow,' seems to mean, as suggested by the pun on the word found in *c,* 'one who makes grow,' i.e. in the context with a broken bone, 'a healer.' In *c, idáṃ,* as Sāyaṇa posits, seems to refer to "a limb flowing with blood" (*srutaraktam aṅgaṃ*). He derives *arundhati* from the root *rudh,* 'to obstruct,' plus *a* and explains it as a goddess who is not overrun by others or who is accustomed to non-obstruction (. . . *anyair anabhibhūte arodhanaśīle vā devi* . . .); but at AVŚ 6.59.1, 2, he glosses it as *sahadevī.* Others, however, understand it to be derived from *arus* plus the root *dha,* i.e. 'wound closing (or healing)' (see Weber, 46–47, and Henry, *La magie,* 180). Vishva Bandhu also considers the first element to be *arus,* but asserts that the second is derived ultimately from *bandha,* i.e. "wound-binding," which fits into his general theory that *arundhatī* = *lākṣā* = a wound-binding sap or lac resin (VIJ, 9: 285; cf. also AVŚ 5.5). Filliozat also understands it to be a resin and bases his interpretation on two observations: 1. The fact that it is associated

---

125; Griffith: "The hymn is a charm, addressed to a plant, to mend a broken bone," *Hymns of the Atharvaveda,* 1: 146; Bloomfield: "Charm with the plant *arundhatī*(*lākṣā*) for cure of fractures," *Hymns,* 19, 384; Weber: "Segen bei Knochenbruch (Charm for a broken bone)," IS, 18: 46; and Whitney-Lanman: "To heal serious wounds: with a herb," *Atharva-veda-saṃhitā,* Pt. 1, 166.

[105] *śastrādyabhighātajanitarudhirapravāhanivṛttaye asthyādibhaṅganivṛttaye ca;* cf. Keśava: *atha śastrādyabhighāte rudhirapravāhe bhaiṣajyāny ucyante.*

[106] *rohiṇy asīti sūktaṃ rātrī māteti śabdasya lākṣāpāryāyatvāt;* see also Bloomfield, *Hymns,* 385, and Whitney-Lanman, Pt. 1, 166; cf. also Caland, AZ, 90.

with the resin *lākṣā́* at AVŚ 5.5.7; and 2. The fact that it exhibits resin-like properties, which, he suggests, are exemplified at AVŚ 5.5 (*La doctrine*, 110–11; cf. also AVŚ 5.5). As we have seen, however, she is rather a plant-goddess, which is also the interpretation of the tradition. The *lākṣā́*-resin, therefore, could have been divinized and made an aspect of the goddess because of its close association with plants. As early as ṚVKh 4.7.5, 6 (see notes to AVŚ 5.5.5, 9), the word *arundhatī́* was considered to have the meaning of 'non-obstructing.' This lends further support to Sāyaṇa's suggested etymology.

VERSE 2

P 4.15.5 reads: *yadi* (K: *yad u*) *śīrṇaṃ yadi* (K: *yad u*) *dyuttam asthi peṣṭraṃ* (K: *peṣṭaṃ*) *ta ātmanaḥ, dhātā tat sarvaṃ kalpayāt saṃ dadhat paruṣā paruḥ*, "If your bone is broken, if your piece of flesh is inflamed, [then] let Dhātṛ set all that in order [and] reunite [it], joint with joint." The major difficulty with the Śau verse lies in the reading *ásti péṣṭraṃ*. For *péṣṭraṃ*, Sāyaṇa reads *préṣṭhaṃ* and glosses: "the most beloved, i.e. another limb (perhaps, the penis) which is broken by means of blows from a mace, etc." (*priyatamaṃ yad anyad aṅgaṃ mudgaraprahārādibhir bhagnaṃ bhavati*). The word, however, seems to be derived from the root *piś*, 'to carve,' and to be related to *piśitá* and *péśi*, 'flesh'; cf. also K's, *peṣṭam*. This, then, would point to the meaning of *péṣṭra* as 'piece of flesh' (see in particular Bloomfield, 387–88; T. Chowdhury, JBORS, 17: 85–86; Alsdorf, *Kleine Schriften*, 24; and Mayrhofer, Wb, 2: 343). Bloomfield has also suggested that the more correct reading of *ásti* is most probably *ásthi* (387–88). This also seems likely as the P has *asthi*, 'bone' (cf. also Alsdorf, *Kleine Schriften*, 24). The mention of the god Dhātṛ in this context of healing is quite unusual. Only in one other place in the AVŚ is there a hint that he may have performed such a function. At 18.4.48, he is called upon to lengthen one's life. His primary role in the ṚV is as a creator or establisher and is often associated with Pūṣan, Savitṛ, Prajāpati and Tvaṣṭṛ who, incidentally, is said to be able to put quickness into horse's feet (AVŚ 6.92.1 = VS. 9.8). In the TB (1.1.9.1), he is mentioned as one of the eight sons of Aditi (see Macdonell, *Vedic Mythology*, 43, 116, 117).

VERSE 3

In *ab*, P 4.15.1 reads as Śau with the omission of *te* in *a*. In *cd*, it has *saṃ te rāṣṭrasya* (?, K as Śau) *visrastaṃ saṃ snāva sam u* (K: *saṃsrāvam astu*) *parva te*, "Let your torn piece of flesh and your joint be flowed together (i.e. be united)" (following K).

VERSE 4

The difficult *pāda c* reads more easily if we emend it, according to P 4.15.3*c*, to *ásṛk te 'snā́ rohatu* (see Alsdorf, *Kleine Schriften*, 25–26; cf. also

Whitney-Lanman, who suggest such an emendation, but are unsure of its strength, 167). Sāyaṇa, however, offers another possible explanation for reading the *pāda* as it is. He suggests, on the strength of *b*, that *c* is elliptical; whereby, *asṛjā* and *asthnā* must be supplied, i.e. "let blood grow with blood; let bone grow with bone" (. . . *carmaṇa carmeti tṛtīyāntasya tatra dṛṣṭatvāt asṛjā asthnā iti tṛtīyāntaṃ padam adhyāhṛtya yojyam. asṛjā asṛj rohatu asthnā asthi rohatv iti. śiṣṭaṃ nigadasiddham*).

VERSE 5

Again *c* reads better if emended according to P 4.15.2b, i.e. *asthnā́ áśthi ví rohatu* (see Alsdorf, *Kleine Schriften*, 26). Sāyaṇa gives the same explanation as in the previous verse. Even with the emendation, *pāda c* seems out of place. *abc* employ the verb in the second person imperative, addressed to the herb, while *c* uses the third person imperative, apparently directed to the patient. It seems, therefore, that *c* should be separated from the rest of the verse, bringing the focus back upon the patient; and it has been so rendered. P 4.15.2–3 offers some interesting variants to these verses: P 4.15.2: *majjā majjñā saṃ dhīyatām asthnāsthy api* (K: *vi*) *rohatu, snāva te saṃ dadhmaḥ snāvnā carmaṇā carma rohatu,* "Let the marrow be united with marrow; let the bone grow forth with bone; we unite your sinew with sinew; let the skin grow with skin" (note that the use of the first person and the addition of *snāvan* in *c* suggest that this *pāda* may have been added). P 4.15.3: *loma lomnā sandhīyatāṃ tvacā saṃ kalpayā tvacam, asṛk te asnā rohatu māṃsaṃ māṃsena rohatu,* "Let the hair be united with hair; make skin join with skin; let your blood grow with blood; let the flesh grow with flesh" (note that the use of the second person in *b* suggests an addition).

VERSE 6

Most translators, basing themselves on Sāyaṇa (*uktam arthaṃ dṛṣṭāntena draḍhayati ratha ityādinā*), assume that there is, in *ab*, an implied comparison which, perhaps, emphasizes the recovery of the victim (see Grill, 18; Bloomfield, 20; Weber, 48; and Whitney-Lanman, 167. Griffith, following Ludwig, renders the line as two separate thoughts, 147). Alsdorf, however, has very astutely noticed an inconsistency in thought between the first and second line. He says that the notion of a good chariot which runs does not correspond with that of an appeal to stand firmly erect (*Kleine Schriften*, 27–28). This objection has led to a complete re-examination of this verse in terms of a healer imploring an animal, perhaps a horse, to stand up and become well. In this way, the implied comparison is no longer needed, and the verse may be read as it is. P 4.15.7 has a variant of this verse which contains many doubtful readings, but may tentatively be presented here: *ut tiṣṭha prehi sam u dhāhi* (Bh.: *samidhāya?*) *te paruḥ saṃ te dhātā dadhātu tanvo viriṣṭam, rathaḥ sucakraḥ supavir yathaiti sukhaḥ sunābhiḥ prati tiṣṭha evam,* "Stand up, advance and become united (?). Let Dhātṛ unite for you your joint [and] what of the body is broken. Like a chariot with strong wheels, rims, axle holes [and] hubs, stand firmly thus." Alsdorf has considered this verse and has suggested that, on the basis of meter, the *pāda* should break between *saṃ te* and *dhātā*, and that *sam . . . dhāhi*, on the basis of Śau verse 5, can only refer to the herb and therefore does not fit with *te paruḥ*. He concludes that *sam u dhāhi te paruḥ* "is not only an interpolation from somewhere else but also corrupt in itself" (*Kleine Schriften*, 27–28). From the above reading we notice that the P seems to support the notion that a simile is present; and, if part of the reading is accepted, Dhātṛ is named as the one who should make the body whole. Unfortunately, like much of the P hymn, this entire verse seems terribly corrupted and, as Alsdorf seems to imply, may be a later interpolation.

VERSE 7

In *d*, Sāyaṇa considers the Atharvavedic *mantra* to be the subject of the verb *sáṃ dadhat* (. . . *evaṃ ātharvaṇo mantro viśliṣṭam aṅgaṃ saṃdadhātīty arthaḥ*). Kuhn (59), Ludwig (508) and Griffith (147) understand that *ṛbhús* should be read here. Kuhn, however, suggests that *ṛbhū́* may be an epithet of *dhātā́* mentioned in verse 2 (59). Grill (126) and Bloomfield (20, 389), on analogy with verse 2, consider Dhātṛ to be the implied subject. This interpretation may also receive support from P 4.15.7 (see previous note). It would be more likely that Tvaṣṭṛ, the mender of horses' limbs who is associated with Dhātṛ, should be understood as the subject. Because of the lack of corroborative evidence, however, this is only conjecture. The most obvious subject seems to be Dhātṛ. Both Grill (126) and Hillebrandt (*Vedachrestomathie*, 48 n) regard this and the previous verse to be later additions. P 4.15.6 presents a rough correspondence to this verse; but, because of the number of obscure readings, it is too difficult to be rendered intelligibly at this time. The text according to Bh., however, is as follows: *yadi vajro visṛṣṭas tv ārakā ṭāt* (?, K: *visṛṣṭa sthārakā jātu*) *patitvā yadi vā viriṣṭam, vṛkṣād vā yad avasad daśaśīrṣaribhūrathasyeva saṃ dadhāmi te paruḥ* (?, K: *vā yadi vāvibhyasi śīrṣarbhūr iti sa evaṃ saṃ dhāmi te paruḥ;* Bar: *yadi vāvyadhyase* or *vā vidhyase*). Is it important to note that the hazards which cause the injury mentioned in the Śau verse seem better to exemplify those which a horse may have encountered, rather than those met by a man.

Notes to 5.5

Most translators agree that AVŚ 5.5 is a charm to a healing plant or to a resin for the cure of wounds.[107] Kuhn mentions verses 8–9 in relation to

[107] Zimmer translates the entire hymn in the course of his discussion of the plant *arundhatī*, *Leben*, 67; Grill renders the hymn under his section, "Krankheit," *Hundert Lieder des Atharva-Veda*, 10, 142; Griffith: "The hymn is a charm, addressed to a Plant, to mend a broken bone," *Hymns of the Atharvaveda*, 1: 195; Bloomfield: "Charm with the plant *silācī*(*lākṣā, arundhatī*) for the cure of wounds," *Hymns*, 20, 419; Weber: "Mistelzweig-Amulett (Mistletoe-

AVŚ 4.12 and the use of Arundhatī to heal the injuries of a horse.[108] The charm is not mentioned in the KauśS; but, according to Dārila, it, along with AVŚ 4.12, is reckoned at KauśS 28.14 in the hymns characterized by the word *lākṣā́(lākṣāliṅga)* and employed in a rite to heal flesh wounds. A variant of the hymn occurs at *Ṛgvedakhila* 4.7 which is inserted after ṚV 10.137 and which, according to BD 8.51, is directed to *lākṣā́*.[109]

VERSE 1

For *rā́trī*, 'the night,' here and at P 6.4.1, ṚVKh 4.7.1 has *bhū́mir*, 'the earth,' which, being more logical, is called *mātṛ́* at AVŚ 6.120.2 and TĀ 2.6.2. In *a*, Vishva Bandhu quite boldly construes *nábhaḥ*, 'cloud,' as a nominative masculine singular in the sense of "day" and emends *ab* to . . . *pítā(tā áryamā) té pitāmaháḥ*, ". . . the day is thy father, Aryaman thy grandfather," arguing that day has to be understood as the common opposite of night and that *pítāryamā́* must be read as five syllables (VIJ, 9: 3–6). His rendering of *nábhaḥ* is suspect, but his proposed emendation is possible. Since Yama is mentioned in verse 8, however, one cannot discount the likelihood that the word is to be read here. In *c*, P(K) has *śilādī*, but O, *śilācī*, the accepted reading for P. At ṚVKh 4.7.1 and P 6.4.8 (see verse 8 below) the reading is *ghṛtā́cī*, 'shining with ghee,' which appears to be the name of a snake or perhaps of a plant (cf. Bloomfield, 608) and which, at AVŚ 19.48 is called *rā́trī* (verse 6) and *mātṛ́* (verse 2). Most western interpreters consider *silācī́* to be a plant, another name for *lākṣā́* and *arundhatī́* (see Weber, 182; Griffith, 195 n; Macdonell-Keith, *Vedic Index*, 2: 450, and Bloomfield, who proposes a connection with *silā́ñjālā*, a creeping plant or weed which grows in grain fields, mentioned at AVŚ 6.16.4 and KauśS 5.16, 450; so also Mayrhofer, who also suggests that both *silācī́* and *silā́ñjālā* may be connected with *śilā*, 'arsenic,' Wb, 3: 470). The derivation from *śilā*, 'stone,' receives support from P and also brings to mind the word *śilājitu* which is a black substance exuding from rocks, used among the people of the Indus Valley and as an āyurvedic medicine (Marshall, *Mohenjo-Daro and the Indus Valley Civilization*, 2: 587–88, and Dutt and King, *Materia Medica*, 95). Filliozat, on the other hand, understands *silācī́*, *lākṣā́* and *arundhatī́* to be names of a resin which exudes and flows down plants (*La doctrine*, 109–11; cf. also AVŚ 4.12.1 n). Vishva Bandhu also maintains that *silācī́* is a resin (VIJ, 9: 1–3). It is difficult to know for sure whether

---

twig-amulet)," IS, 18; 181; Whitney-Lanman: "To a healing plant, *lākṣā*," *Atharva-veda-saṃhitā*, Pt. 1, 228; Vishva Bandhu: "An Atharvan hymn to Lac(*lākṣā́*)—AV V.5," VIJ, 9 (1971): 1–20; 281–89; see also an earlier version of the hymn rendered by Vishva Bandhu in *Siddha-Bhāratī or The Rosary of Indology* (Hoshiapur, 1950), 201–13.

108 "Indische und germanische Segenssprüche," KZ, 13 (1864): 61.

109 See Isidor Scheftelowitz, *Die Apokryphen des Ṛgveda* (1906; rpt. Hildesheim, 1966), 120, and L. C. Barret, "Three versions of an atharvan hymn" (J. D. C. Pavry, ed., *Oriental Studies in honour of Cursetji Pavry*, London, 1933), 26–28; cf. also A. A. Macdonnell, *The Bṛhad-Devatā*, Pt. 2 (1904; rpt. Delhi, 1965), 306–307.

these obscure words refer to a plant or to a resin found on the plant. It does seem apparent, however, that they have a vegetal connection and, in fact, may be different aspects of a female divinity, the characteristics of whom become manifested quite distinctly in the verses of this charm.

VERSE 2

For *bhartrī*, 'protectress,' P 6.4.2 has *dhartrī* 'female supporter', and ṚVKh 4.7.2 reads *trātriṇī*, 'protectress,' 'savioress' (from the root *trā*; note the pun on *trāyase* in *b*). P continues *cd* with the possible reading: *ca śaśvatām asi śaśvatāṃ ca nyañcanī* (K manuscript: *tyanvañcanīṃ*, Edgerton: *tv anvañcanī*). Similarly ṚVKh: *śáśvatām asi śáśvatāṃ samyáñcanī*. Vishva Bandhu speculates that the second *śáśvatāṃ* may have been a scribal error; or perhaps, being derived from the root *śas*, 'to cut,' it could mean "wounded ones," specifying the *jánānāṃ* of the Śau (VIJ, 9: 12). This latter explanation is appealing, but much too speculative to be considered seriously. For the corrupt *tyanvañcanīṃ* in K, he posits the possible reconstruction: *adhyanvañcanī*; and for *samyáñcanī* in the ṚVKh, he proposes *samayañcanī*. Both emendations, like *nyáñcanī*, may then be derived from the root *vañc*, 'to cover'; and in this way, the resinous *silācī* could be considered as covering over a wound (ibid., 10–11). This is an interesting hypothesis. It should be pointed out, however, that the primary Vedic meaning of the root *vañc* is 'to move in a waving manner,' 'to stagger.' It is more likely that *nyáñcanī* is from the root *añc*, 'to bend' and with the prefix *ní* has the sense of a place where one could hide by crouching, i.e. 'a refuge' (cf. ṚV 8.27.18, AVŚ 4.36.6, Kuiper, IIJ, 2: 158, and Mayrhofer, WB, 3: 748).

VERSE 3

For *ab*, ṚVKh 4.7.4. has: *vṛkṣáṃvṛkṣaṃ sáṃ patasi vṛ́ṣāyantīva kanyánā*, " You, like a mannish young girl, fly unto each and every tree." p 6.4.5 (=7.12.6.) reads as Śau, but has *vṛṣaṇyantīva* in b. *jáyantī*, 'triumphant,' has later come to designate a particular plant. The word *spáraṇī* is uncertain, but appears to be derived from the root *spṛ*, 'to release from.' Vishva Bandhu again quite boldly conjectures that it is from *spaś*, 'to stick' and renders *d* as " 'seizer' by name thou art, indeed" (VIJ, 9: 12–13). P 6.4.5 (7.12.6) reads *saṃjayā*, 'subduing' and similarily ṚVKh has *saṃjeyā*, 'overpowering'? The tradition, therefore, seems to have understood a different word whose meaning is quite similar to that of *jáyantī*. *spáraṇī*, therefore, may have the sense of subduing with the purpose of releasing one from difficulty or disease. Filliozat mentions this verse in support of his theory that resin is referred to: "Il est dit en effet qu'elle grimpe aux arbres (AV 5.5.3) mais les traînées de résine courent sur l'écorce comme des tiges de lianes auxquelles on peut comparer" (*La doctrine*, 110 n). The verse seems to suggest a goddess who, perhaps in the form of resin, mounts the trees; and because of that, she came to be known as a conquerer who adheres to the trees and who has the power to extricate or disentangle one from difficulty.

VERSE 4

hárasā is questionable but may be derived from the root *hṛ,* 'to take,' i.e. 'by force,' 'by violence' or from *hṛ,* 'to flame,' i.e. 'by fire' or 'by a flame.' Since specific, rather than general, means for causing injury are mentioned, the rendering 'by a flame' is more acceptable (cf. Mayrhofer, Wb, 3: 579, and Vishva Bandhu, VIJ, 9: 14). *níṣkṛtiḥ* has the primary meaning 'eradicator(feminine)' or 'healer(feminine)'; but in the context of broken limbs it has the sense of 'mender(feminine).' In *cd,* P 6.4.3 reads: *tasya tvam asi bheṣajī niṣkṛtir nāma vā asi,* "You are the medicine of (for) that [limb], indeed you are mender, by name"; and ṚVKh 4.7.3 has *tásya tvám asi níṣkṛtiḥ sā̃nau níṣkṛtya óṣadhīḥ,* "Being removed at ground level, you, O herb, are the mender of the [limb]." This half-verse suggests a ritual process of removing plants from the ground and indicates that a herb or plant is to be used in the healing rite. The entire verse shows that healing or mending is one of the auspicious qualities of the goddess (see verse 6 below).

VERSE 5

P 6.4.4, like ṚVKh 4.7.5, reads the plants in the locative, but has *bhadrā,* in *a, c,* and *plakṣeṇa,* in *a.* In *ab,* ṚVKh has *nís tiṣṭhā̃śvatthé;* in *c, parṇé nyagródhe* and in *d, sā̃ mā̃ṃ rautsī̃d arundhatī̃,* "[For] that Arundhatī has covered me" (note that the play on the words *rautsī̃d* and *arundhatī̃* suggests that *arundhatī̃* is from the root *rudh,* 'to cover,' 'to obstruct'). The idea expressed by *nís tiṣṭhasy,* "You arise out of," hints at the notion of a resin (see Filliozat, *La doctrine,* 110 and note; cf. also Vishva Bandhu who renders it as "steadfast" which presumably refers to the resin which sticks on the trees, VIJ, 9: 15–16).

VERSE 6

A parallel to this verse is not found in the ṚVKh. For *hiraṇyavarṇe,* 'O golden one,' P 6.4.7 reads *hiraṇyabāhu* (O: *hiraṇyabāho*), 'O golden armed' which, in the Epic, refers to Śiva (cf. Vishva Bandhu who takes *bāhu* in the sense of "hue," VIJ, 9: 16–17); for *cd,* P has the much easier reading: *rutaṃ gacchāsi niṣkṛdhi* (Raghu Vira: *niṣkṛte*) *semaṃ niṣkṛdhi pūruṣam,* "May you go to the fracture. Mend [it]; indeed, mend this man"; O reads differently: *rutaṃ gacchati niṣkṛtiḥ sedaṃ niṣkṛdhi bhadrayā,* which may tentatively be rendered as "The mender goes to the wound; indeed, by means of the auspicious lady, mend this (one)." Filliozat mentions that the golden color expressed in this and the next verse can be correctly applied to resins, but not to the red lac (*La doctrine,* 110–11). It could also refer to the foliage of trees.

VERSE 7

For *híraṇyavarṇe,* 'O golden one,' ṚVKh 4.7.7 reads *híraṇyaparṇe,* 'O golden-winged (or leaved) one' which draws us back to the plant *parṇá* mentioned in verse 5; or, as Barret points out, it could merely be a graphic error involving the letters *v* and *p* ("Three versions . . . ," 28). For *śúṣme,* 'fiery (fire-colored)' (see, Bloomfield, 421, and ZDMG, 48: 565 ff.), it has *sókṣme,* from *sūkṣma,* meaning perhaps 'delicate.' For *lómaśavakṣaṇe,* 'O hairy-sided one,' P(K) 6.4.6 has *lómaśamakṣaṇe,* 'visibly hairy(?),' emended by Edgerton and Barret to read as Śau; O has, in *a, yuva te*(?), suggesting a binding action, and *lomasuvakṣane* (=Śau?), in *b.* Vishva Bandhu ascribes the epithet, "sister of the waters," to the fact that when the resin first appears, it is in the form of "viscous honey-like drops" and therefore, is liquid like water. For *d,* he renders: "The wind, verily, became your solidifier" and explains: "The exposure of 'the sister of the waters' to the air causes its encrustment. This seems to be referred to by the description of *vātá-* as its *ātmán-*, 'solidifier, one that makes it a compact mass' " (VIJ, 9: 18, 20). Such an explanation seems to be very unlikely. While it is possible that the initial liquid nature of a resin could be meant by "sister of the waters," it also suggests a plant which is found living in or near ponds or lakes. To read *ātmán* as "solidifier," however, is completely out of the question. Nowhere in the Vedic literature has such a meaning been testified. It could refer to a tree's wind-stirred leaves or branches which bear witness to the wind's presence.

VERSE 8

For *silācī,* P 6.4.8 has *ghṛtācī* (cf. ṚVKh 4.7.1 and verse 1 above); for *'jababhru, 'jababhrū* and for *táva,* P(K) has *bhava,* Bar. and O read as Sau. In *d,* it reads *ukṣitā;* and O has *śāvas,* in *c.* In *ab,* Grill emends *kānīnó* to *kānīná,* and *ájababhru* to *ajábabhruḥ* and renders: "Silācī ist ein Jungfernkind, dein Vater braunrot, wie des Bock. . . ." He further equates these with the father and mother mentioned in verse 1 (11, 143; cf. also Zimmer, 67). This is a possible interpretation; but, as Bloomfield points out, it is problematic (421). In *c,* the *pada*-text reads *āsnā,* 'by the mouth,' for *asnā,* 'with the blood.' Most translators read *asnā* because, as Grill (145) and Bloomfield (423) suggest, a similar notion is found in German mythology and a reference to Yama's bloody mouth occurs at TĀ 4.29. The idea seems to be that *silācī* has absorbed the divine animal's blood with which she has been sprinkled and has, therefore, gained from it her power, virtue and color. There is, however, a problem with *silācī.* Previously, it has been understood as a feminine. Here, however, the word must be conceived as a masculine, i.e. the father, brown in color and born of a young girl. Vishva Bandhu conjectures that on account of the mention of brown-colored lac, the similarly colored *śilājit* (bitumen) must be meant as the father. He therefore posits, phonetically, the reading *śilācit* (VIJ, 9: 281). We may arrive at a similar conclusion if we understand *silācī* to be a nominative masculine singular from *silācín* (cf. Weber, 184). Although the problem cannot be settled with certainty, it is clear that the poet wished to speak of the male counterpart or producer of the female *silācī,* a word which in turn is a variant of the name *silācī.* Vishva Bandhu goes on to discount the reading *ájababhru* as "goat-brown," and based on the K reading, asserts that it is actually to be understood as two words: *átha bábhru.* This is possible; however notice Barret emends to Śau. *ajabahrū* is, nevertheless, found in K and O. For *kānīnó,* Vishva Bandhu renders, "mine-born," stating that it is merely a phonetic variant of *khanī,* 'mine.' This explanation seems forced and the meaning is not at all clear in the context. In *d,* he prefers the reading *āsnā* (cf. above) and renders *ukṣitā* as "carried" which, he says, may ultimately be derived from the root **vakṣ,* i.e. *vah,* 'to carry' (VIJ, 9: 282–83). The reading of *āsnā* for *asnā* is a matter of opinion and the meaning of *ukṣitā* as "carried" is unlikely.

VERSE 9

This is an extremely obscure verse. ṚVKh 4.7.6 reads: *áśvasyā́sṛk saṃpatasi tát parṇám abhi tiṣṭhasi, sarát pataty arṇasi* (Vishva Bandhu proposes the emendation: *sarā patatriṇī asi,* VIJ, 9: 285) *sā́ mā́ṃ rautsīd arundhatī,* "You, O horse's blood, stream forth [and] tread upon that *parṇá*-tree. You are [as] a winged stream (following Vishva Bandhu). [Therefore,] that Arundhatī has covered me." P 6.4.9 has *parṇam* in *b* (O also has *śiṣyadaḥ*?), and in *d, sarā patatriṇy asi,* "you are a winged stream." For *asnáḥ,* Whitney-Lanman (229) and Vishva Bandhu (VIJ, 9: 283) read *āsnáḥ,* which makes better sense; but, as noticed in ṚVKh, "blood" seems to be the intended meaning. One can only surmise that the poet wished to make an indirect comparison, i.e. streaming as horse's blood; or perhaps, he had in mind the red color of the blood which could be conceived as streaming from it. It may also point to a mythological episode in which the goddess became a specific tree-divinity. The notion of a "winged-stream" is also encountered at ṚV 10.97.9 and seems to reflect the sense of speed (cf. Vishva Bandhu, VIJ, 9: 284). K has two additional verses which, Barret states, are most probably later additions ("Three versions . . . ," 27, 28): 10. *ghṛtācake vāmarate vidyatparṇe arundhati, yāturaṃ gamiṣṭhāsi tvam aṅganiṣkary asi.* 11. *yat te 'jagrabhaṃ piśācais tat tarhāpy āyatāṃ punaḥ, lākṣā[yā] tvā viśvabheṣajī[r] devebhir trāyatāṃ saha.* These are wanting in the Orissa manuscripts, thereby lending support to Barret's contention.

Notes to 2.3

Most translators agree that AVŚ 2.3 is a charm against bodily discharges, perhaps produced by a wound.[110] Sāyaṇa prescribes it, along with AVŚ

---

[110] Weber: "Wundenbalsam (Wound-balsam)," IS, 13: 138; Ludwig: "Heilendes Waszer (To healing waters)," *Der Rigveda,* 3: 507; Grill renders it under his section: "Durchfall und Wundkrankheit (Diarrhea and wound-disease)," *Hundert Lieder des Atharva-Veda,* 17, 79; Griffith: "The hymn contains a charm in which water is used to cure disease," *Hymns of the Atharvaveda,* 1: 43; Bloomfield: "Charm against excessive discharges from the body, undertaken with spring water," *Hymns,* 9, 277; and Whitney-Lanman: "For relief from flux: with a certain remedy," *Atharva-veda-saṃhitā,* Pt. 1, 40.

1.2, for use in a rite against "fever, diarrhoea, excessive flow of urine, and [discharges caused by] a wound to the (blood) vessels (or fistula)"[111] at KauśS 25.6–9. Although it was ultimately used in a healing rite, it appears, from the context, that the charm may have originally been recited while the healer was preparing his remedy.

VERSE 1

P(K) 1.8.1 has part of *cd* only: . . . *bheṣajaṃ subheṣajaṃ tad u kṛṇomi bheṣajam.* Bh., however, has the entire verse: *amuṣmād adhi parvatād avatkam asi bheṣajam, bheṣajaṃ subheṣajaṃ yat te kṛṇomi bheṣajam,* "You are the medicine, flowing from yonder mountain. [Thus,] I make for you medicine, the medicine which [is] an effectual medicine." For the difficult *avatkám,* in *b,* Sāyaṇa, based on the *Sūtra,* understands the tips of the *muñja*-grass which protect by removing disease (*vyādhiparihāreṇa rakṣakaṃ muñjaśiraḥ*). Rather, it seems to be a present participle from the obscure root *av,* 'to move' (see T. Chowdhury, JBORS, 17: 35) and may thus be rendered as 'gliding' or 'flowing,' suggesting water. Bloomfield also understands water to be meant and, relating the word to *avatá,* 'spring,' translates: "spring water" (9, 278; cf. also Grill, 17, 79 and Weber, "Brünnelein," 138). Whitney-Lanman, on the other hand, suggest that it is a present participle from the root *av,* 'to favor,' formed like *ejatká* at AVŚ 5.23.7 and thus render: "aiding" (40). The exact sense of the second line is uncertain. It appears that the healer recited this verse while preparing a remedy which, with the addition of mountain stream water, becomes very potent (cf. Weber, 138; Griffith, 43 n, and Bloomfield, 278). Ludwig emends to *súbheṣajo,* making it adjectival to the subject of *ásasi,* i.e. "so that you may have good medicine." In this way both *te,* in *c,* and the subject refer to the patient (507). This receives support from P (Bh).

VERSE 2

In *ab,* P 1.8.2 has: . . . *śataṃ yā*(K:*yad*) *bheṣajāni te sahasraṃ vā ca yāni te,* which may tentatively be rendered: ". . . [of those] which are your hundred medicines or [of those] which are your thousand [medicines]. . . ." In *b,* however, Bh. has *te sahasraṃ vāghajāni te,* ". . . or your thousand [medicines] born of sin," which is absurd (cf. Renou, JA, 252: 425). *cd* reads as Śau, except, K has *ārohaṇam,* 'ascending?' for *árogaṇam* (Bh. reads as Śau). *ab* is also found at P(K) 20.33.8 which has in *cd:* [*śreṣṭham āsrāva-bheṣajaṃ*] *vasiṣṭhaṃ roganāśanam,* "[you are] the best medicine against *āsrāva* [and] the most excellent destroyer of the affliction"; O has *teṣāṃ asi tvam uttamam* (=K 20.33.8*a*) *śreṣṭhatamāsrāvabheṣajaṃ vasiṣṭhaṃ roganāśanam,* "You are the best of them, the very best medicine against *āsrāva* [and] the

---

[111] *jvarātīsārātimūtranāḍīvraṇeṣu,* cf. Keśava: *atha jvarātisārabhaiṣajyāny ucyante* and Dārila: "This is a cure for diarrhoea because that is the meaning of the word *āsrāva*" (*atisārabhaiṣajyam āsrāvaśabdasya tadvāditvāt;* cf. also Bloomfield, AJPh, 7: 468).

most excellent destroyer of the affliction" (cf. AVŚ 6.44.2 and notes, 78 and 211). Sāyaṇa considers *āsrāvá* (root *sru* plus *ā́*) to be 'the discharges beginning with diarrhoea, excessive urine-flow and [that caused by] a wound to the (blood) vessels (or fistula)' (*āsravantīti āsrāvāḥ atīsārātimūtranāḍīvraṇādayaḥ*) and *rogaṇa* as 'the disease rooted in them' (*tanmūlaroga*). Sāyaṇa may be correct, for at AVŚ 1.2.4 and 6.44.2, affliction (*róga*) and *āsrāvá* are found together. They represent the bodily affliction or flesh-wound with its symptoms. In this case, the symptoms are the discharges; and the wound is simply known as the affliction. Bloomfield points out that *a* is to be understood as a rhetorical question (279).

VERSE 3

For P 1.8.3*cd*, see AVŚ 6.44.2 n, 211, below. P 19.30.9 reads *ab* (=manuscript 'P' *cd*) as Śau *cd*. In this verse, the medicine (*bheṣajá*) appears to refer to the trickling water (*avatká*) (see verse 1 above and AVŚ 19.30.8). P 20.43.4*cd* and 20.54.3*ab* read as Śau *cd*. At 20.54.3, there is a reference to medicine derived from the mountains and from the sea and which is also employed against *takman* (20.54.1, 2). These numerous occurrences of the phrase suggest that it may be formulaic, at least, in P. The word *arusrā́ṇam* 'treatment for wounds' (Roth-Whitney read: *arussrā́ṇam* or *aruḥsrā́ṇam*, see Whitney-Lanman, 41) is difficult. In *b*, Sāyaṇa, reading *aruḥsrā́ṇam*, suggests that it is either the place where the wound ripens, i.e the head of the sore; or, it is the medicine which brings about the sore's ripening (. . . *vraṇasya pākasthānam. vraṇamukham ity arthaḥ. . . . aruḥ srāyati pakvaṃ bhavati upaśamanonmukhaṃ bhavati aneneti. . . . idam mahat auṣadhaṃ* . . .). At P(K) 1.8.3, 4 (see below), the word is read as *aruspānam*, 'wound-protector.' Bh., however, has *arusthānam* which Renou, recalling the sense of *sthāna* in the medical texts, renders: "le lieu (de traitement) des blessures" (JA, 252: 425–26). Most translators understand *aru(ḥ)srā́ṇa* to be a healer of wounds (see Weber, 138; Grill, 17, 80; Griffith, 44; Bloomfield, 9, 279–80; and Whitney-Lanman, 41). In light of the discrepancy in the P readings, one is forced to accept the Śau which, in itself, suggests a remedy (*bheṣajá*) which brings about the suppuration of wounds [*aru(ḥ)srā́ṇa*] i.e. a treatment for wounds. The medicine buried by the *ásuras* refers to *pippalī́* (see AVŚ 6.109.3, below, 213).

VERSE 4

For *upajī́kā*, in *a*, P(K) 1.8.4 has the Pāli form *upacīkā;* and for *cd*, it reads *aruspāno 'sy ātharvaṇo rogasthānam asy ātharvaṇam*, "You are the wound-protector belonging to the Atharvans; you are the disease receptacle belonging to the Atharvans." Bh. reads *ab* as Śau; and for *c*, he has *arusthānam asy* (cf. notes to verse 3 and Renou, JA, 242: 426). Sāyaṇa glosses *upajī́kā* as "female termites issuing from a termites' nest" (*valmīkaniṣpādikā vamryaḥ*). Weber renders the word as "Wassernixen." On the basis of KauśS 25.6–9, however, he has suggested that it may have the sense of *upadīkā* (a species of ant); although, he finds it hard to see a connection between

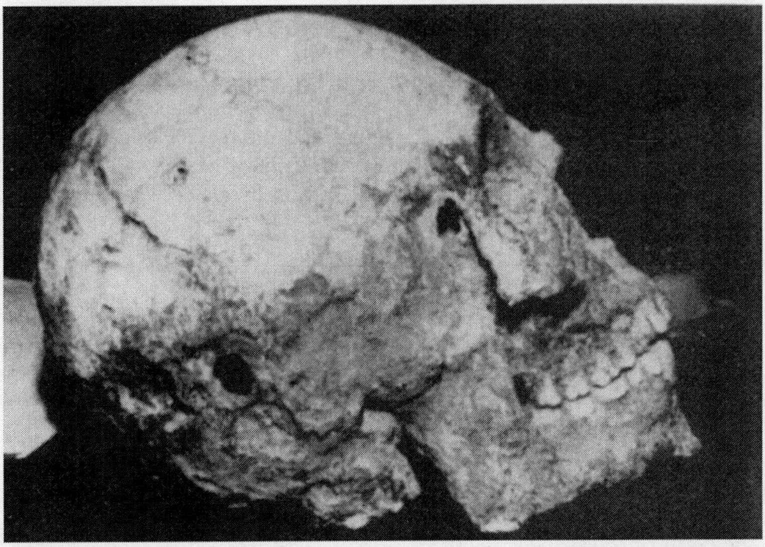

FIG. 7. Questionable trepanation. Skull of adult, #H 796B. Harappa. 3rd–2nd millennium B.C.

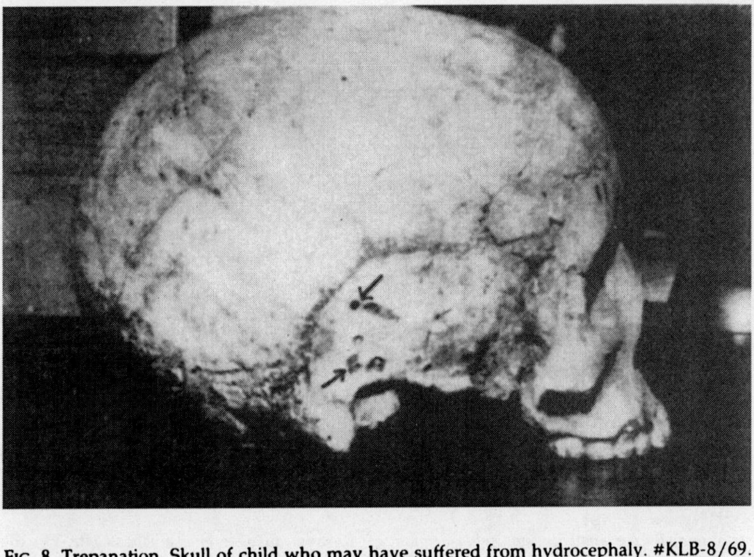

FIG. 8. Trepanation. Skull of child who may have suffered from hydrocephaly. #KLB-8/69. Kalibangan (Rajasthan). 3rd–2nd millennium B.C. Arrows indicate holes and burn marks.

ants and the sea (139–40). Bloomfield has confirmed the derivation of *upajīkā* from *upadīkā* and has shown that these (white) ants were thought to be endowed with the quality of producing water which was beneficial in healing (AJPh, 7: 482–84; see also Grill, 81; Griffith, 44 n; and Whitney-Lanman, 41; cf. also AVŚ 6.100.2 where *upajīkās* are connected with water). Sāyaṇa, following KauśS 25.7, considers that the medicine has the form of clay from a termites' nest (*valmīkamṛttikārūpam auṣadham*). Rather, it appears to be medicine derived from the third source, the sea or large lake, i.e. water.

VERSE 5

For *arusrā́ṇam*, in *a*, P(K) 1.8.3 has *aruspānam* (Bh., *arusthānam*, see above; Raghu Vira: *aruspānam*, see Hoffmann, IIJ, 11: 4 n6). Sāyaṇa understands this to be a reference to the medicine which has the form of clay from the field and which, being a styptic for the wound, was extracted from a marshy field (. . . *vraṇasya pācanaṃ* . . . *kedārādikṣetrarūpāyāḥ sakāśāt*. . . . *uddhṛtam*. . . . *yad* . . . *auṣadhaṃ kṣetramṛttikārūpam* . . .). This verse may refer back to verse 3, in which the plant remedy was dug up from the ground. Cf. also AVŚ 1.24.4 where a dark plant (*śyāmā́*) is said to be taken up from the earth (*pṛthivyā́ ádhy údbhṛtā*).

VERSE 6

A parallel in P is wanting. In this verse, we notice that the two types of remedies or medicines are clearly defined as water and plants. Also we have a hint that the cause for the bloody discharge may have been arrows sent by demons or enemies. Cf., in particular, AVŚ 1.2, 6.44 and 6.109.

Notes to 6.44

Translators agree that AVŚ 6.44 is a medical charm. They are, however, not unanimous in their views concerning the disease to be removed. Bergaigne-Henry, Griffith and Whitney-Lanman consider it to be generally remedial;[112] while Florenz specifies it as against "Durchfall (Diarrhea)"[113] and Bloomfield as "against excessive discharges from the body."[114] Sāyaṇa prescribes its use "in a rite to heal deteriorated wind (or slander)"[115] at KauśS 31.6.

VERSE 1

ab are found with slight variants at AVŚ 6.77.1*ab* (*d* concludes with making horses stand in their station), at P 3.40.5*ab* (*d* concludes with re-

[112] Bergaigne-Henry: "Conjuration en appliquant un remède," *Manuel*, 151; Griffith: "A charm to remove disease," *Hymns of the Atharvaveda*, 1: 268; and Whitney-Lanman: "For cessation of a disease," *Atharva-veda-saṃhitā*, Pt. 1, 312. Cf. also Ludwig who entitles it simply: "*viṣāṇakā́*," *Der Rigveda*, 3: 509.

[113] BB, 12: 314.

[114] *Hymns*, 10, 481.

[115] *apavāta* (or *apavāda*) *bhaiṣajyakarmaṇi*; cf. Keśava: *apavāde bhaiṣajyam ucyate*. On the variant reading see Bloomfield, *Hymns*, 481–82, and Caland, AZ, 99 n4.

questing desire to stand still), at P 19.23.9*ab* (*cd* concludes with the statement that the danger of poison has stood still and that adversity has become, as it were, feeble) and at P 20.56.3*ab* (*d* concludes with the healer proclaiming that he has put an end to the patient's red color?). Because of the repetition of these two *pādas* in verses culminating with various requests, there is a strong suggestion that they are formulaic (cf. Bloomfield, 483). *cd* is found unchanged at P 20.33.7*ab* (cf. note 2, below). Sāyaṇa describes *rógo,* in *d,* as that "characterized by the flow of blood" (*rudhirasrāvātmakas*). Bloomfield, however, does not wish to limit the flow or discharge merely to blood and, on the basis of KauśS 25.6–9 and its commentaries, considers that it indicates excessive discharges in general (234–35, 277–78, 483). In *c,* Bergaigne and Henry suggest the unlikely reading *ūrdhvásvapnas* which, when construed with *rógo,* means a disease which causes insomnia (151 n and 210; see also Henry who says the treatment in this verse is only clear enough to enable one to appreciate its serene absurdity, *La magie,* p. 196). The affliction or wound (*róga*), as at AVŚ 2.3, appears to be that which has a discharge of blood as its major symptom. The healer, therefore, implores the blood-flow to stop (cf. AVŚ 1.17, 80 and 213–17).

VERSE 2

P 20.33.7*ab* reads as Śau verse 1*cd* (above) and in *d,* it has *saṃbhṛtāni,* 'collected' for *sáṃgatāni.* For *cd,* P 20.33.8*cd* reads as Śau (see AVŚ 2.3.2 n, 207–208, above). Sāyaṇa glosses the difficult word *sáṃgatāni,* in *b,* as 'attained (or produced)' (*saṃprāptāni*). It means literally: 'those gone together' (root *gam* plus *sáṃ*) and seems to reflect the sense of 'collected' (as P; see also Bloomfield, 10) or 'brought together.' At ṚV 1.24.9 Varuṇa's medicines (or physicians) are enumerated as one hundred and one thousand (*śatáṃ te rājan bhiṣájaḥ sahásram . . .*). The hundred *bhiṣájs,* however, may refer to the *śatabhiṣak nakṣatra,* associated with Varuṇa at TB 3.1.2.9 [see Paul-Emile Dumont, "The Iṣṭis to the Nakṣatras (or Oblations to the Lunar Mansions) in the Taittirīya-Brāhmaṇa," *Proceedings of the American Philosophical Society,* 98(3) (1954): 204–23]. Understanding the hundred and thousand *bhiṣájs* as perhaps stars in lunar mansions avoids the problem of translating *bhiṣáj* (physician) as medicine (*bheṣajá*). Cf. also AVŚ 2.3.2–5.

VERSE 3

For *cd,* P 19.31.12*cd* reads: *pṛthivyāṃ niṣṭhitam asi viṣāṇā nāma vātīkṛtabheṣajī,* "You, the medicine for *vātīkṛta, viṣāṇā,* by name, are situated on the earth." Similarly at AVŚ 19.32.3*ab* there is: *diví te tū́lam* [*or mū́lam*] *oṣadhe pṛthivyā́m asi níṣṭhitaḥ,* "Your panicle [or root], O herb, [is] in heaven [and] you are situated on the earth," referring in this instance to the *darbha*-grass. This strongly suggests that *viṣāṇā* (feminine) in the P was a plant, and so also *viṣāṇakā́* in the Śau, may be considered as such (cf. also Zimmer, *Leben,* 389; Florenz, 304; Griffith, 268 n; and Bloomfield who identifies it with *viṣāṇikā* of the later medical texts, 483). Sāyaṇa, however, glosses it as 'cow-horn' (*gośṛṅga*) and Whitney-Lanman suggest that it "points to the use of a horn as such is indicated in the *Kauśika*" (p. 313). Cf. also Mayrhofer, Wb, 3: 228–29. Although *viṣāṇakā* is derived etymologically from *viṣāṇā*, 'horn,' the evidence seems to point to a plant which, along with water, as suggested by Rudra's urine, constitutes one of the two principal ingredients in the cure. These two are the same remedial elements mentioned in the treatment for such a malady at AVŚ 2.3.6. The notion of the fathers' root is obscure. It may suggest the root or stalk of the plants from which the stems and leaves were cut and used in the treatment. Cf. AVŚ 7.74(78).1 where the root of the divine sage is used to destroy *apacíts*. Bloomfield equates Rudra's medicine, *jālāṣá* with urine (19; see also AJPh, 12: 427–28; cf. AVŚ 6.57.2 n); cf. chapter on *jālāṣá*, 93–95, above. On "the navel of immortality," cf. TUp 3.10.6 and MahānārUp 9.12. The exact meaning of *vātī́ kṛta* remains questionable, but literally is translated as 'that which is made to become wind,' and may indicate a type of stomach or intestinal upset (see Filliozat, *La doctrine*, 140). Cf. also AVŚ 6.109.3 and 9.8.20.

Notes to 6.109

Most translators consider AVŚ 6.109 to be a charm to heal wounds.[116] Sāyaṇa prescribes its use in a rite "for the purpose of quieting all wind-disorders beginning with *dhanurvāta* (perhaps, tetanus) and thrown-weapon-caused wind-disorders"[117] at KauśS 26.38. It is also mentioned along with numerous other hymns at KauśS 26.33 and is listed among the *gaṇakarmāgaṇa* at AthPariś 32.24.

VERSE 1

In *cd*, P 19.27.9 reads: . . . *akalpayan* (manuscript 'P': *atalpayann?*) *alaṃ jīvitavā* (K manuscript, manuscript 'P': *jīvātavā*) *iti;* and from this, *iti* has been employed in our rendering. Sāyaṇa understands *kṣiptabheṣajī́* to be "other medicines which are cast . . . or else the medicine is the remover of that sent, i.e. of the particular wind disease" (. . . *kṣiptāni tiraskṛtāni anyāni bheṣajāni. . . . yadvā kṣiptasya vātarogaviśeṣasya bheṣajī nivartikā*) and *atividdhabheṣajī́* as "other medicines which have pierced completely,

---

[116] Ludwig: "Heilende Frucht (Healing fruit)," *Der Rigveda*, 3: 509; Zimmer translates the hymn under his discussion of *vātīkārá* (*vātīkṛta*), disease caused by wounds, *Leben*, 389; Griffith: "A charm to heal punctured wounds," *Hymns of the Atharvaveda*, 1: 305; Bloomfield: "The pepper-corn as a cure for wounds," *Hymns*, 21, 516; Bergaigne-Henry: "Conjuration contre les blessures," *Manuel*, 154; and Whitney-Lanman: "For healing: with *pippalī́*," *Atharva-veda-saṃhitā*, Pt. 1, 359.

[117] *dhanurvātakṣiptavātādikṛtsnavātavyādhiśāntyarthaṃ;* cf. Keśava: *atha vātavikāre bhaiṣajyam ucyate*, including *vātavikāre dhanurvātagulme vātaśūle kṣiptavātapradoṣe karmakṛte vāte utpanne sarvavyādhivikāré*. . . . Dārila states simply that it is "for the healing [of wounds from] missiles" (*kṣiptabhaiṣajyam*).

i.e. have struck . . . or else *atividdhā* means pierced through, i.e. afflicts every disease" (. . . *atiśáyena viddhāni tāḍitāni bheṣajāntarāṇi. . . . yadvā kṛtsnaṃ rogam atividhyati nipīḍayatīti atividdhā*). In both instances, Sāyaṇa's rendering of these compounds seems very unlikely. Although it goes against the general rules governing accent, it appears more correct to translate them as *tatpuruṣas* rather than *karmadhārayas* (cf. Bloomfield, 516).

VERSE 2

a is found at ṚV 10.97.22, with the variant: *óṣadhayaḥ sáṃ vadante . . . ,* "The herbs converse with . . ." and *cd* occurs at ṚV 10.97.17, etc. For *pūruṣaḥ,* 'man,' P 19.27.8 has *pauruṣaḥ*. Whitney-Lanman, based on ṚV 10.97.17*ab,* suggest that the true reading in *ab* may be *avadann āyatīs:* "Coming, they conversed . . ." (360, see also ṚV 10.97.17 n, 246, below).

VERSE 3

For *a,* P(K) 19.27.10 reads: *asurās te ni khanantu,* "Let the *asuras* bury your [medicine?]." Manuscript 'P' is as Śau; and for *cd,* P 15.15.9 has the interesting variant: *vātīkṛtasya bheṣajy āgan devy arundhatī,* "Let the goddess Arundhatī, the medicine for *vātīkṛta,* approach." Here we notice *arundhatī* is called a goddess and the medicine for *vātīkṛta,* which suggests an equation between *arundhatī* and *pippalī.* At P 15.16.2, she is called the queen of all herbs [*rājñī sarvāsām* (O: . . . *hi vasvāsām*) *asy oṣadhīnām arundhati*]. At AVŚ 2.3.3, and *ásuras* are said to have buried a wound treatment which is a medicine for *āsrāvá* and injury; and at AVŚ 6.44.3 *viṣāṇakā,* is called the destroyer of *vātīkṛta.* It is clear that in each case a plant having the name *pippalī, arundhatī* or *viṣāṇakā* is meant and that this plant was noted for being a specific against the discharge of blood caused by a wound as well as against *vātīkṛta* which may be a symptom manifested by a victim of a wound and which suggests a type of dyspepsia (cf. AVŚ 6.44.3 n, 212, above). Sāyaṇa, in *c,* glosses *vātīkṛtasya* as "the body burdened with wind-disease" (*vātarogāviṣṭaśarīrasya*) and *kṣiptásya* as "a kind of wind-disease called 'convulsion' which habitually [has as a symptom] the repeated throwing of a limb" (*muhurmuhuravayavakṣepaṇaśīlasya ākṣepakanāmno vātarogaviśeṣasya*).

Notes to 1.17

Most translators consider AVŚ 1.17 to be a charm to stop the flow of blood from the body.[118] Sāyaṇa prescribes its use in a rite for "the cessation

---

[118] Weber: "Zur Blutstillung (For stopping the flow of blood)," IS, 4: 411; Ludwig: "Blutfluss (Blood-flow)," *Der Rigveda,* 3: 508; Grill: "Blutung (Bleeding)," *Hundert Lieder des Atharva-Veda,* 16, 76; Griffith: "The hymn is a charm to be employed when venesection is performed," *Hymns of the Atharvaveda,* 1: 21; Bloomfield: "Charm to stop the flow of blood," *Hymns,* 22, 257; Whitney-Lanman: "To stop the flow of blood," *Atharva-veda-saṃhitā,* Pt. 1, 18; and Henry: "Les blessures et l'hémorrhagie," *La magie,* 197. Cf. also Filliozat: "Une conjuration contre les hémorragies," *La doctrine,* 130.

of excessive menstrual flow and of the flow of blood caused by the stroke of a sword, etc."[119] at KauśS 26.9(10)–13.

VERSE 1

P(K) 19.4.15 reads: *amūr yā yantu jāmayaḥ sarvā lohitavāsasaḥ, abhrātara iva yoṣitas* (K manuscript: *yoṣas,* cf. Nir 3.4: *yoṣās*) *tiṣṭhanti hatavarcasaḥ,* "Let all those sisters, who have blood-stained garments, proceed. Like brotherless young women, they stand with their beauty drained." Another close variant occurs at Nir 3.4: in *ab,* it reads as K; in *c: yoṣās* and in *d: hatavartmanaḥ* 'with their path obstructed.' Yāska explains that the simile in *cd* means the prohibition of marrying a brotherless maiden (*ity abhrātṛkāyāḥ anīrvāhaḥ aupamikaḥ;* cf. *Manu* 3.11 and *Yājñavalkya Smṛti* 1.53). Note the rather close similarity between K and the *Nirukta.* It is evident from these two variants that a menstruating woman is being described. Both read *sarvā* for the difficult *hirā́* which Sāyaṇa glosses as "bodily vessels (*sirāḥ*), i.e. tubes for carrying away impurities (menstrual discharges)" (*rajovahananāḍyaḥ*). Similarly, most translators, based on Sāyaṇa and other Vedic texts, consider them to be 'veins' or more generally, 'small blood vessels' (Filliozat, *La doctrine,* 128; see also, in particular, Weber, 411; Grill, 16; Bloomfield, 22; Whitney-Lanman, 18; and Henry, *La magie,* 197). Based on K, *Nirukta* and Sāyaṇa, it appears that these *hirā́s* may refer to those vessels directly involved with menses. Symbolically, therefore, the vessels may have been described in terms of young, menstruating women.

VERSE 2

For *cd,* P(K) 19.4.16 reads: *kaniṣṭhikāsi tiṣṭhās tiṣṭhād id dhamanir mahī,* "[Since] you are the smallest, [therefore,] you should stop; indeed, the *dhamani*-[blood] vessel should [also] stop." In *ab,* Sāyaṇa understands that the *dhamáni* are bodily vessels (*sirā*) distinguished according to the place of residence (*pūrvārdhe pratyakṣeṇa dhamanīnāṃ sthānabhedabhinnānāṃ prārthanā kṛtā*); and in *cd,* they are indicated with respect to size (*adhunā parimāṇato bhinnānāṃ tāsām eva pārokṣyeṇa* [!] *prārthanā kriyate*). In this way, *kaniṣṭhikā́* refers to the "more minute tubes" (*sūkṣmatarā . . . nāḍī*) and *dhamánir* to "the larger (or thicker) bodily vessels" (*mahatī sthūlatarā . . . sirā*). Such a description, along with verse 3, led Filliozat to posit the explanation that the *hirā́s* were blood vessels which were small in size and numerous; while, the *dhamánis* were blood vessels larger in size and fewer in number (*La doctrine,* 124, and 130–31).

VERSE 3

At AVŚ 7.35(36), a charm against a rival woman, verse 2 contains information which may help us to understand this verse and hymn: "With

[119] *śastraghātādijarudhirapravāhasya strīrajasaḥ ativartanasya ca nivṛttaye;* cf. Keśava: *atha lohitaṃ vahati śarīramadhye bahiśca . . . karmāṇy ucyante.*

a stone, I have closed the aperture of all those your hundred *hirā́*-[blood] vessels and thousand *dhamáni*-[blood] vessels" (*imā́ yā́s te śatáṃ hirā́ḥ sahásraṃ dhamánīr utá, tā́sāṃ te sárvāsām ahám áśmanā bílam ápy adhām*). Here, Sāyaṇa explains the hundred *hirā́s* as a hundred tubes which are small and situated inside for the purpose of sustaining the embryo (. . . *śatasaṃkhyākā* . . . *nāḍyaḥ garbhadhāraṇārtham antaravasthitāḥ sūkṣmā yā nāḍyaḥ santi* . . .) and the thousand *dhamánis* as a thousand tubes which are large (or thick) and which lean against the womb (. . . *sahasrasaṃkhyākā* . . . *dhamanyaḥ garbhāśayaḥ avaṣṭambhikā bāhyāḥ sthūlā yā nāḍyaḥ santi* . . .). Cf. SuŚāSth 3.10 where the *dhamanis* are defined as the vessels which carry the menstrual fluid to the uterus. It is interesting to note that Sāyaṇa, based on the later medical tradition, considers these to be vessels located in the womb or uterus. The closing of the aperture with a stone could, therefore, refer to the plugging of the uterus at the vagina. Also, the relative numbers of the two types of vessels are opposed to those mentioned at AVŚ 1.17.3. In *a*, P(K) 19.4.13 reads: *śatasya te;* in *b: hirāṇāṃ te;* and in *c*, it replaces *imāḥ* with *vā*. Sāyaṇa considers the hundred *dhamánis* to be the hundred principal tubes going to the heart, citing KaṭhUp 6.96 as support (. . . *śatasaṃkhyānāṃ* . . . *hṛdayagatānāṃ pradhānanāḍīnām*), and the thousand *hirā́s* as the thousand bodily vessels [or] branched tubes, citing PraUp 3.3 as support (. . . *sahasrasaṃkhyākānāṃ* . . . *sirāṇāṃ śākhānāḍīnām*). The discrepancy between the quantities of these two vessels according to the places where they have occurred leads one to the conclusion that their numbers were considered to be very large and that a distinction between them with respect to quantity is quite uncertain (cf. also AVŚ 6.90.2, where a hundred *dhamánis* are mentioned). Their definition according to size, and location in the uterus, however, appears to be possible. In the light of AVŚ 7.35(36).2, *pāda-d* could refer to the blocking or stopping of the blood-flow which issued from the uterus. In *d*, Whitney-Lanman propose the emendation of *ántyās*, 'the end ones' for *ántā* (18). Sāyaṇa reads *antā́* and understands them as "all the final, i.e. remaining, tubes" (*antimā avaśiṣṭāḥ sarvā nāḍyaḥ*). From the context, it would appear that Whitney-Lanman's emendation is justified.

VERSE 4

pāda-c is found unaltered at ṚV 1.191.6. P(K) 19.4.14 reads: *pari vas sikatāmayī dhanūs sthirā śaras sthiraḥ* (Raghu Vira: *sthirāḥ*), *tiṣṭhatelayatā su kam*, "Around you the bow-like (shaped) bank made of sand is firm, the layer of reeds(?) is firm. Stop remain perfectly still." Sāyaṇa considers *ab* to be a reference to a type of tube which is the bladder and which is bent like a bow. This tube contains dirt [or impurities]; or else, it is a type of disease with the name gravel, from which the sandy tube originates (. . . *sikatāḥ rajāṃsi tadvatī tadādhārabhūtā nāḍī. yadvā aśmaryākhyo vyādhiviśeṣo yasmād utpadyate sā nāḍī sikatāvatī.* . . . *dhanurvad vakro mūtrā-*

śayo nāḍīviśeṣaḥ). Rather, it appears that this could be a reference to the practice of sprinkling sand on the place of bleeding in order to help the blood to coagulate (see below). Or, if we consider the blood flow to be that of menses, the sand (K; sand and layer of reeds) could suggest a type of sanitary napkin. In this way, the difficult *dhanū̃r* may be understood as a 'sandbank' or 'dike' (see Bloomfield, 22; Whitney-Lanman, 18; and Henry, *La magie*, 197) shaped like a bow. Weber suggests that it may be a reference to a type of bandage filled with wet sand to make it harder and cooler (411) and Grill considers the verse to be a later addition (76). In the light of the medical practices suggested in verses 3, 4, it seems appropriate to include here a tentative rendering of P 1.94 which is also concerned with stopping the flow of blood and which may help us to understand some of the references in this hymn (the text follows that of Bh. and for the translation, cf. Renou, JA, 252: 33):

Verse 1. *yās te śataṃ dhamanayaḥ sahasrāṇi ca viṃśatiḥ, babhror aśvasya vāreṇāpi nahyāmi tā aham*, "With the tail of the brown horse, I tie up those your *dhamani*-[blood] vessels which number a hundred, a thousand and twenty."

Verse 2. *śatasya te dhamanīnāṃ sahasrasyāyutasya ca, dṛteḥ* (K: *tṛtes*) *pādam iva sārathir api* (K: *iva sārathim api*) *nahyāmi yad bilam*, "I tie up the aperture of your hundred *dhamani*-[blood] vessels, [your] thousand and [your] ten thousand, as a charioteer [ties to the chariot] the foot of a [water-carrier's] skin" (for *c*, cf. *Manu*, 2.99 and Renou).

Verse 3. *paramasyāṃ parāvati* (K: *parāvataś*) *śuṣko bhaṇḍuś ca tiṣṭhataḥ* (K: *abhy arugnaś ca tiṣṭhatu*), *tataḥ śuṣkasya śuṣmeṇa tiṣṭhantu lohinīr apaḥ* (Bar.: *lohinir apa;* Raghu Vira: *lohiṇīr apa*), "[Since] the *śuṣka* and *bhaṇḍu* stop in the remote distance, therefore, by the impulse of *śuṣka*, let the red-waters stop" (according to Bh., *śuṣka* and *bhaṇḍu* are parts of the human body, xxvii).

Verse 4. *pari vaḥ sikatāmayam arumbile vapāmasi, daka cid asravīt purā taka cid aśramīd idam* (K: *akaśadaśvavait purā takaś ca daśamīm idam*), "We strew much sand around you at the wound-opening. To be sure, [some] liquid flowed before; but now, that small amount has stopped (?)" (cf. Renou).

From verses 1, 2, we notice that the quantity of *dhamani*s is inconsistent and seems merely to reflect a large number. The particular type of blood flow appears to be that which could have been caused by a wound (verse 4); and the method for stopping it involved the tying off or closing of the vessels, perhaps by a type of ligature using horse's hair, and the sprinkling of sand on the wound in order to help the blood to coagulate. The latter technique may be the same as that mentioned at AVŚ 1.17.4; however here, it is more clearly defined and may point to a later and more generalized use of the charm (cf. KauśS 26.9–13, 79, above).

Notes to AVŚ 1.23, 24

Most translators, based on Sāyaṇa, consider both AVŚ 1.23 and 24 to be charms against a type of leprosy.[120] Sāyaṇa prescribes their use in a rite "for the removal of cutaneous whiteness"[121] at KauśS 26.22–24. TB 2.4.4.1–2 preserves only five of the original eight verses of these charms: the first four are close variants of 1.23 and the fifth is a variant of 1.24.3.

AVŚ 1.23

VERSE 1

P 1.16.1 reads as Śau (K is corrupt; Hoffmann has noted that Bh.'s *naktaṃ jātā* should be read as *naktaṃjātā*, IIJ, 10: 9). TB 2.4.4.1 reads as Śau. In *ab*, Sāyaṇa understands four plants to be expressed: *óṣadhi* is the herb called *haridrā; rā̃mā* is the herb called *bhṛṅgarājā; kṛ́ṣṇā* is called *indravāruṇī;* and *ásiknī* is called *nīlī.* At TB, however, he considers there to be one herb (*oṣadhe*) called *nīlī* with the quality of blackness represented by the other vocatives in the line (*tathāvidhe he nīlyākhyauṣadhe . . .*). In *c*, he understands *rajani*, '(female) colorer,' from the root *rañj*, 'to color,' to be representative of the four herbs and to be expressive of their coloring or dyeing quality (*pūrvam oṣadhiśabdena nirdiṣṭāya haridrāya jananakriyāsaṃbandhitvena kuṇṭhitaśaktitvāt rañjanakriyāyam api saṃbandhaṃ darśayituṃ punarāha rajanīti . . . rañja rāge . . .*). At TB, he glosses it simply as "the herb capable of dyeing with its own color" (*. . . svakīyena varṇena rañjanakṣama oṣadhe . . .*). In *d*, he explains *kilā̃saṃ* as the limb affected with *kuṣṭha* (skin disease) ([*kilāsaṃ*] *kilāsaḥ kuṣṭharogaḥ tadyuktam aṅgaṃ . . .* ; cf. to TB: *śvetarogagrastam aṅgaṃ . . .*). Filliozat argues that there is one herb, *rajanī*, signified here and that it is the indigo plant (*La doctrine*, 102–103). This viewpoint is supported by the commentary to TB. The fact remains, however, that we cannot be sure whether *rajanī* refers to a specific plant or whether it is merely an epithet of a dark plant or a plant used for tincturing purposes. Being derived from the root *rañj* plus the suffix *anī*, it means 'the coloring one,' or in the feminine, '(the female) colorer.'

VERSE 2

In *ab*, P 1.16.2 reads as Śau. In *c*, based on TB 2.4.4.1, which reads: *ā̃ naḥ svó aśnutāṃ várṇaḥ*, "let our own color pervade us," the editors of P(K)

---

[120] Weber: "Gegen Aussatz (Against leprosy)," IS, 4: 416, 417; Ludwig: 1.23 is untitled and 1.24 is called "Sāmā," *Der Rigveda*, 3: 506 and 509 respectively; Grill: "Aussatz," *Hundert Lieder des Atharva-Veda*, 19, 77; Griffith: "The hymn is a charm against leprosy," *Hymns of the Atharvaveda*, 1: 27, 28; Bloomfield: "Leprosy cured by a dark plant," *Hymns*, 16, 266, 268; and Whitney-Lanman: "Against leprosy; with a healing herb" and "Against leprosy," *Atharva-veda-saṃhitā*, Pt. 1, 23, 24. Bergaigne-Henry have 1.23: "Conjuration contre la lèpre blanche," *Manuel*, 135. Cf. Henry, *La magie*, 191.

[121] *śvetakuṣṭhāpanodanāya;* cf. also Keśava: *atha śvetakuṣṭhabhaiṣajyāny ucyante.*

emend *c* to *ā tvā svo 'śnutāṃ,* "let your own color pervade you" (so also Bh.). *d* is wanting in the P(K). TB has *párā śvetāni pātaya,* "make the white colors fly away." Bar. and Raghu Vira restore the K according to Śau. Bh., however, reads according to TB, a reading which Renou prefers (JA, 252: 427). For *pṛ́ṣat,* 'the spotted one,' Sāyaṇa reads *pṛ́thak,* 'separately' (*pṛthak-kṛtya*). At TB, however, he reads *pṛ́ṣat* and glosses it more correctly as *citrarūpaṃ* 'multi-formed (or variegated).' Syntactically, *pṛ́thak* would be easier. As Whitney-Lanman point out, however, it receives very little support in the manuscript traditions (24). Likewise, since TB reads *pṛ́ṣat* (and Sāyaṇa agrees with it), it would appear that it is the true reading. Sāyaṇa assumes a digression in *c* directed to the patient rather than to the herb (. . . *he rugṇa* . . .). This is also supported by the TB. Henry, however, considers it to be directed to the herb and renders: " 'Que ta couleur propre t'impregne,' et conséquemment pénètre avec toi dans le sujet" (*La magie,* 191 n. 1; see also Bergaigne-Henry, *Manuel,* 135 n). Filliozat also understands it to be addressed to the plant, but for different reasons. He suggests that the purpose of the charm is to make the white spots pass into the black plant and to be absorbed by it. Therefore, he translates: "Que la couleur qui est sienne (la couleur de ce qui est blanc) te pénètre" (*La doctrine,* 102–103 and 105). One would think rather that it is a question of the white color being overpowered by the black; in which case, the healer would implore the natural dark color to enter the patient in order to drive away the unnatural whiteness. Thus, the sympathetic association of like colors is demonstrated in this verse.

VERSE 3

P 1.16.3 reads as Śau. TB 2.4.4.1–2 has, in *a, ásitaṃ te niláyanam,* "black [is] your abode." In this verse, Sāyaṇa considers the indigo plant to be singled out and to be addressed (*anayā nīlīm eva avayutya prārthayate- he nīli* . . . ; cf. TB, where he indicates that merely the herb is addressed, *he oṣadhe*). For *praláyanam,* 'bed,' he glosses "the place of birth" (*utpattis-thānam;* cf. his gloss of *niláyanam* at TB: *layaprāptisthānam aṅgam,* "the limb, i.e. the place of the attaining of dissolution") and for *āsthā́nam,* 'site,' he understands "[that] having the form beginning with a throwing-instrument (?)" (*prakṣepaṇabhājanādirūpam;* cf. to TB, *vastirūpaṃ,* 'having the form of a dwelling'). Filliozat, however, basing himself on Bergaigne-Henry, understands these two words to refer to the plant both in its living and dead state and renders: "Dépourvue de blanc est ta solution, ta station est dépourvue de blanc, . . ." (*La doctrine,* 102). The word *praláyanam,* being derived from the root *lī* plus *prá,* 'to dissolve oneself,' indicates, according to Bergaigne-Henry "solution" or "decoction." This then represents the dead state of the plant which is opposed to the living one represented by *āsthā́nam,* 'station (on the stalk).' Thereupon, whether the plant is dead or alive, it is always black (*Manuel,* 135–36 n). Filliozat mentions in a footnote that he finds this interpretation uncertain and proposes an alternative rendering: " 'dépourvue de blanc (quand) ta position est couchée . . . ,' ce qui d'ailleurs revient à dire 'morte (arrachée) ou vivant (encore debout) tu es noire' " (*La doctrine,* 102–103 n.5). These scholars' interpretation of *praláyanam* is questionable, since both the TB's alternate reading and the commentary understand it to be a place. The notion of the plant having a station on the stalk, i.e. growing, is a possible meaning of *āsthā́nam;* but again, station has the sense rather of place or location than of a state. The suggestions of Bergaigne, Henry and Filliozat, therefore, raise doubts. Even in the alternative translation proposed by Filliozat, the concern is with the plant in its living and dead condition. Weber (416), Bloomfield (16) and Whitney-Lanman (24) render *praláyanam* in the sense of a resting or hiding place and *āsthā́nam* as a station or dwelling place. It would appear that a concrete locality rather than a condition or state is indicated. One might suspect that the poet-healer was referring to the herb's ecological habitat: the "site" could have been the general "community" which, being in dense growth hidden from the sun, is dark, and the "bed" or, as Sāyaṇa suggests, birthplace, might refer to its soil or ground which can be dark, even black (cf. 1.23.3, 4). In *d,* Sāyaṇa again reads *pṛ́thak* (at TB, however, *pṛ́ṣat,* i.e. *bahuvidhaṃ,* 'manifold').

VERSE 4

P(K) 1.16.4 has only *bcd,* which read as Śau. Bh. reads the entire verse as Śau. In *c,* TB 2.4.4.2 reads: *kṛtyáyā kṛtásya . . . ,* 'caused by magic.' In *b, yát tvací,* is literally, 'which [is] in the skin'; and, being neuter, refers to the 'white mark' (*lákṣma śvetám*). For the difficult word *dū́ṣyā,* in *c,* Sāyaṇa understands: 'the magical act produced by an enemy' and derives it from the causative of the root *duṣ,* 'to defile,' i.e. it injures living beings (. . . *dūṣayati prāṇinaṃ hinastīti dūṣiḥ śatrūtpāditā kṛtyā*). On the basis of the TB and Sāyaṇa, it would appear to signify a magical action produced and sent by a foe, i.e. a curse. Cf. Henry, who suggests that *tvací dū́ṣyā kṛtásya* may be rendered as one unit: "déposée sur la peau par une femelle malfaisante" (*La magie,* 191). Because of the disruption of the syntax, however, one would cast a suspicious eye on this interpretation.

AVŚ 1.24

VERSE 1

In *c,* P 1.26.1 reads: *tad āsurī yudhā jitā,* "then, the *āsurī,* overpowered in battle" (K: *tavāsurī jighāṃsitā?*); and in *d,* K has *vanaspatiḥ;* cf. also Whitney-Lanman, 24. For the difficult *pādas cd,* Sāyaṇa glosses *jitā́* with *jitavatī,* 'conquered' and understands that the *āsurī́,* after having made battle with the bird, conquered and seized its gall, which she made into the form of a tree (*suparṇena saha saṃgrāmaṃ kṛtvā . . . jitavatī . . . jayena labdhaṃ tat pittaṃ . . . oṣadhyātmanā sevyam ākāram akārṣīt*). On the basis of this explanation, Bloomfield, hesitatingly, proposes the emendation of *jitā́* to *jitvā́* and renders: "The Āsurī having conquered this (gall) gave it to the trees for their color" (16; 268–69). Although one cannot be sure, it

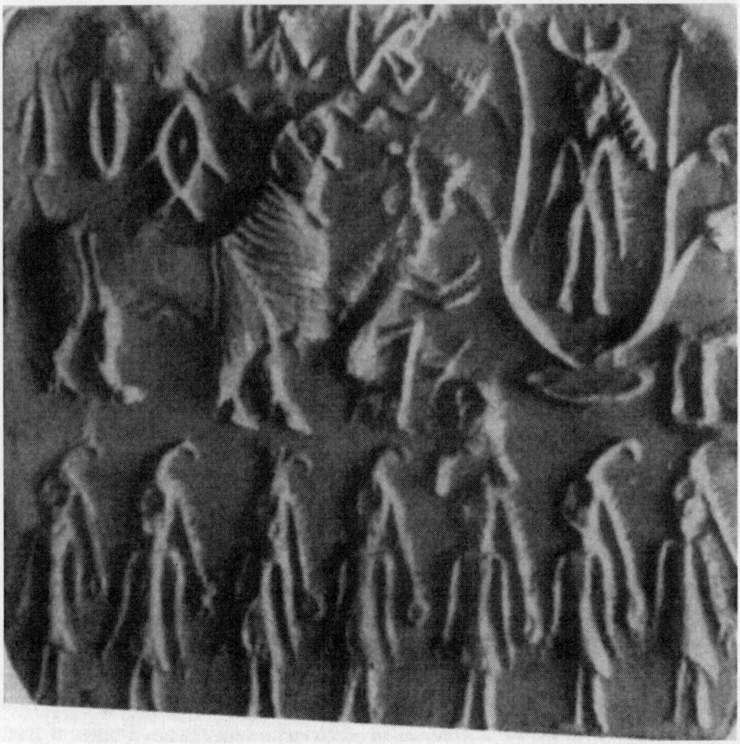

FIG. 9. Tree-goddess and seven devotees. Perforated seal. Mohenjo-Dāro. 3rd–2nd millennium B.C.

seems rather to refer to a mythological episode in which a certain female *ásura* was defeated in battle; and the gall from her torn-asunder abdomen gave the trees their color which, in *b*, appears to be that of greenish yellow gall or bile (cf. Weber, 417 and Whitney-Lanman, 24). As Sāyaṇa points out, *rūpáṃ* refers to the appearance to be inhabited with a herbal nature (. . . *oṣadhyātmā sevyam ākāram akārṣīt*), i.e. a vegetal color (cf. also Bloomfield, 417). The use of the root *kṛ* with the double accusative suggests that one of the nouns has a dative sense, i.e. "gave form (color) to the trees." Cf. the mention of *ásura* in healing charms at AVŚ 2.3.3, 6.100.3 and 6.109.3. Later, *āsurī* came to signify a division of surgical medicine and a plant.

VERSE 2

Throughout P(K) 1.26.2, *surūpām* occurs in place of *sárūpām;* Bh. reads as Śau. For *ab*, Sāyaṇa understands that the *āsurī* was the first of the healers of *śvitra* ('morbid whiteness of the skin') and made the indigo-plant, etc., which was fashioned from the eagle's gall, the *śvitra*-removing medicine (*āsurī . . . śvitracikitsakanām ādibhūtā . . . suparṇapittena nirmitaṃ nīly-ādikaṃ . . . kilāsasya śvitrasya nivartakam auṣadhaṃ . . . kṛtavatī*); and for *sárūpam*, he explains: "having the same color because the skin is devoid of *śvitra*" (*śvitrahitatvacā samānavarṇām*). Cf. also Grill, 19, 78; Griffith, 29; Bloomfield, 16; and Henry, *La magie*, 191. In *d*, Sāyaṇa considers "the medicine beginning with indigo" (*tad nīlyādyauṣadhaṃ*) to be the subject of both *ánīnaśat* and *akarat*.

VERSE 3

P 1.26.3 reads as Śau, except for K's *surūpā*. This verse is also found at TB 2.4.4.2 which has in *c*: *sárūpāsy oṣadhe*, "you, O herb, are even-colored." Sāyaṇa, suggests that the herb's mother and father are the earth and sky, respectively (*he oṣadhe . . . tava . . . jananī bhūmiḥ . . . tathā . . . tava pitā dyauḥ*). At TB, however, he explains that the herb's mother is the earth and its father is a type of seed (*he oṣadhe . . . tava mātṛsthānīyā bhūmiḥ . . . tava pitṛsthānīyo bījaviséṣaḥ*, so also at the Śau, as an alternative explanation). It is possible that the mother is the earth, since at verse 4, the earth or soil is mentioned as the birthplace of the dark plant. The question of its father, however, is uncertain. It could be a dark, rain-threatening sky or even the night (cf. AVŚ 1.23.1, 3). In *d*, *idáṃ* seems to refer to the skin (*tvácam*) mentioned in the previous verse. Sāyaṇa, however, understands it to be "the limb ruined by the *śvitra*-disease" (*śvitrarogadūṣitam aṅgaṃ*; cf. TB: *śvetarūparogagrastaṃ śarīraṃ*, "the body afflicted with the disease of white-color"). P inserts a verse (1.26.4) which tentatively is as follows: *yat tanūjaṃ yad agnijaṃ* (Raghu Vira: *asthijaṃ*) *citraṃ kílāsaṃ jajñiṣe, tad astu sutvak* (K: *sukṛtaṃ*, K manuscript: *sukṛtas*) *tanvo yatas tvāpa nayāmasi*, "Since we dispel you far away, [therefore,] let that *kilāsa*, who is body-born, fire-born [and] born variegated, be(come) the body's beautiful skin (?)" (cf. AVŚ 1.23.4, TB 2.4.4.2 and Renou, JA, 252: 429–30).

VERSE 4

In *a*, P 1.26.5 is as Śau, except for *surūpaṃ*, in *a*. In *b*, Sāyaṇa reads: *pṛthivyā́ ádhy údbhṛtā* and renders; "You were produced over the earth . . ." (. . . *tvam . . . bhūmer upari . . . utpāditā*). For *c*, he quite correctly explains: "You, O herb, aptly make the limb, attacked with *kilāsa*, free from disease" (. . . *he oṣadhe tvam . . . kilāsākrāntam aṅgaṃ . . . suṣṭhu rogavinirmuktaṃ kuru*). One might, however, understand the skin, as in verse 3, rather than the limb. The action of "taking up from the earth" suggests the uprooting of the plant.

Notes to 6.25

Most translators consider AVŚ 6.25 to be a charm against sores which afflict the neck and shoulders.[122] Sāyaṇa prescribes its use in a rite "for the

---

[122] Florenz: untitled; but he adds: "Es ist nicht ganz sicher, ob dieser Zauber gegen Krankheit gerichtet ist, obgleich nicht gut etwas anderes zu verstehen ist . . . Hier vielleicht einer hitzige Krankheit mit Hautausschlägen auf Nacken und Schultern zu verstehen?" "Das sechste Buch

purpose of the cessation of scrofulous neck-swellings"[123] at KauśS 30.14–16.

A. Kuhn has included a translation of this charm in his discussion of "Siebenundsiebzigerlei Krankheit" (Seventy-sevenfold disease) which in the Germanic tradition commonly referred to fever.[124] He has presented one interesting example of a north German charm which mentions seventy-seven Zahnrose.[125] Most of the article, however, is taken up with a discussion of numbers in general and specifically those enumerations which are associated with divinities.

VERSE 1

This verse has a parallel at P 8.16.3 and 19.5.6. In *b,* P 8.16.3 has *cārūḍhā vakṣaṇānu,* "who are raised up [and spread] over the abdomen"; and 19.5.6 replaces *mányā* with *skandhyā,* 'shoulders.' In *c,* 8.16.3 reads as Śau, but the K manuscript begins with *yadas;* 19.5.6 has *adas,* (K manuscript: *yadas*) *tās sarvā.* In *d,* K 8.16.3 has the unintelligible *anuttāḥ pratthajño mayaḥ* (O: *muttāḥ putthajño mayā*) and 19.5.6 reads as Śau. Sāyaṇa explains the first line: "The scrofulous neck-swellings amounting to fifty-five, i.e. the (blood) vessels (=*manyā*) situated on the upper part of the neck, permeate everywhere" (*pañcādhikapañcāśatasaṃkhyākā . . . gaṇḍamālāḥ . . . galasyordhvabhāge sthitā dhamanīr manyāśabdavācyā*[!] . . . *sarvato vyāpnuvanti*); and for *d,* he interprets: "The defilements which are to be referred to, are repelled, and are destroyed as when one obtains an adored and virtuous wife" (. . . *vacanīyā doṣāḥ . . . pūjitāṃ pativratāṃ striyaṃ prāpya yathā parāhatā naśyanti tathety arthaḥ;* note: he derives *apacít* from the root *ci* plus *apa,* 'to honor'). Bloomfield quite rightly calls his explanation of *d,* "the low water-mark of his hermeneutical capacity" (473). In *d,* the difficult word *vākā̆* seems to refer to particular types of noises commonly associated with insects (cf. also Whitney-Lanman, 299). Kuhn has rendered it "swarm" (138); Florenz, "buzzing" (280); and Whitney-Lanman, "noises" (298). Because of its apparent discontinuity with his understanding of *apacít* as "swelling," Bloomfield has suggested its emendation to *pākā̆* "pustules" (19, 473), an appealing but unsupported reading. From the P readings it appears that the tradition understood these *apacít*s to be raised bumps or swellings which covered the abdomen or shoulders. Their characterization as noisemakers, however, suggests rather an insect. Perhaps the poet-healer is presenting us with a clue to their description as raised bumps or pustules similar to those produced by insects' bites. The disappearance of the buzz-

---

der *Atharva-saṃhitā:* übersetzt und erklärt," BB, 12: 280, 281; Griffith: "A charm against *apacíts,* pustules or scrofulous swellings," *Hymns of the Atharvaveda,* 1: 258; Bloomfield: "Charm against scrofulous sores upon the neck and shoulders," *Hymns,* 19, 472; and Whitney-Lanman: "For relief from pains(?) in the neck and shoulders," *Atharva-veda-saṃhitā,* Pt. 1, 298.

[123] *gaṇḍamālānivṛttyartham;* cf. Keśava: *atha gaṇḍamālābhaiṣajyam ucyate.*

[124] "Indische und germanische Segenssprüche," KZ, 13 (1864): 128–35.

[125] Ibid., 128.

ing-sound created by these vermin as they leave their victim could, therefore, indicate the removal of the disease or at least the agents of the disease. In this way, the *apacíts* may have been looked upon as both the disease or skin-affliction itself and its cause. The numerical sequence fifty-five, seventy-seven and ninety-nine, while referring to an indeterminately large number, suggests an increase in the severity of the rash as it moves down the neck to the shoulders.

VERSE 2

Parallels to this verse are found at P 8.16.2 and 19.5.5. In *b,* 8.16.2 reads as 8.16.3 and 19.5.5 is as Śau. In *cd,* 8.16.2 is as 8.16.3; and at 19.5.5, *cd* as Śau. Sāyaṇa renders *a* as "The scrofulous neck-swellings amounting to seventy-seven, i.e. the vessels on the neck, permeate on both sides" (*saptādhikasaptatisaṃkhyākā . . . gaṇḍamālāḥ . . . grivāsu bhavā nāḍīḥ . . . abhito vyāpnuvanti*).

VERSE 3

Parallels to this verse occur at P 8.16.1 and 19.5.4. In *b,* 8.16.1 reads as 8.16.3 and 19.5.4 has *manyā* (K manuscript: *manyābhiḥ*) for *skándhyā.* In *cd,* 8.16.1 is as 8.16.3 and 19.5.4 like 19.5.6. Sāyaṇa translates *a* as "The scrofulous neck-swellings amounting to ninety-nine, i.e. the (blood) vessels in the region below the necks (=*skándhyā*), permeate on both sides" (*navottaranavatisaṃkhyākā . . . gaṇḍamālāḥ. grīvābhyo 'dhaḥpradeśaḥ skandhaḥ. tatra bhavā dhamanīḥ . . . abhito vyāpnuvanti*).

Notes to 6.83

Most translators agree that AVŚ 6.83 is a charm against *apacíts* or scrofulous sores.[126] Sāyaṇa prescribes it, along with AVŚ 7.76(80), for use "in a rite for the healing of scrofulous neck-swellings"[127] at KauśS 31.16–17. Verse 3*cd* is mentioned at KauśS 31.20 in a rite for the healing of the same basic malady and verse 4 is cited at KauśS 31.21 in a ceremony against scrofulous neck-swellings arising from an unknown source.[128]

---

[126] Ludwig: "*Apacit,*" *Der Rigveda,* 3: 500; Griffith: "A charm against sores and pustules," *Hymns of the Atharvaveda,* 1: 290; Bloomfield: "Charm for curing scrofulous sores called *apacit,*" *Hymns,* 17, 503; and Whitney-Lanman: "To remove *apacíts,*" *Atharva-veda-saṃhitā,* Pt. 1, 342.

[127] *gaṇḍamālābhaiṣajyakarmaṇi;* cf. Keśava: *atha gaṇḍamālābhaiṣajyam ucyate.*

[128] Caland entitles the *sūtra* as such, based on internal evidence; and Dārila calls it *ajñātakaraṇaṃ ajñātāruḥ . . .* (AZ, 102; cf. also Bloomfield, *Hymns,* 504). At KauśS 31.21, Keśava defines it as *atha gardabhādyuruṃgaṇḍabhaiṣjyam ucyate,* "the healing of large boils on an ass etc. (?)"; similarly, Sāyaṇa: *catuṣpādgaṇḍabhaisajyārthaṃ,* "for the purpose of healing the neck boils of the four-footed ones (?)" Clearly, Keśava and Sāyaṇa understand the charm to be used in a rite of veterinary medicine.

VERSE 1

P 1.21.2 reads as Śau. In *d,* however, we may, along with Bar., emend K to *candram ā vo'poccatu,* "Let [the sun], with its light, drive you off towards the moon." This may, against the *pāda*-text, also apply to the Śau text. Sāyaṇa derives *ápacit* (note change of accented syllable) from the root *ci* plus *apa,* 'being heaped up from behind because of the "humors," ' and defines it: "scrofulous neck-swellings beginning at the throat and extending downward" (*doṣavaśād apāk cīyamānāḥ galād ārabhya adhastāt prasṛtā gaṇḍamālāḥ . . .*). For *b,* a similar notion is found at P(K) 19.13.9 in a charm against *balā́sa* (see AVŚ 6.14.3 n, 135, above). The phrase, "as an eagle from its nest," in the context of bodily *apacít*s, suggests a type of parasitic insect which resides in its host's head of hair; and the sight of which, when forced to depart, may resemble that of a bird flying from its nest.

VERSE 2

pāda-c is found at ṚV 1.191.13*c.* P 1.21.3 reads as Śau. Sāyaṇa explains the import of the verse as follows: "By this [verse], through mentioning the names of the [different] kinds of *apacit*s, their departure is requested" (*anayā apacitprabhedānāṃ nāmagrahaṇena tāsām apagamanaṃ prārthyate*). This notion of seizing (i.e. knowing) and of reciting the names (i.e. descriptions) of the disease entities is very important and occurs frequently in the Vedic medical charms.

VERSE 3

For *cd,* P 1.21.4 has: *glaur itaḥ pra patiṣyati sa galanto na śiṣyati* (K: *sakalaṃ tena śudhyati,* "Therefore, he [?] is completely cleansed"), ". . . The oozing does not remain," or better, "The oozing will perish" (*naśiṣyati,* see Renou, JA, 252: 428). Sāyaṇa explains *asū́tikā,* 'barren' as "not producing a pus-flow, i.e. that having a period of prolonged ripening" (*pūyasrāvam ajanayantī. ciraparipākety arthaḥ*). For *rāmāyaṇī́,* 'the black one's daughter,' he understands a tube (*nāḍī*), "i.e. that (which has) the nature of a wound" (*vraṇātmakety arthaḥ*). It is more likely that the barren *apacít* refers to a single sore just before it suppurates or better after it has done so. For *c,* which includes the difficult *gláur,* Sāyaṇa suggests: "The loss of sexual desire, caused by the sore, will fly forth from the limb, i.e. with the departing of the disease, the perception of the pain produced by it will go away; or else, *glauḥ* is the moon who will cause the *apacít* to go forth from here . . ." (. . . *vraṇajanito harṣakṣayaḥ . . . asmād aṅgāt pra patiṣyati vyādhyapagame tajjanitaduḥkhānubhavo 'pi prakarṣeṇa nirgamiṣyatīti arthaḥ. yadvā glauś candramāḥ itaḥ asmād . . . apacitaṃ pra patiṣyati . . .*). He probably bases his first interpretation on CaCiSth 3.36, where *glāni,* 'exhaustion,' is found in connection with mental fever. Bloomfield (503), however, relates it to *gilāyu* (Wise: *gīlin,* 311) which Suśruta defines as a glandular swelling in the throat about the size of a stone of the fruit of the *āmalaka*-plant and whose treatment requires surgery (NiSth 16.58 and CiSth 22.66). Mayrhofer suggests the meaning: "round lump, wen-like excrescence" (Wb, 1: 354–55; cf. also MWSED, 374, col. 3). The notion of a round lump could have then given rise to Sāyaṇa's second suggestion, "the moon." Filliozat states that the word cannot seriously be defined as a disease (*La doctrine,* 106). It is difficult to know precisely what *glaúr* means. Most translators, however, accept the idea of "boil" (see, in particular, Griffith, 290; Bloomfield, 17; and Whitney-Lanman, 343). For *galuntó,* Sāyaṇa explains: "the excrescences on the neck born everywhere in the joints of the hands and feet, etc. by the affliction produced by the scrofulous neck-swellings" (. . . *gaṇḍamāl-odbhavavikāreṇa tatra tatra hastapādādisaṃdhiṣu udbhūtān gaḍūn tasyati upakṣapayatīti gaḍuntaḥ;* cf. Whitney-Lanman, 343). Griffith defines it as a "morbid growth" (290); Bloomfield, "swelling" (17); and Whitney-Lanman, as an ablative from *gala,* i.e. "from the neck" (343). Filliozat again casts doubt on any definite meaning for it (*La doctrine,* 106; cf. Mayrhofer, Wb., 1: 330). It appears to be derived from the root *gal,* 'to ooze,' and may refer to the suppuration or pus from the *gláu,* if we accept that *gláu* means 'boil' (see T. Chowdhury, JBORS, 17: 67–68). For *naśiṣyati,* Sāyaṇa glosses "does not remain" (*nāvaśeṣayati*); cf. P 1.21.4 at AVŚ 6.83.3 n (224, above). Such an interpretation is possible. One tends, however, to favor the reading as a future, since the other verbs in the verse are in that tense. Nevertheless, with either reading the meaning remains much the same, i.e. the *galuntá* will go away. T. Chowdhury, however, has proposed another possible reading for *d: ságalantas naśiṣyati,* "[The boil will fly forth from here and] will disappear together with the pus" (JBORS, 17: 68). This is quite possible and, in light of P 1.21.4, helps to elucidate the meaning. In this case, the second line may refer to a type of suppurating boil or sore which will be removed by washing or cleansing.

VERSE 4

A variant of this verse is found at K 19.5.9(10) which breaks after *manasā svāha,* and concludes: *svāha manasā yad idaṃ kṛṇomi,* "When I make this [offering] with the mind, [saying:] '*svāhā.*' " Sāyaṇa considers the subject, "you" of the verb *vīhí* to be "the god who lays claim to the *vraṇa* (sore or wound)-disease" (*he vraṇarogābhimānin deva tvaṃ* . . .). Although the verse appears to be an intrusion into the hymn (Whitney-Lanman, 343), it does suggest an interesting practice in the medical ritual which, as Bloomfield points out, bears a relationship to the rite found at KauśS 31.21 (505). The performance of a mental offering and oblation to a divinity is not common in the medical charms and may well be an elaboration of the more common practice of appeasing the demon and winning it over by means of praise. Nevertheless, it indicates a definite ritualistic activity. It is perhaps significant to note that P 1.21.5 is different: *apeto apacitvarīr indraḥ pūṣā ca* (K: *tu*) *cikyatuḥ, apetv asya grīvābhyo apa padbhyāṃ vijāmataḥ,* "Let the supporter of the *apacits* depart, [for] both Indra and Pūṣan are attentive [to the problem]. Let [her] depart from the nape of his neck, from [his] feet [and] from [his] *vijāman*-joint" (cf. Renou, JA, 252: 228–29, and see also AVŚ 7.76[80].2 and ṚV 7.50.2 on *vijā́man*).

Notes to 7.74(78)

Although this hymn contains a total of four verses, only the first two, which have specific reference to *apacít*, have been presented. The remaining two are concerned with completely different topics: verse 3 is against jealousy and verse 4 is to Agni.[129] Most translators agree that verses 1 and 2 are against *apacíts*.[130] Sāyaṇa prescribes its use in a rite "for the purpose of healing scrofulous neck-swellings"[131] at KauśS 32.8–10.

VERSE 1

In *a*, P(K) 19.36.2 has *arjunīnām apacitāṃ*, 'of the white *apacits*'; in *b*, *śuśrotha*, 'you have heard'; manuscript 'P' has *sūsrava* (=*susrāva*, or better, *śuśrava*) and in *d*, *chinadmi*, 'I cut off.' Sāyaṇa derives *apacít* from the root *ci*, 'to gather,' plus *apa:* 'being heaped up from behind by means of the "humors" ' and defines them as "scrofulous swellings clinging to the neck [and] scattered downward in the place beginning with the armpits; or else, they gather up the strength of the man" (*doṣavaśād apāk cīyamānā galād ārabhya adhastāt kakṣādisaṃdhisthāneṣu prasṛtā gaṇḍamālāḥ apacitaḥ. yadvā apacinvanti puruṣasya vīryam . . .*). He speculates that "by the root of the *múni*, the god," there is meant an arrow which is fashioned from the root of a certain tree having the nature of a reed (i.e. by the *múni*, to god, *vanaspati* is meant) or which gains its efficacy by being shot from a bow fashioned from the *veṇudārbhūṣa*-tree (cf. KauśS 32.8) (. . . *muner devasya iti padadvayena śaraprakṛtibhūto vṛkṣaviśeṣa ucyate. muner . . . devasya devarūpasya vanaspateḥ . . . tasya mūlena mūlavat sārabhūto yo vṛkṣasyāṃśas tannirmitena mūlapradeśanirmitena vā śareṇa . . . atha vā muner devasya iti padadvayena dhanuḥprakṛtibhūto veṇudārbhūṣasaṃjñako vṛkṣa ucyate. tasya mūlena sāmarthyādhāyakena śarena. . . . adhijyasya hi dhanuṣaḥ sāmarthyam iṣuvisarjanena gamyate iti tasya mūlabhūtaḥ śara ity uktam*). He goes on to state that "others proclaim that the divine (or zealous) *muni* . . . is Rudra

---

[129] See Bloomfield, *Hymns*, 18–19, 577, and Whitney-Lanman, Pt. 1, 439.

[130] Henry: "Guérison des écrouelles," *Le livre*, VII, 30, 99 (see also *La magie*, 194, where he renders verses 1, 2 in his section: "Les Affections cutanées"); Griffith: "A charm to cure pustules or scrofulous tumours," *Hymns of the Atharvaveda*, 1: 363; Bloomfield: "A charm for curing scrofulous sores called *apacit*," *Hymns*, 18, 557; and Whitney-Lanman: "Against *apacíts*," *Atharva-veda-saṃhitā*, Pt. 1, 439.

[131] *gaṇḍamālābhaiṣajyārthaṃ*. He also, following Keśava, rubricates this hymn rather than AVŚ 6.83 which begins with *apacítaḥ*, to KauśS 31.16 for the same purpose. Keśava to KauśS 32.8 proposes the first two verses of this hymn along with verses 1, 2 of AVŚ 7.76(80) for use in that rite "for the purpose of healing scrofulous neck-swellings" (*atha gaṇḍamālābhaiṣajyam ucyate. apacitām lohinīnām iti dvābhyām ā susrasa ity . . .*). This, as Bloomfield points out, is quite unusual, but nevertheless possible (*Hymns*, 558 n; see also Caland, AZ 105 n).

and that this arrow, being effective by the piercing of the swellings, is not a worldly arrow but an arrow connected with Rudra, the destroyer of the *asuras'* cities"; after citing TS 6.2.3.1, 2 to support this notion, he renders the last line as follows: "I, the maker of the medicine, do not pierce the swellings, divinely produced by evil, with a worldly arrow but with Rudra's arrow" (*kecid āhuḥ- muneḥ manyumataḥ devasya. . . . rudrasya ity arthaḥ. . . . gaṇḍamālāvedhanasādhanabhūto 'yaṃ śaraḥ laukikaḥ śaro na bhavati kiṃ tu asurapuranirbhedakasya rudrasya saṃbandhī śaro 'yam. . . . pāpadevatān-iṣpāditā gaṇḍamālā ahaṃ bhaiṣajyakartā laukikena śareṇa na vidhyāmi kiṃ tu rudrasya śareṇeti*). It is obvious that Sāyaṇa is merely guessing at the meaning of the phrase in *c*. Henry, however, has pointed to the fact that Rudra may be the *muní*, the god (*La magie*, 194; cf. also Whitney-Lanman, 440). This interpretation receives further support from the fact that at AVŚ 6.44.3 the fathers' root (*pitṝṇā́m mū́lād*) is mentioned in connection with Rudra's urine. The root itself may be the root of a plant or perhaps a penis. On the general notion of *múni* as "medicine-man," see Macdonell-Keith, *Vedic Index*, 2: 167.

VERSE 2

For *vídhyāmy*, 'I prick,' in *ab*, P 19.36.3 has *chinadmy*, 'I cut off'; and in *c*, it has the easier reading *uto*, 'and also' (manuscript 'P' *atho*, 'likewise') for *idā́ṃ*, 'now.' Sāyaṇa states that the scrofulous swellings are of three types, distinguished by the (respective) preponderance, equality, or deficiency of the (three) "humors" (*doṣaprakarṣasāmyālpatvabhedena gaṇḍamālās trividhāḥ*). It is more likely that the three refer to the location of the *apacíts*, i.e. those which accumulate on the nape of the neck, about the neck and on the shoulders (AVŚ 6.25.1–3) and those which occur on the neck, along the sides and on the *vijā́man*-joint [AVŚ 7.76(80).2]. Sāyaṇa glosses *stúkām* as *ūrṇāstukā*, 'tuft of wool.' It may also refer to a tuft of hair [see Bloomfield, AJPh, 11: 324; later, however, "flake (of wool)," *Hymns*, 18; and Griffith, 335] or to any tuft or flake (see Henry, 29; and Whitney-Lanman, 440). The verse appears to point to a medical practice similar to that which present-day doctors perform when they lance a boil. First the healer pricks the pustule to let the pus ooze out; then, after the pus has drained, he cuts it off level with the skin.

Notes to 7.76(80)

This charm, like AVŚ 7.74(78), can be divided into sections: the first two verses are concerned with *apacít*; verses 3–5, with the disease *jāyā́nya* and verse 6 is to be recited at the midday pressing of Soma.[132] Sāyaṇa prescribes

---

[132] Bloomfield divides the hymn into three sections: "A. Charm for curing scrofulous sores calld *apacit*; B. Charm for curing tumors called *jāyā́nya*; C. Stanza sung at the midday pressure of Soma," *Hymns*, 17, 559; Whitney-Lanman also notices a division: "Against *apacíts* and *jāyā́nya*; etc.," *Atharva-veda-saṃhitā*, Pt. 1, 441 (verse 6, they say, "is wholly independent"); Ludwig: the entire charm is against "*apacit*," *Der Rigveda*, 3: 500; Henry considers the hymn

verses 1–2 for use "in a rite for the healing of scrofulous neck-swellings"[133] at KauśS 31.16–17.

VERSE 1

For *a*, P 1.21.1 reads: *mā saṃ srasan svayaṃ srasan*, "[The *apacits*] do not drop off together, [they] do not drop off individually" (cf. Renou, JA, 252: 428). Sāyaṇa quite rightly points out that "because of the name in the subsequent verse, *apacits* are also referred to here" (. . . *uttaramantre 'bhidhānād atrāpi apacita evocyante)*. He understands *ab* quite differently however: "[since] these *apacits* flow excessively everywhere, i.e. are accustomed to discharging pus, etc., therefore, let such swellings called *apacits*, which are hindering (=*ásattarāḥ*), be accustomed to flowing, totally and completely (reading: *ā́ susrásaḥ* as one word, *ā́susrásaḥ*) from those hinderings, i.e. from the manifestations of the disease (=*ásatībhyo*)" (*atyarthaṃ sravantyaḥ sarvadā pūyādisravaṇaśīlāḥ. . . . ata eva . . . satīviruddhā asatyaḥ bādhikā rogavyaktayas tābhyo 'pi asattarāḥ atyartham asatyo bādhikā evaṃvidhā apacinnāmikā gaṇḍamālāḥ . . . ā samantād niravaśeṣaṃ sravaṇaśīlā bhavantu*). This rendering seems to be mere guesswork in an effort to explain a difficult textual reading. Henry, distressed by the apparently unattached *ā́* at the beginning of *a*, suggests the reading: *ā́ asisrasas*, "tu as fait tomber," stating: "Le conjurateur s'addresse à son remède, et suppose le problème résolu, comme il le fait souvent, ou bien encore il se sert de l'aoriste d'habitude" (30, 97). While it is often the case that a preterite verb form is used when a healer, desiring a result which has not yet occurred, states it as if it has; nevertheless, in this case, as Bloomfield points out, the context would demand a comparative adjective. He therefore suggests the accepted emendation: *ā́ susráso susrástarāḥ* (559–60; see also AJPh, 11: 324; cf. Griffith, 364–65; and Whitney-Lanman, 441). The function of *ā́* in *a*, as Whitney-Lanman suggest, might be to strengthen the ablative force of *susráso* or it may be an interjection of contempt or disgust (ibid.). Our rendering implies the former. For the difficult word *séhor*, Sāyaṇa reads *śéhor*, and glosses: "a dispersed (injured?) limb by that name which is completely sapless (worthless) and which has the form of a tuft of wool, etc." (*śehur nāma viprakīrṇāvayavaḥ atyantaṃ niḥsāras tūlādirūpaḥ*). The word is found along with *plīhā*, 'spleen,' at KS 34.12, suggesting that it refers to a part of the body which Filliozat defines as an "undetermined internal organ" (*La doctrine*, 127). In *c*, Henry has offered the unacceptable emendation: *arasā́d arasátarā*, stating that it fits well with the opposition to wet in *d* (98). Whitney-Lanman suggest that the addition of *ā́* at the beginning of *c*, as in *a*, would rectify the meter (441). Rather, the word seems to be related to

---

(with the exception perhaps of verse 6) as "Guérison des écrouelles," *Le livre*, VII, 29, 95; likewise, Griffith: "A charm to cure scrofulous pustules," *Hymns of the Atharvaveda*, 1: 364 (verse 6, he states, "has no apparent connexion with the object of the charm").

[133] *gaṇḍamālābhaiṣjyakarmaṇy*; see also notes to AVŚ 7.74(78), 226, above.

sebhu, 'mucus,' 'spittle' (Mayrhofer, Wb, 3: 502, 504). In order to correct the meter, Hoffmann has proposed the reading: *ásehor arasátaraḥ,* "saftloser als ein Speicheloser" (*Aufsätzer,* 2: 451 n). Although dog's saliva is prescribed in the Kauśika ritual (KauśS 30.15) it is merely secondary; the notion of spit or saliva in the hymn is literary. Hoffmann's emendation, therefore, more closely reflects the original. *víkledīyasīḥ,* from the root *klid,* 'to be wet,' plus *ví,* has the primary meaning 'more moist.' Although the exact meaning of the last *pāda* is uncertain, it may be looked on as more descriptive than comparative. One might suppose that salt was sprinkled on the sores; as they began to ooze the salt would absorb the exudation and become dissolved, leaving wet pussy matter, at the same time causing the scabby *apacíts* to fall off as if they were insects. Although this would, of course, be very painful for the patient, it would, nevertheless, have beneficial results. Sāyaṇa, again merely guessing, makes a comparison between the salt which, when placed anywhere, disperses in a flowing manner, and the very moist nature of the suppurating *apacits* (*vikledīyasīḥ atiśayena vividhaṃ kledanavatyaḥ. yathā lavaṇo yatra kutrāpi nihito 'pi sarvadā sravati tasmād api . . . sarvāṅgasaṃdhiṣu pūyādisravaṇaśīla bhavati. etādṛṣyo 'pacitaḥ āsusraso bhavantv iti saṃbandhaḥ*).

VERSE 2

A parallel to this verse is not found in the P. For the difficult word *upapakṣyā̀ḥ,* in *b,* Sāyaṇa glosses: "being under the shoulder, near the shoulder, under the armpit" (*upapakṣe pakṣasamīpe upakakṣe bhavā*). Henry, likewise, understands it to mean the armpits: "de l'aisselle" (98); Griffith: "upon the shoulder-joints" (365); Bloomfield, originally rendered: "upon the breast" (AJPh, 11: 324), but then changed his mind and translated: "upon the shoulders" (*Hymns,* 17). Being derived from *pakṣá,* 'wing' plus *upa,* i.e. 'under the wing,' it could have the meaning: 'under the armpits,' or more generally, 'along the sides' (cf. Whitney-Lanman, 442; and Filliozat, *La doctrine,* 91–92, 122). If the *apacíts* are as numerous as AVŚ 6.25 would have us believe, it would seem that their localization under the armpits would be much too confining. It is more likely, therefore, that the poet-healer was defining their position as along the sides, including under the armpits. Sāyaṇa derives the obscure *vijā̃mni* from the root *ja,* 'to be born,' plus *ví,* 'exceedingly' and understands it to be the concealed region, i.e. the [region of the] thigh-joint characterized by the pudenda (*viśeṣeṇa jāyate apatyam atreti vijāmā guhyapradeśaḥ. . . . vijāmni guhyapradeśe tadupalakṣite ūrusaṃdhau*). Whitney-Lanman merely follow Sāyaṇa (442). Likewise, Filliozat considers this as a possible meaning (*La doctrine,* 126). The word occurs again at ṚV 7.50.2 alongside *párus,* 'joint' and appears to refer to a type of joint. It is also found at ŚB 3.6.1.2, where Eggeling renders: "the Dhiṣṇya-hearths, forsooth, are other than its (sacrifice's) congeners" (*vijā̃māno háivāsya dhíṣṇyā̀ḥ; The Śatapatha Brāhmaṇa,* 2: 148–49). Along these lines, Henry (30, 98) and Griffith (365) render: "on the two-fold limbs." Bloomfield states simply that it is a part of the body (17, 560) and Ludwig guesses the ankle (nöchel) (500). Being derived from the root *jā*, plus *ví*, and having the principal meaning, 'related,' it seems to refer to the parts of the body which are related or symmetrical to each other, such as joints, starting from the shoulders and moving downward.

Notes to 6.21

Translators generally agree that AVŚ 6.21 is a charm to improve the condition and growth of one's hair.[134] Whitney-Lanman considered it rather to be directed "To healing plants."[135] Sāyaṇa prescribes its use in a rite for "one desiring the growth of hair"[136] at KauśS 30.8–10. It is clear from the context that medicinal plants or simples, perhaps the *nitatnī* plants, after having been consecrated with the charm, were used ritually to strengthen and to promote the growth of hair.

VERSE 1

For *a–c*, P 1.38.1 reads as Śau. In *d*, P has *sam u jagrabhaṃ* (Bh.: *jagrabha;* cf. Renou, JA, 252: 934) *bheṣajam*. For *ab*, Sāyaṇa suggests that the three earths are the three worlds beginning with earth; or else the three worlds beginning with the earth, divided singly into three parts, citing ṚV 2.27.8 and AB 2.17 as support (*pṛthivyādyās trayo lokāḥ santi. yadvā pṛthivyādayas trayo lokāḥ pratyekaṃ tridhā bhinnāḥ*). Although it implies a cosmology which is found in the Mbh. and the Purāṇas, there is the possibility that the three earths refer to: 1. the earth's surface; 2. the *nāgaloka* or *pātāla*, the realm of the *nāgas* which is under the earth; and 3. the *naraka*, the infernal region. In this way, the ground (*bhūmi*) may be considered as the most beneficial, the best (see Grill, 160; Bergaigne-Henry, 150 n; Griffith, 256; and Bloomfield, 471; cf. also Florenz, 275) or simply the topmost (*uttamā*). In *cd*, therefore, the "skin" (*tvacó*) is equated to the ground or soil (cf. Sāyaṇa: . . . *pṛthivīnāṃ . . . tvag iva upari vartamānā yā bhūmiḥ tasyā . . . upari prarūḍhaṃ . . . vyādhinivartakam auṣadham . . . saṃgṛhṇāmi*). There seems, therefore, to be a symbolic association, as Grill suggests, between the earth's surface on which the plants grow and the skin, the body's surface, on which hair grows (160; cf. also Bloomfield, 470).

VERSE 2

In *ab*, P. 1.38.2 reverses *bheṣajānām* and *vīrudhānām* (Bh. has the preferable *vairudhānām;* cf. Renou, JA, 252: 434); and in *c*, it has *yajño bhaga*

---

[134] Florenz: "Haarzauber (Hair-spell)?" "Das sechste Buch der Atharva-saṃhitā," BB, 12: 275; Grill: "Haarwuchs (Hair-growth)," *Hundert Lieder des Atharva-Veda*, 50, 160; Bergaigne-Henry: "Conjuration pour faire pousser les cheveux, " *Manuel*, 150; Griffith: "A charm to strengthen hair and promote its growth," *Hymns of the Atharvaveda*, 1: 256; and Bloomfield: "Charm to promote the growth of hair," *Hymns*, 30, 470.

[135] *Atharva-veda-saṃhitā*, Pt. 1, 295.

[136] *keśavṛddhikāmaṃ*; cf. Keśava: *atha keśavṛddhikaraṇe kośapatane bhaiṣajyam ucyate.*

iva (K manuscript, Bar.: *eva*), ". . . as the sacrifice, Bhaga . . ."(?). For *c*, Sāyaṇa explains: "There, on account of his excellence, the example is Soma. . . . When the divisions of day and night are to be determined, the moon [=*sóma*] and sun [=*bhága*] are mentioned, from the fact that they bring about divisions of time. Thus the meaning is 'you are the best' " (*tatra śraiṣṭhyena . . . dṛṣṭāntaḥ—somaḥ iti. . . . ahorātrabhāgeṣu . . . somaḥ candramāḥ bhagaḥ sūryaś ca kālāvacchedahetutvena praśastau tadvat śreṣṭham asīty arthaḥ*). His gloss of Soma as the moon seems acceptable (cf. Macdonell, *Vedic Mythology*, 107, 112–13). His understanding of *bhága* as the sun is possible, for in the ṚV, it is one of the Ādityas which in later literature are enumerated as the twelve sun-gods (ibid., 43–44, 45). In this way, a later cosmology, as suggested in verse 1, may also be implied in this verse. It may, however, simply designate a god who dispenses wealth or general good fortune (ibid., 45; cf. Grill 106). *yā̃meṣu* is also a difficult word. Its basic meaning is 'moving' and thus could signify "wandering stars" or "planets" (see Florenz, 275; Grill, 160–61; and Griffith, 256; cf. Bergaigne-Henry, 150 n). At *Manu* 7.145, it occurs in the context which suggests that it means a watch or division of time (about three hours) (*utthāya paścime yāme*, "having arisen at the last watch"; cf. Kullūka Bhaṭṭa's gloss: . . . *rātreḥ paścimayāma utthāya* . . .). On the basis of this passage and its commentary, and because it occurs with Soma in the verse, Bloomfield (30) and Whitney-Lanman (296) suggest that it refers to the night watches. Rather, it appears to have the more general meaning, as Sāyaṇa implies, the watches in general, those which occur during the night (Soma) as well as during the day (Bhaga). Bergaigne and Henry suggest yet another, less likely, explanation: *somabhā̃g iva yāmeṣu*, " 'comme celui qui a part au Soma (Indra) parmi Dieux qui marchent (les Dieux actifs guerriers),' par contraste avec [*pāda d*] comme Varuṇa parmi les Dieux (souverains, immobiles, en repose, etc.)" (150 n). In this verse, therefore, there seems to be a reference to a plant which, as well as being the most excellent of the medicines, is also equal with Soma (the moon and plant) and Bhaga (the dispenser of light and perhaps of health) among the watches of the day and night and with Varuṇa (the first) among the gods.

VERSE 3

This verse again appears to be directed to the simples (Sāyaṇa: *oṣadhayaḥ*, cf. also Florenz, 276). In *ab*, P 1.38.3 has the easier reading: . . . *anādhṛṣṭāḥ siṣāsantīḥ siṣāsatha* (K: *siṣāsata*), "You . . . O unassailed [and] gracious [plants] be generous [to us]" (cf. Renou, JA, 252: 434). In *cd*, P reads: *etāḥ stha keśavardhanīr atho stha keśadṛṃhaṇīḥ* (Bh. cites the Mahantipura, Orissa, manuscript reading: *keśavṛṃhaṇīḥ*, 'means for increasing [the thickness of] the hair'). The meaning is unaltered from that of the Śau. In *a*, Sāyaṇa glosses *ánādhṛṣaḥ* as "not injured by anything" (*kenacid api ahiṃsitāḥ*). This is the meaning adopted above (cf. however, Bloomfield, who renders it: "irresistible," 30; and Whitney-Lanman, who translate it with more of an active sense: "doing no violence," 296). The two desideratives from the root *san*, as Bergaigne and Henry point out, have the sense of both 'to conquer' and 'to be generous' (150 n). In this way, the plants may be considered as conquerors of malady and benevolent bestowers of health (cf. Sāyaṇa: . . . *sanitum ārogyaṃ dātum icchantyaḥ yūyaṃ;* cf. also the notion of Soma and Bhaga in verse 2) in the form of strong, thick hair. At AVŚ 6.30.3, we notice that the plant *śamī* is requested to be gracious to hair (*mṛḍa kéśebhyaḥ śami*). P 1.38 adds another verse (4) which is a variant of AVŚ 6.137.3 below.

Notes to 6.136 and 137

Translators generally agree that AVŚ 6.136 and 137 are charms to promote the growth of hair.[137] Sāyaṇa prescribes their use in a rite for "one desiring the promotion of hair-growth"[138] at KauśS 31.28.

6.136

VERSE 1

P(K) 1.67.1 reads as Śau, with the following word order: *devī devyāṃ jātāsi pṛthivyām adhy oṣadhe.* In *c*, Bh. has *tvam* in place of *tā́m*. For *oṣadhe*, in *b*, Sāyaṇa glosses: "that beginning with the *kācamācī*" (*kācamācīprabhṛtike*), which is equated with *nitatnī* (see Caland, AZ, 103 n), glossed in *c*, as "O down growing one, i.e. the herb, accustomed to growing forth in a downward direction" (. . . *nitanvāne nyakprasaraṇaśīle oṣadhe*). The word *nitatnī* occurs in later Vedic literature as a personification of one of the bricks used in the fire altar (TS 4.4.5.1; KS 40.4, *Viṣṇu Smṛti* 67.7) and as a star of the constellation *kṛttikā* (TB 3.1.4.1). Griffith suggests that it is a "plant with deep roots and therefore supposed to strengthen the root of the hair" (321 n). Being from the root *tan* plus *ní*, 'to stretch down,' it appears to refer to the entire plant rather than just to its roots. Whitney-Lanman consider it to be an epithet rather than an actual name of a plant (383). Since it is a feminine in *ī*, it is more probable that it signifies a plant whose very name may describe it as a hanging vine or perhaps a symbiotic plant which grows downward from other vegetation. Note, therefore, its symbolic association with long cranial hair.

VERSE 2

P 1.67.2 reads: *indras tvā khanat* (K: *khanatu*) *prathamo varuṇasya duhitṛbhyaḥ, dṛṃha jātāñ janayājātāṃ ye jātās tān u varṣīyasas* (Bar: *ye jās tān*

[137] Zimmer translates the charms in his discussion of *nitatnī*, a plant used against hair which falls out, *Leben*, 68; Grill: "Haarwuchs (hair-growth)," *Hundert Lieder des Atharva-Veda*, 50, 176; Griffith (both): "A charm to promote the growth of hair," *Hymns of the Atharvaveda*, 1: 321; Bloomfield (both): "Charm with the plant *nitatnī* to promote the growth of hair," *Hymns*, 31, 356, 357; and Whitney-Lanman (both): "To fasten and increase the hair," *Atharva-veda-saṃhitā*, Pt. 1, 383.

[138] *keśavṛddhikaraṇakāmaḥ;* cf. Keśava: *keśavṛddhikaraṇe bhaiṣajyam ucyate.*

varṣīyasas; Raghu Vira: *ye jā[tā]s tān varṣīyasas) kṛdhi,* "Indra uprooted you first from Varuṇa's daughters. [Therefore,] you strengthen the born, beget the unborn [and] make those which have already been born, long lasting" (cf. Renou, JA 253: 16 and AVŚ 6.137.1 below). The first two *pāda*s, apparently lost in the Śau but preserved in the P, have increased our knowledge of the mythology surrounding this plant.

VERSE 3

In *a,* P 1.67.3 has *vatataḥ,* 'stretched down' (K: [*a*]*vatataḥ;* see Renou, JA, 253: 16) in *b, vṛścyate,* 'is pulled out,' confirming Whitney-Lanman's emendation of the Śau reading (383). K has *dṛśyate,* 'is seen,' which is possible, but seems out of place in the context. In *c,* P has *sarvaṃ taṃ.* Although *vṛścáte* (*vṛścyáte*), being from the root *vraśc,* 'to cut,' 'to hew,' literally means, 'is cut(down),' common sense would dictate that it predicates the hair which is "pulled out by its roots," as opposed to that which "falls out naturally" (*avapádyate*)—one cannot "cut off" the roots of the hair without scalping the individual. *sámūlo* has perhaps the sense of 'by the roots,' 'completely,' as in Classical Sanskrit. Because something is said to be sprinkled over the hair, Zimmer speculates that it may be the sap of the plant (68). KauśS 31.28, however, prescribes that the plant's fruit, which usually hangs from it and appears to grow downward, should be used and implies that this fruit is to be decocted before it is poured over the affected area. Although the exact part or parts of the plant are not specified in the hymn, it would seem reasonable to assume that, as in the KauśS, originally a decoction made with the plant was sprinkled over the patient suffering from the loss of hair whether by natural causes or by accident.

6.137

VERSE 1

P has no parallel to this verse. Sāyaṇa explains that *jamádagni* is a "great *ṛṣi*" (*maharṣiḥ*); *vītáhavya* is "the name of a great *ṛṣi*" (*vītahavyākhyo maharṣiḥ*); and *ásita* is "a sage who has black hair" (*kṛṣṇakeśasya etatsaṃjñasya muner*). Jamadagni is mentioned at AVŚ 2.32.3 as a destroyer of worms (*krími*); and at AVŚ 5.28.7, his triple lifetime is mentioned. Vītahavya is, according to the *ṚV-Sarvānukramaṇī,* the *ṛṣi* of ṚV 6.15, whom Griffith considers to be thought of as a magician like Virgil in the Middle Ages (321–22 n). Whitney-Lanman, along with the *AV-Anukramaṇī,* suggest that the word should be understood as an epithet, "after the god has enjoyed his oblations" (Pt. 1 383). Nothing further is known about the word. At AVŚ 1.14.4, there is a reference to a spell authored by Asita who, Sāyaṇa says, is a *ṛṣi* (*etan nāmna ṛṣeḥ*). Although the name of the herb (Sāyaṇa: *oṣadhiṃ*) is not expressed in the verse, it is likely that it is *nitatnī* mentioned at AVŚ 6.136.1.

VERSE 2

P 1.67.4 puts everything in the singular. In *ab,* it reads: *astu viyāmenānumeyaḥ* (K: *vyāmenānumeyaḥ;* cf. Renou, JA, 253: 16); and in *c,* it has *naḍa iva* (K: *na na tvair*). Sāyaṇa renders *ab:* "First your hairs, O one desirous of hair-growth, where to be measured by finger-breadths, i.e. to be measured by four and six finger-breadths, then they were to be measured by the length of two extended *hastas* (i.e. about 36 inches)" (*he keśābhivṛddhikāma tvadīyāḥ keśāḥ prathamam. . . . aṅgulināmaitat. . . . aṅgulibhiḥ. . . mātavyāś caturaṅgulāḥ ṣaḍaṅgulā ity evaṃ paricchedyā. . . . tato . . . prasāritahastadvayaparimāṇena . . . anu paścāt meyāḥ mātavyā āsan*); for *cd,* he understands the meaning to be: "As those [*naḍá*-plants], born on the edge of the water of a tank, being closely joined and growing quickly, become longer, so also, let the hairs grow" (*te yathā taṭākodakaprānteṣu utpannāḥ saṃhatāḥ santaḥ śīghraṃ vardhamānā drāghīyāṃso bhavanti tathā keśā api vardhantām ity arthaḥ*). In *a,* the difficult word *abhīśu* has the basic meaning, 'rein,' and some translators have chosen to render it so (see Grill, 51; Griffith, 322; and Whitney-Lanman, 383). According to *Nighaṇṭu* 2.4.3, 5, however, it can have the meaning "arm" (*bāhu*) in the dual and "finger" (*aṅguli*) in the plural (cf. Bloomfield, 537). The latter meanings make better sense if, like Sāyaṇa, we consider that initially the hairs were a finger breadth in length and after the treatment with the medicinal herb, they were found to have grown to a length equal to that of two *hastas*. In *ab,* the Śau reading implies a continuation of the mythological episode mentioned in verse 1; in which case, it was Jamadagni's daughter's hairs which were measured. P however, avoids this connection by reading *astu* to agree with *vardhatām* in *c.*

VERSE 3

In *b,* P 1.38.4 has: *yaccha . . . yamayauṣadhe* (K: *yacchā madhyaṃ yāmayauṣadhe*); and in *cd,* it reads: *keśavardhaṇam asy ātharvaṇaṃ keśadṛṃhaṇaṃ asy ātharvaṇam,* "You are the hair-promoters belonging to the Atharvans [and] you are the hair-strengtheners belonging to the Atharvans" (cf. AVŚ 4.3.7, 6.21.3*cd,* P 1.8.4 to AVŚ 2.3.4, 208, above, and Renou, JA, 252: 434). The sequence of three requests found in *ab,* reminds one of the three demands of the *nitatnī*-plant mentioned at AVŚ 6.136.2.

Notes to 6.24

There is disagreement among translators concerning the import of AVŚ 6.24. Florenz[139] and Grill[140] consider it to be generally against "disease." Griffith calls it: "A hymn to the Rivers";[141] Bloomfield, basing himself on KauśS 30.13, entitles it: "Dropsy, heart-disease and kindred maladies cured

---

[139] "Das sechste Buch der Atharva-saṃhitā," BB, 12: 279.
[140] *Hundert Lieder des Atharva-Veda,* 13, 161.
[141] *Hymns of the Atharvaveda,* 1: 258.

by flowing water";[142] and Whitney-Lanman: "To the waters: for blessing." [143] Sāyaṇa prescribes its use "for the purpose of quieting the diseases of jaundice, dropsy and derangement of the 'humors' in the region of the heart" [144] at KauśS 30.13.

VERSE 1

In this verse the patient is speaking. In *ab*, K 19.7.8 reads: *himavataḥ pra sravata tās sindhum upa gacchata*, "Let that [water] flow from the Himavant [and] approach the Sindhu." In *cd*, P 3.17.6 reads quite differently: *tā āpaḥ sarvāḥ saṅgatya cakṣuḥ prāṇañ ca dhatta naḥ* (K: *prāṇaṃ dadhatu naḥ*), "When all those waters have come together, let [them] bestow on us eye[-sight] and *prāṇa*-breath." In both of the above verses, the first line is similar to that of the Śau, which suggests that it may be formulaic, being recited when consecrating the water to be used in the rite. In *b*, *samaha*, 'somewhere,' may also have the sense of 'somehow' (cf. Grill: "weiss nicht wie?" 13). In *d*, Sāyaṇa explains *hṛddyotabheṣajám* as "[that] well-known medicine which ceases the heat in the heart" (*prasiddhaṃ . . . hṛdayadāhanivartakam auṣadhaṃ . . .*). It seems to refer to the waters which are themselves the medicine for such an ailment.

VERSE 2

In this verse the patient appears to be speaking. K 19.7.9 reads quite differently: *akṣibhyām ādidyota pārṣṇibhyāṃ hṛdayena ca, āpas tat sarvaṃ niḥ karan tvaṣṭā riṣṭam ivānaśat*, "As Tvaṣṭṛ removed the injury [so also] may the waters eradicate all that [which] has afflicted [my] two eyes, two heels and heart." At P 8.8.4, *cd* is as P 19.7.9*cd* (O has *taṣṭāriṣṭam ivānas[ś?]aḥ[t?]*, in *d*); but *ab* reads: *yad aṅgair apaḥ*(?) *paspṛśe, yac chīrṣṇā yac ca pṛṣṭibhiḥ*, ". . . [all that] which has afflicted the action(?) of the limbs, of the head and of the ribs." Again P *cd* appears to be formulaic, referring to the waters. At P 8.8.4, *paspṛśe* 'has afflicted' (root *spṛś*, 'to touch') has replaced *ādidyóta* whose meaning as 'afflicted' may be confirmed by the replacement. Sāyaṇa understands *ādidyóta*, in *a*, to be "[that], born of disease, causes inflammation, i.e. causes pain, in my two eyes" (. . . *rogajātaṃ . . . mama akṣṇoḥ . . . ādīpayati vyathayati*), suggesting rather a symptom than a proper disease. The pun on *ādidyóta* in *a*, and *hṛddyotá* in verse 1*d*, may, as Grill suggests, distinguish "äussere Verletzung nach der inneren Krankheit" (161). The notion of that which afflicts the two heels and the

---

[142] *Hymns*, 12, 471.

[143] *Atharva-veda-saṃhitā*, Pt. 1, 298.

[144] *hṛdayadoṣa-* (Śankar Pandit: *dṛṣyadoṣam*, 'visible derangement of the "humors" ') *jalodarakāmalarogaśāntyartham*; cf. Keśava: *atha hṛdayadāghe* ('heart-affliction') *jalodare kāmale ca bhaiṣajyāny ucyante* and Dārila who considers it to be only for one suffering from dropsy (*jalodariṇam abhiścotate*).

front of the two feet suggests the demonic foot-*rápas* (cf. ṚV 7.50 and the chapter on *rápas,* 25–28, above).

VERSE 3

In this verse, either the patient or the healer could be speaking. The verse appears to be a general incantation to the waters for benefit. In *a,* K 19.7.10 merely reverses the order of *síndhupatnīḥ síndhurājñīḥ*. In *c,* Sāyaṇa explains *tásya bheṣajáṃ* as medicines which remove our disease (. . . *asmākaṃ . . . rogasya . . . nirvartakam auṣadhaṃ . . .*); and in *d, bhunajāmahai* (root *bhuj,* 'to enjoy,' 'to consume') seems to have a more pregnant sense, as suggested by Sāyaṇa: "through [that] medicine, we eat [those things] connected with you, i.e. after having subdued the disease, we are dependent on the strength-producing elements, food, drink, etc." (. . . *auṣadhena . . . yuṣmākaṃ saṃbandhino vayaṃ bhunajāmahai. nivṛttarogāḥ santaḥ annapānādi balakaraṃ vastu upajīvāma*). In this way, *bhunajāmahai* implies an enjoyment which is derived from the waters' benefits after their consumption, i.e. after drinking the water we hope to obtain its benefits (cf. Florenz, 280; Bloomfield, 12–13; and Whitney-Lanman, 298).

Notes to 6.57

Translators are not unanimous in their understanding of AVŚ 6.57. Griffith calls it: "A charm for a wound or bruise";[145] Bloomfield, basing himself entirely on KauśS 31.11–15 and its commentaries, entitles it: "Urine (*jālāṣa*) as a cure for scrofulous sores";[146] and Whitney-Lanman, more generally: "With a certain remedy against disease." [147] Sāyaṇa prescribes its use "for the purpose of healing the sore without an opening,"[148] at KauśS 31.11–15. Verse 3 is found in the list of purificatory rites (*bṛhacchāntigaṇa*) at AthPariś 32.26 and with AVŚ 6.19, etc. in a rite for welfare at KauśS 41.14. The context points to a charm for the consecration of Rudra's watery medicine to be used for the healing of sores.

VERSE 1

In *d,* P 19.10.3 reads *apabruvan* (Raghu Vira: *apabruvat*). Sāyaṇa explains that *bheṣajám,* in *b,* is "the medicine for the removing of this (or his) sore" (. . . *asya vraṇarogasya nivartakam auṣadham*); and for *apabrávat,* in *d,* he reads: *upabrúvat* and glosses: "he recited" (*prāyuṅkta*). It, therefore, appears that Sāyaṇa understands *upabrúvat* to be an imperfect without augmen-

---

[145] *Hymns of the Atharvaveda,* 1: 276.
[146] *Hymns,* 19, 488.
[147] *Atharva-veda-saṃhitā,* Pt. 1, 323.
[148] *mukharahitavraṇabhaiṣajyārthaṃ;* cf. Keśava: *akṣatavraṇabhaiṣajyam ucyate,* 'healing of unbroken sores'; on the reading *akṣata* in place of the printed *akṣita,* see Bloomfield, *Kauśika Sūtra,* xliii, and Whitney-Lanman, 323.

tation. On analogy, P's *apabruvan* could be also an imperfect in the third person plural. It is preferable, however, to take it to be a subjunctive (cf. Bloomfield, 19; and Whitney-Lanman, 323). The arrow mentioned here is probably the disease sent by Rudra; and the remedy is also given by Rudra.

VERSE 2

For *cd*, P(K) 19.10.4 has a slightly easier reading: *jālāṣé bhadráṃ bheṣajáṃ tásya no dehi jīváse* (text accented), "O *jālāṣá*, bestow on us his (its?) auspicious medicine so that we may live"; manuscript 'P': *jālāṣam ugraṃ bheṣajaṃ tasya*(?) *no dehi*(?) *jīvase*, "Bestow on us his powerful medicine, *jālāṣa*, so that we may live." Sāyaṇa following KauśS 13.11–15, prefaces his comments to this verse by saying that (Ṛgvedic) *jálāṣa*, which he reads throughout for *jālāṣá*, is mentioned in the *udakanāman* (water-rite?) in which it is characterized by the foam of cow's urine (*jalāṣam iti udakanāmasu paṭhitam. atra ca viniyogānusāreṇa gomūtraphenalakṣaṇam*). He, then, renders *ab*: "Oh, attendants run towards the sore with it and then rinse near to (or around) the sore with it" (*he paricārakāḥ tena . . . vraṇam abhitaḥ prakṣālayata. . . . tathā tenaiva . . . vraṇasamīpa*[*e*?] *prakṣālayata*). Rather than 'to rinse' (root *kṣal*), the root *sic*, has the sense of 'to sprinkle.' In *c*, he glosses *ugráṃ* as *tīkṣṇaṃ*, 'sharp,' 'pungent,' which brings to mind both the smell of urine and the points of the arrows. In the Vedic context, *ugrá* generally conveys a sense of fear and power, which, when applied to Rudra's medicine would signify to the listener a medicine which is so potent that its effect is positively frightening. Perhaps, "powerful," therefore, is the best translation for the reading *ugráṃ*. The first line suggests a ritualistic procedure which entailed the sprinkling of liquid on to the area affected by sores or wounds caused by Rudra's arrow.

VERSE 3

b occurs at ṚV 9.114.4*cd* and AVŚ 10.5.23*d*. The formulaic expression *kṣamā̃ rápo* is found at ṚV 8.20.26; 10.59.8–10. For *cd*, P(K) 19.10.5 reads: *kṣamādhamo*(?) *viśaṃ no 'stu bheṣajam*, "To the ground [let] the *adhama* (vileness?) [go]; let there be medicine for us"; manuscript 'P' reads as Śau: *kṣamā rapo . . .* , which is the correct reading. Sāyaṇa considers the medicines in the last line to be both the sentient and non-sentient beings as well as every action, in fact, everything (. . . *samastaṃ sthāvarajaṅgamātmakaṃ . . . asmākaṃ . . . auṣadham astu. . . . kṛtsnaṃ karma . . . asmākaṃ bheṣajaṃ astu*). Not knowing of what the Vedic materia medica was composed, Sāyaṇa included nearly everything. As we have noticed, plant and animal products are often used as medicines; but "action" is not. The last verse appears to be a benediction recited to increase the overall efficacy of the *jālāṣá*-medicine. Cf. ṚV 5.42.11 where Rudra is said to be the master of every medicine (. . . *yó víśvasya kṣáyati bheṣajásya*).

Notes to ṚV 10.97

Most translators consider ṚV 10.97 to be a hymn in praise of medicinal herbs and plants.[149] Sāyaṇa, referring to the *Sarvānukramaṇī*, mentions that the *ṛṣi* is Bhiṣaj, the *ātharvaṇa* (son of the Atharvan), that the hymn's meter is *anuṣṭubh*, and that it encompasses the praise of herbs by the physician. Ritually, he states that when the consecrator succumbs to a disease such as fever, he should be purified by this *sūkta* and quotes ĀśvŚS 6.9 as example: "after having washed [him], one should rub [him] down, while reciting the *oṣadhisūkta*."[150] At BD 7.154, it is said that the hymn is in praise of herbs and that the hymn of *Bhiṣaj* is used for the destruction of *yakṣma*.[151]

VERSE 1

For *a*, TS 4.2.6 verse 1 reads: *yā̄ jātā̄ óṣadhayo* and for *c*, *mándāmi babhrū̄ṇām ahám*, "I celebrate . . . of the brown ones." MS 2.7.13 verse 1 and KS 16.13 verse 1 have *yā̄ óṣadhayaḥ prathamajā̄ḥ*, in *a*; similarly, KapS 25.4 verse 1, but *prathamajā*. In *c*, KS, KapS begin with *manaí*; and MS begins with *manvé*. VS 12.75 reads as ṚV. *triyugáṃ* has been understood by Sāyaṇa to be either "the three ages beginning with the *kṛta*" (. . . *kṛtādiyugatrayamuktaṃ* . . .) or else, following ŚB 7.2.4.26, the three seasons, i.e. in the spring, in the rainy season and in the autumn (. . . *vasante prāvṛṣi saradi cety arthaḥ*; so also Sāyaṇa to TS and Mahīdhara to VS; cf. Eggeling, SBE, 41: 339–40). It appears rather to be a reference to a mythical event which occurred in the distant past; and the standard translation of "age" seems best (cf. Renou, EVP, 16: 155). Both Sāyaṇa to TS and Mahīdhara to VS understand *babhrū̄ṇām* to be "those herbs reddish-brown by maturity or fit for the nurturing of living beings" [. . . *prāṇi*- (Mahīdh: *jagajjana*-) *bharaṇasamarthānāṃ paripākena* (Mahīdh: *pākena*) *piṅgalavarṇānāṃ vā tāsām oṣadhīnāṃ* . . .]. Sāyaṇa to ṚV, however, states that they are "the brown colored herbs beginning with Soma" (. . . *babhruvarṇānām somādyoṣadhīnām* . . . ; cf. Geldner, 306). The brown color probably refers to plants which are naturally so, or to those plants or herbs which, when dried, turn brown. There is some disagreement about the exact meaning of the last *pāda*. At ŚB 7.2.4.26 the hundred *dhā̄man*s are said to be the direct result of living a hundred years, of having a hundred merits and of

---

[149] See, in particular, Roth: "Das Lied des Arztes, Rigveda 10.97 (The hymn of the doctor. . .)," ZDMG, 25: 645–48; the same translation is given by Grassmann, *Rig-Veda*, 2: 378; Hillebrandt: "An die Pflanzen (To the plants)," *Lieder der Ṛgveda*, 107; Griffith: "Praise of Herbs," *Hymns of the Ṛgveda*, 2: 533; Geldner: "*Lob der Heilkräuter* (Praise of the healing-plants)," *Der Rigveda*, 3: 306; and Gonda: "An address of a 'doctor' to his herbs," "The so-called secular, humorous and satirical hymns of the *Ṛgveda*," *Selected Studies*, 3: 388; cf. also Renou: "Louange des Plantes," EVP, 16: 155, notes only.

[150] Anu: *yā oṣadhīs tryadhikātharvaṇo bhiṣag oṣadhistutir ānuṣṭubham;* Sāyaṇa: *atharvaṇaḥ putrasya bhiṣaṅ nāmna ārṣam. . . . dīkṣitānāṃ jvarādyupatāpe saṃjāte 'nena sūktena mārjayet. sūtritaṃ ca—'oṣadhisūktena cāplāvyānumṛtjet' iti* (ĀśvŚS 6.9; see also MŚS 38.3).

[151] . . . *yā oṣadhīstavaḥ, prayoge bhiṣajas tv etad yakṣmanāśāya kalpate;* cf. Macdonell, *The Bṛhad-Devatā*, Pt. 2, 292.

having a hundred energies; and seven refers to the seven vital airs in the head (see, Eggeling, SBE 41: 340; also cited by Sāyaṇa to ṚV). Yāska at *Nirukta* 9.28, however, considers it to be either 107 species of plants or else 107 (or 700, depending on the meaning of *saptaśataṃ*) vulnerable spots (*marman*) of the body, on which the herbs are placed (. . . *dhāmāni trayāṇi bhavanti. sthānāni nāmāni janmanīti. janmāny atrābhipretāni. saptaśataṃ puruṣasya marmaṇāṃ. teṣv enā dadhatīti vā;* cf. also L. Sarup, *The Nighaṇṭu and The Nirukta,* 148 n. 6). Sāyaṇa to ṚV glosses *dhā́māni* as "refuge station" (. . . *āśrayabhūtāni sthānāni* . . . ; one of Yāska's choices). This idea of location is followed by Hillebrandt (107). Although the usual meaning of *dhā́man* is station or location, it seems more likely, as Yāska points out, that it refers to the 107 varieties, types or species of brown herbs (see in particular, Geldner, 3: 306, Renou, EVP, 16: 155, and Gonda, *The meaning of the Sanskrit term dhāman,* 54); and in the light of verse 2 and AVŚ 8.7, where numerous types of plants and herbs are extolled, the mention of the 107 kinds of herbs points to an already developed pharmacopoeia, in which only the most efficacious plants are included.

VERSE 2

In *c,* TS 4.2.6 verse 2 and MS 2.7.13 verse 2 read *áthā;* MS and KapS 25.4 verse 2, *śatakrato* and KS 16.13 verse 2 and VS 12.76 follow the ṚV. Sāyaṇa to ṚV glosses the obscure word *śatakratvo* as "whose actions are a hundredfold" (*śatakarmāṇaḥ*). Although the etymology of the word *krátu* is disputed, it seems to have had the early meaning 'power,' in this context, 'healing power' (see Mayrhofer, Wb. 1: 276; cf. also Renou, 155). Mahīdhara to VS explains that the disease or poison (*gada*), from which the patient, i.e. the sacrificer, suffers is that of the six waves of existence beginning with hunger and thirst (. . . *yajamānam agadaṃ kṣutpipāsādiṣaḍūrmirogarahitaṃ* . . .). *amba,* as Mayrhofer notices, is a "Lallwort" for mother (Wb. 1: 45, cf. Geldner, 306) and so may be best expressed by the colloquialism "mama." The later application of the word to the goddesses Durgā and Kālī implies more fear and respect than love and compassion. This also seems to be inherent in its utterance in this verse.

VERSE 3

For *ab,* AVŚ 8.7.27 reads: *púṣpāvatīḥ prasū́matīḥ phalínīr aphalā́ uta,* "[let] the flowering [and] shoot-bearing [herbs] as well as [those] bearing fruit and [those] not bearing fruit . . . ," which also occurs at KS 16.13 verse 3 and KapS 25.4 verse 3. TS 4.2.6 verse 3 and MS 2.7.13 verse 3 read similarly, but *prasū́vatīḥ* replaces *prasū́matīḥ*. At the end of *d,* TS, KS and KapS have *pārayiṣṇávaḥ*. VS 12.77 reads as ṚV; cf. also TS 4.1.4.4 and VS 11.47. In *a,* Sāyaṇa construes *óṣadhīḥ* as a vocative (*he* . . . *oṣadhayaḥ*); Ludwig, Griffith (533) and Hillebrandt (107) render it as an accusative, "rejoice at the herbs"; and Geldner as a nominative (see, *Der Rigveda,* 3: 306). If *óṣadhīḥ* is translated as a vocative, the words in *b* must also be considered as such and if, along with the words in *b*, it is rendered as an accusative, the subject of the verb in *a* is obscure. Perhaps, following Geldner, it is best to construe it as a nominative, so also in *b*. The implied meaning of *pārayiṣṇaváḥ*, as Sāyaṇa to ṚV notices, is making the patient pass from the point of disease (. . . *rugṇaṃ puruṣaṃ pārayantyo rogāt*).

VERSE 4

This verse is quite obscure. For *cd*, TS 4.2.6 verse 4 and MS 2.7.13 verse 4 read: *rápāṃsi vighnatī́r ita rápaḥ cātáyamānāḥ*, "go, destroying the *rápas*, dispelling the *rápas*." The apparent redundancy is corrected in KS 16.13 verse 4 and KapS 25.4 verse 4, which replace *rápaḥ* by *rákṣaś*. VS 12.78 reads as ṚV. Sāyaṇa to ṚV understands *íti* to refer to the entire second line: "This is to be said to your adjunct physician: 'I, having the herbs as purpose, give to you, O physician, a horse, a cow, fine muslin, in short myself' " (. . . *yuṣmākaṃ saṃbandhinaṃ bhiṣajaṃ . . . vakṣyamāṇam iti ittham . . . upa bravīmi. . . . oṣadhyartham aham aśvaṃ gāṃ . . . aṃśukaṃ kiṃ bahunā ātmānam api he . . . cikitsaka . . . tubhyaṃ . . . dadāmi*). Mahīdhara to VS also follows this line of interpretation, but replaces *cikitsaka* by *yajñapuruṣa*. There are three basic problems with this explanation: 1. In the verse, *ātmā́naṃ* refers to the man (*pū́ruṣa*) not the speakers; 2. the verb *sanéyam* has the more usual sense of 'obtain,' 'get' (root *san*); and 3. the syntactical placement of *íti* in the verse is an argument against its reference to the entire second line. The verse seems to indicate the rewards which the healer will obtain if the herbs he is using perform their designated healing function; and he is appealing to these divine mothers (cf. verse 2) to restore the man's life (self) so that he may gain his just reward. This latter function of the herb implies that she was believed to have activities other than just healing and was looked on as a general luck-bringer (cf. Hillebrandt, 107; and Geldner, 106); cf., however, AVŚ 8.7.11 where the herbs are requested to rescue a similar list of items. *pāda-d* occurs at verse 8*d*, below.

VERSE 5

In *a*, MS 2.7.13 verse 5 has *nivéśanaṃ*; in *c*, *gobhā́jā*; and in *d*, along with KS 16.13 verse 5, it reads *sanávātha*. TS 4.2.6 verse 5, KapS 25.4 verse 5 and VS 12.79 read as ṚV. Sāyaṇa to ṚV glosses *parṇá* by *palāśa* and cites TB 1.1.3.10 which points to the relationship between the *parṇá*-tree and Soma. Concerning the two trees, Mahīdhara to VS, citing *Nirukta* 2.5 as support, mentions that *aśvatthé* and *parṇé* are to be understood in a derivative sense, i.e. the wooden ladles for the purpose of making an oblation by the *adhvaryu* are made from their wood (. . . *adhvaryuṇā homārthaṃ juhvāṃ sthāpanāt aśvatthaparṇaśabdābhyāṃ* . . .). Along similar lines, Roth suggests that a small box in which the healer carries the prepared aromatic herbs was made from the wood of these plants (645; cf. Geldner, 306). It appears rather to be an allusion to the healing-plant goddess Arundhatī who, at AVŚ 5.5.5, is said to arise out of, among other trees, the *aśvatthá* and *parṇá,* or perhaps to the *kúṣṭha*-plant who was acquired from the seat of the gods the *aśvatthá*-tree (see AVŚ 5.4.3; 6.95.1; 19.39.6), or yet, as Sāyaṇa implies, to the Soma plant. Because the herbs are personified (see verses 2, 4, 6, etc.), they are entitled to a human gift, cows, given presumably in the form of a sacrifice.

VERSE 6

For *ab,* TS 4.2.6 verse 7 reads: *yád óṣadhayaḥ saṃgácchante rā́jānaḥ sámitāv iva.* MS 2.7.13 verse 6 follows TS, but has *sámitā*(?), in *b;* and in *c, kávī,* 'poet,' replaces *bhiṣág.* KS 16.13 verse 7 reads as TS, but has *samágamata* in *a;* and, likewise, KapS 25.4 verse 7 follows TS. VS 12.80 reads as ṚV. Sāyaṇa to ṚV glosses the difficult *sámitāv* as "in battle" (*saṃgrāme,* to TS; *yuddhe*). Likewise, Mahīdhara to VS glosses it as "in battle" (*yuddhe*). The translators, however, based on the occurrences of the word in the ṚV, tend to favor the meaning "at the council" (see in particular, Roth, 646; Hillebrandt, 107; and Geldner, 306; cf. also Renou, 155). Against the native tradition, therefore, the preferred meaning is "council." In *c,* Sāyaṇa to ṚV considers *vípraḥ* to be a wise Brāhmaṇa (*prājñaḥ brāhmaṇaḥ*), thus anticipating verse 22 (cf. Geldner, 306; and Renou, 156). At the TS, however, he explains him more fully as the wise man who is skilled in the production of the (herbs') juices and strengths (. . . *vipro medhāvī rasavīryabhāvanābhijño yaḥ puruṣaḥ* . . .). Mahīdhara to VS understands the word to refer to "an honored servant" (*bhavadāśrito*). Such a person may be called a "healer," or based on the etymology of the word (i.e. from the root *vip,* 'to shake'), a "shaker." It is interesting to note that the MS replaces *bhiṣág* with *kávī,* suggesting that a healer is one skilled in the use of words rather than herbs, as Sāyaṇa suggests. [Cf. Geldner's rendering of *vípraḥ,* "der Redekundige (Brahmane)," 306.] It seems likely, therefore, that a physician was considered to be one who possessed skill in the preparation and application of medicinal herbs as well as knowledge and mastery of the recitation of charms and incantations.

VERSE 7

In *a,* TS 4.2.6 verse 14(!) and MS 2.7.13 verse 8 read *somavatīm;* and in *c,* MS has *ā́yukṣi,* 'I have brought together,' which fits better in the context of the preceding verse. KS 16.13 verse 6, KapS 25.4 verse 6 and VS 12.81 follow ṚV. Sāyaṇa to ṚV considers there to be four different types of principal herbs (*aśvāvatyādayaḥ pradhānabhūtā oṣadhayaś catasraḥ*); and at TS, he explains them in detail: "a certain type, *aśvāvatī,* horses are in it, i.e. where there is affluence [obtained] through herbs, horses are obtained by means of wealth (i.e. by purchase); another type of herb is *somavatī,* the Soma-sacrifice is in it, i.e. where there is the affluence [obtained] by grain, the Soma-sacrifice is able to be made; another is *ūrjayatī.* It makes strength or actions of life; another kind is *udojas,* it has the form of the eight elements and causes the bodily elements to thrive by means of food" (*kācid oṣadhijātir aśvāvatī, aśvā asyāṃ santīty aśvāvatī, oṣadhisamṛddhau satyāṃ dhanadvāreṇāśvā labhyanta ity arthaḥ. anyā kācid oṣadhijātiḥ somavatī somayāgo 'syām astīti somavatī, dhānyasamṛddhau satyāṃ somayāgaḥ kartuṃ śakyata ity arthaḥ. aparorjayantī, ūrja balaṃ prāṇaceṣṭāṃ vā karotīty arthaḥ. anyā jātir udojāḥ, utkṛṣṭayojo 'ṣṭamadhāturūpaṃ yasyāḥ sodojāḥ annadvāreṇa śarīradhātūn poṣayatīty arthaḥ*). Mahīdhara to VS on the other hand, makes them attributes of herbs (*óṣadhīr*) (see Geldner, 307). This is in accordance with the general context of AVŚ 8.7 and seems the most plausible way of understanding the words. It is difficult to know exactly to what *aśvāvatīṃ* refers. Literally, it means '[the herb] possessed of horses.' It may signify, therefore, as Sāyaṇa to TS suggests, "that which obtains horses" (cf. Geldner, 307); or perhaps a better explanation is "that which has the power of horses" (see Gonda, 389). Roth emends the word to read *apjāvatīm*, "Des wässrige" (646) and Hillebrandt leaves it, as well as the other words, in *ab*, untranslated (107). Cf. AVŚ 8.7.6 and 27, below.

VERSE 8

TS 4.2.6 verse 10, MS 2.7.13 verse 10, KS 16.13 verse 8; KapS 25.4 verse 8 and VS 12.82 read as ṚV. Sāyaṇa to ṚV glosses *śúṣma* as "strengths" (*balāni*). This is the primary meaning of the word; yet, as Roth notices, it also has the sense of "odor" (646). This sense may fit in this context; but elsewhere "power," "force," "strength," etc. is more suitable (cf. Renou, 155).

VERSE 9

In *a*, TS 4.2.6 verse 8 reads *níṣkṛtir;* in *b, sáṃkṛtīḥ;* in *c, sarā́ḥ patatríṇīḥ* and in *d, níṣkṛta.* In *b*, KS 16.13 verse 12 reads: *átho tvá asi níṣkṛtiḥ* and in *c, sarā́h* and *stha.* Similarly, MS 2.7.13 verse 7 has *áthā tvám asi sáṃkṛtiḥ,* in *b* and *sarā́ḥ* in *c.* On the other hand, KapS 25.4 verse 12 reads, in *b: atho yūyaṃ stha niṣkṛtīḥ;* in *c, sīrāḥ . . . sthana* and in *d, niṣkṛtha.* VS 12.83 follows ṚV. It is clear that the words *íṣkṛtir, níṣkṛtīḥ* and *sáṃkṛtiḥ* were considered to be almost synonymous (cf. Geldner, 307, and Renou, 115–16). For the difficult word *sīrā́ḥ*, Sāyaṇa to ṚV glosses "those accustomed to flowing (or moving quickly)" (*saraṇaśīlāḥ*); and to TS, he explains *sarā́h patatríṇīḥ* as "the winged destroyers of that beginning with hunger" (*sarā́ḥ kṣudhādīnām apavārayitryaḥ* . . . , cf. Mahīdhara, below). Mahīdhara, however, offers three possible explanations: They exist with fluidy drink and food; or they are the destroyers of [misfortunes] beginning with hunger; or else *sīra* means a plough (. . . *sīrāḥ saha irayā annena vartanta iti sīrāḥ . . . yadvā sīrāḥ kṣudhādīnām apasārayitryaḥ. yadvā sīraṃ halaṃ* . . .). It is clear that Mahīdhara is merely guessing. At AVŚ 5.5.9*c*, we read: *sarā́ patatríṇī,* 'winged stream,' as a description of the goddess Arundhatī and at AVŚ 5.5.6, she is called *niṣkṛti.* These parallel occurrences suggest that the poet of this Ṛgvedic passage had in mind this plant-goddess and her various forms when he composed the verse. Based on this and the fact that the majority of parallel passages from the Yajurvedic texts read *sarā́ḥ* in place of *sīrā́ḥ*, the more correct reading appears to be *sarā́ḥ*. *sīrā́ḥ*, as Geldner suggests, could therefore, be a scribal error (307).

VERSE 10

In *b,* P(O) 11.7.1 has *akramīt*. In *c,* TS 4.2.6 verse 11, KS 16.13 verse 9 (accents wanting), MS 2.7.13 verse 11, KapS 25.4 verse 9, and P(O) read *óṣadhayaḥ*. In *d,* TS has *tanúvāṃ* and KS, *kiṃcit tanvo*. VS 12.84 follows ṚV.

VERSE 11

In *a,* TS 4.2.6 verse 6(!), KS 16.13 verse 11 and KapS 25.4 verse 11 reverse the position of *imā́* and *ahám*. MS 2.7.13 verse 9 and VS 12.85 follow ṚV. Sāyaṇa to ṚV understands *vājáyann* to mean "making the diseased one strong" (. . . *rugṇaṃ balinaṃ kurvan*), which is followed by Renou (156). Hillebrandt renders: "siegreich" (168) and Geldner: "nach dem Siegerpreis (Gewinn) verlangend" (307). The same notion of holding herbs in the hand in order to cure a patient occurs at AVŚ 4.13.6. In *d,* Yāska at *Nirukta* 3.15, unfortunately, does not explain the difficult *jīvagṛ́bho*. Sāyaṇa to ṚV, however, glosses it as: "As because of a seizer of living beings beginning with birds, i.e. as because of a hunter, lives perish" (*jīvānāṃ śakunyādīnāṃ grāhakādvyādhādyathā jīvā naśyanti tadvat*), but also offers the alternative: "just as life is taken away in the presence of death" (*yadvā. jīvagṛbho mṛtyoḥ sakāśāj jīvo 'pahriyate tadvat*). Similarly, at TS, he glosses it: "the seizer of beings beginning with hares" (. . . *jīvasya śaśāder grahaṇāt* . . .). Mahīdhara's explanation is that the *jīvagṛ́bh* is an executioner and the *yákṣma* is the life of a condemned man in his presence. Roth (646), Hillebrandt (108) and Geldner (307 n) understand it in a similar way, i.e. "Häscher." The idea of *cd* appears to be that when the healer holds the herbs in his hand and, presumably, strokes or waves them over the body of the patient, the essential power of the demonic disease perishes, just as a living being's life disappears in the presence of one who takes its life, where the analogy is between a beast of prey and a healer (cf. verse 13 below).

VERSE 12

AVŚ 4.9.4 has, in *a, yásyāñjana prasárpasy* (P 9.9.2: *yasya yava;* P 13.13.6: *yasyauṣadhayaḥ*) and in *c,* . . . *bādhasa* (P 8.3.11: *tasmād yakṣmām vibādha tvam;* P 9.9.2: *tasmād viṣaṃ vi bādhasa;* P 13.13.6: *tásmād yákṣmaṃ ví bādhadhvam,* unaccented in O). TS 4.2.6 verse 12 reads differently: *yā́ḥ ta ātasthúr ātmā́naṃ yā́ āviviśúḥ páruḥparuḥ, tā́s te yákṣmaṃ ví bādhantām ugró madhyamaśī́r iva,* "Let those [herbs], who have ascended your self (body) [and] who have entered [your] every joint, drive away your *yákṣma* as an impartial law-enforcer." KS 16.13 verse 10 (unaccented) and KapS 25.4 verse 10 follow TS, but omit *yā,* in *b.* MS 2.7.13 verse 12 reads as TS, but reverses *ātasthúr* and *āviviśúḥ*, in *ab.* VS 12.86 follows ṚV. The numerous occurrences of the verse suggest that it is formulaic. For *d,* which includes the difficult word *madhyamaśī́r,* Sāyaṇa to ṚV explains: "Just as a king, having raised his strength (*ugró*), being in a neutral position, drives away, step by step, the enemies causing trouble immediately contiguous to [him]" (*ugraḥ udgūrṇabalaḥ . . . madhyamasthāne vartamāno rājā yathā upadravakāriṇaḥ samanantaraśatrūn pade pade vibādhate tadvat*). A similar gloss is given to AVŚ 4.9.4, where he cites the definition of *madhyamaśī́r* from the *Nītiśāstras* (i.e. "*arir mitram arer mitram*"; cf. Geldner, 370). At TS, however, he understands the word slightly differently: the king who lies in [or] adheres to the middle, i.e. the impartial path which conforms to the *śāstras* (. . . *madhyamena svakīyaparakīyapakṣapātarahitena śāstrīyamārgeṇa śete vartata iti madhyamaśī́ḥ. tādṛśo rājā* . . .). Mahīdhara to VS, in his typically eloquent manner, derives "*śī́r*" from the root *śṝ,* 'to crush' and considers *madhyamaśī́r* as well as the *pāda* as follows: "as one who crushes, i.e. injures in the middle, in the middle of the body; being in the middle, the spot of the vulnerable (or vital) points [of the body]. Thus as a superior *kṣatriya,* bruising the vulnerable (or vital) point, with his sword raised [and] with his (finger protectors called) Godha and Aṅgulitra fastened on, removes the enemies; or else the powerful Rudra who crushes with the middle, i.e. the middle part of the trident, (and) removes people at the end of the age" (. . . *madhye dehamadhye bhavaṃ madhyamaṃ marmabhāgaṃ śṛṇāti hinasti madhyamaśī́ḥ. . . . marmaghātaka ugra utkṛṣṭo baddhagodhāṅgulitrāṇa udgūrṇaśastraḥ kṣatriyo yathā śatruṃ bādhate. yadvā ugro rudro madhyamena triśūlamadhyabhāgena śṛṇātīti madhyamaśī́ḥ yathā yugānte janad bādhate* . . .). The native commentaries, therefore, notice a definite military or political image in the last *pāda,* so also most translators (see especially, Roth, 646; Hillebrandt, 108; Geldner, 307; and H. P. Schmidt, "Ṛgvedic *madhyāyú* and *madhyamaśī́,*" *Annals of the Bhandarkar Oriental Research Institute* [Diamond Jubilee Volume] [1977–1978], 309–17; cf. also Renou, 156). Rather than construing *madhyamaśī́r* as a noun, it may be possible to render it as an adjective, meaning, "residing in the middle," i.e. "impartial." *ugró,* therefore, could be a substantive, referring to a type of "policeman," who enforces the king's will (see Macdonell-Keith, *Vedic Index,* 1: 83; and Rau, *Staat und Gesellschaft,* 114–15). The idea seems to be that as an impartial law-enforcer enters a dispute to put an end to it, just so the herb, ointment or barley enters between the disease-demon and the victim in order to eradicate the bodily malady. This may have been carried out ritually when the healer held the herb in his hand or applied the ointment, etc. (cf. verse 11). Cf. T. Chowdhury who has suggested a clever but unconvincing derivation of the word *madhyamaśī́r,* i.e. *mádhyam* (accusative singular) and *aśī́r* (nominative singular), i.e. "as a sharp boring instrument [drives away] the middle part (of anything by cutting a hole)" (JBORS, 17: 89–90).

VERSE 13

In *b,* TS 4.2.6 verse 13 has *śyenéna,* 'with the hawk' and MS 27.13 verse 13 reads: *cāṣeṇa kikidīvyā.* KS 16.13 verse 13, KapS 25.4 verse 13 and VS

12.87 follow ṚV. For *cā̃ṣeṇa* and *kikidīvínā*, Sāyaṇa to ṚV understands two birds (. . . *atiśīghram patatā cāṣākhyena pakṣiṇā saha. tathā kikidīvinā pakṣiṇā ca saha*). At TS, however, he considers *śyenéna* and *kikidīvínā* to be two diseases: *śyená* is a disease born of *pitta* (bile), because of its hawk-like conquering nature, and *kikidīví* is a disease born of *śleṣman* (phlegm), because *kiki* is onomatopoeic for a throat obstructed by phlegm (*śleṣmāvaruddhakaṇṭhajanyadhvaner anukaraṇārtho 'yaṃ kikiśabdas tena kikinā dhvaniviśeṣeṇa dīvyati vyavaharatīti rogaviśeṣaḥ kikidīviḥ, sa ca śleṣmajanyaḥ śyenavattīvrataratvāt pittajanyo rogaḥ śyenaḥ*). Mahīdhara to VS, on the other hand, understands *kikidīvínā* to be the sound made by the *cā̃ṣa*-bird (. . . *kimbhūtena cāṣeṇa. kikidīvinā. kikīti śabdānukaraṇam. kikīti śabdena dīvyati krīḍatīti kikidīvis tena. cāṣas tavocitaḥ sārthaḥ*). He, like Sāyaṇa, explains the two words in *b*, as diseases and adds for *vā̃tasya dhrā̃jyā*, the disease of the wind (*vātarogaḥ*). Although their meanings are obscure, the context would suggest that *cā̃ṣa* and *kikidīví* most probably refer to birds: the *cā̃ṣa* is a blue jay and the *kikidīví* is closely related to it (see Meulenbeld, *The Mādhavanidāna*, 464). In *d*, for the difficult *nihā̃kayā*, Sāyaṇa to ṚV glosses: "with the varan" (*godhikayā*). At TS, he does not comment upon it; Mahīdhara to VS defines it as "pain in all limbs" (*sarvāṅgavedanā*). Previously in his comment to this verse, Mahīdhara equated it with "destruction, serious misfortune" (*nirṛtiḥ kṛchrāpattis*). Mayrhofer notices a connection with the word *nīhārá*, 'snow or blizzard,' and thus offers the meaning "storm" or "rainshower" (Wb, 2: 170; 3: 744; cf. Geldner, 307; and Renou, 156). It may, like *kā̃hābāha* at AVŚ 9.8.11, be onomatopoeic for flatulence which is suggested by the phrase *vā̃tasya dhrā̃jyā*, 'with the force of the wind.' Roth considers that the actual hymn concludes with this verse and that the remaining verses were added later as adornment (647).

VERSE 14

In *c*, P 13.13.7 has *oṣadhayaḥ saṃvidānā* and TS 4.2.6 verse 9(!) reads: *tā̃ḥ sárvā óṣadhayaḥ saṃvidānā̃*; and in *d*, P(K) has *idaṃ me pra tiratā vacaḥ*, ". . . must increase this my charm" (O as Śau); and MS 2.7.13 verse 14 has *óṣadhayaḥ prā̃vata vā̃caṃ me*. KS 16.13 verse 14 (unaccented in *b*), KapS 25.4 verse 14 and VS 12.88 follow ṚV. In this verse, the coming together or combination of herbs seems to be implied. On the repetition of the root *av*, see Renou, 156.

VERSE 15

cd is repeated unchanged at AVŚ 6.96.1*cd* and at P 13.13.9 (O: 11.7.5, 6). In *b*, KS 16.13 verse 16 reads: *akośā̃ḥ kośínīś ca yā̃ḥ*, "which are sheathless and which have a sheath." Similarly, MS 2.7.13 verse 15 has *akośā̃ . . . kośínīḥ*. TS 4.2.6 verse 15 and VS 12.89 follow ṚV. KapS omits the verse. Roth considers this verse to be the words of the sick man and his family (647). *bṛ̃haspátiprasūtās* implies that the power of the herbs are increased by the words of the poet-healer. Cf. also verse 3 above.

VERSE 16

This verse occurs unaltered at AVŚ 6.96.2. A close variant of *cd* is found at AVŚ 8.7.28, which has *víśvasmād,* in *d.* TS, KS, MS and KapS omit the verse; and VS 12.90 follows ṚV. In *a,* Sāyaṇa to ṚV understands *śapathyā̀d* as "the evil produced by a curse" (. . . *śapathasaṃjātād enasaḥ* . . . ; cf. to AVŚ 6.96.2: . . . *śapathajanitād brāhmaṇākrośajāt pāpād* . . .) and *varuṇyā̀d* as "[evil] caused by Varuṇa" [. . . *varuṇasaṃbhavāt* . . . ; cf. to AVŚ: . . . *varuṇakṛtād anṛtavadanādijanitāt pāpād* . . . , "the evil born from speaking lies (and) caused by Varuṇa"]. Thieme, however, renders *ab* slightly differently: "May they (the plants used in a particular spell) free me of the shackle [that was put upon me] by an oath (*śapátha*), and also of the shackle [that was put upon me] by a true speech (like a vow, etc.) [or, by God True-Speech] . . . ," commenting "the side by side of 'oath' and 'Varuṇa' shows them to be related, but not identical" (*Mitra and Aryaman,* 63–64). He is quite correct in understanding that it is from the harmful bodily effects of the "oath" or "vow" and from those imposed by Varuṇa that the herbs are requested to release the victim (cf. Geldner, 307). In other words, it refers, therefore, to bodily damage connected with the two punishing gods Yama and Varuṇa and with the infringement of the cosmic order in accordance with the "oath" (*śapátha*) of the gods. Rather than "an evil committed by the gods" (Sāyaṇa to ṚV and AVŚ: *devaiḥ kṛtāt pāpān*), *devakilbiṣā̀t* refers to the "sin committed against the gods" (cf. Geldner, 307). This is the last verse of the hymn rendered by Hillebrandt (108). Roth, as in the previous verse, considers this one to be the words of the victim and his family (647).

VERSE 17

This entire verse is found unchanged at P 13.13.8. *cd* occurs at AVŚ 6.109.2*cd,* where the Arundhatī-related *pippalī̀*-plants are specified as having spoken the words. For *b,* KS 16.13 verse 15 reads: *divo antebhyaḥ pári* (?) (unaccented in middle of *ab*) and KapS 25.4 verse 15 follow this (note: there is an apparent misprint in *a,* i.e. *avapatantīr* should be read for *apavatantīr*). TS 4.2.6 verse 17, MS 2.7.13 verse 16 and VS 12.91 follow ṚV, except MS has *aśnávāmahe,* in *c.*

VERSE 18

ab occurs at P 13.13.9. TS 4.2.6 verse 16 reads differently: *yā̀ḥ óṣadhayaḥ sómarājñīḥ práviṣṭāḥ pṛthivī̀m ánu, tā̀sāṃ tvám asy uttamā̀ prá ṇo jīvā̀tave suva,* "You are the choicest of those herbs whose king is Soma [and] who have entered the earth; [therefore,] urge us to long life." KS, MS and KapS omit this verse, and VS 12.92 follows ṚV. Sāyaṇa to ṚV glosses the difficult *śatávicakṣaṇāḥ* as "having many appearances" (*bahudarśanā* . . .), which is similar to Renou's contention that it is a superlative form of the adjective *vicakṣaṇá* and a common epithet of Soma (156). Mahīdhara suggests that it means the herbs who are "clever or [those] who have many strengths or yet [those] of whom there are a hundred praises" (. . . *śatamasaṃkhyaṃ vicakṣaṇāś caturāḥ bahuvīryā vā śataṃ vicakṣaṇāḥ stotāro yāsām iti vā* . . . ; cf. Geldner, 308). The compound word appears to point to the herb's characterization of being multi-skilled, that is to say, its ability to perform functions other than healing (verses 2, 4, above). Cf. AVŚ 5.4.9 and 19.39.4, where the Soma related *kúṣṭha* plant is known as the "choicest" (*uttamá*, masculine!) among the herbs.

VERSE 19

TS 4.2.6 verse 16 has *ab* only (see verse 18 n above). KS, MS and KapS omit this verse; and VS 12.93 follows ṚV. In *c*, Sāyaṇa to ṚV understands *asyaí* to refer to "the body of the diseased man" (*rugṇatanve*). Mahīdhara, on the other hand, glosses it: "the herb held by me" (. . . *oṣadhyai madgṛhītāyai* . . .). Either interpretation can be correct. Since the most obvious feminine noun is, however, *óṣadhi*, the subject of the entire hymn, Mahīdhara's explanation is perhaps more likely to be correct (cf. verse 21, below, Roth, 647 and Geldner, 647). Cf. verse 15 n above.

VERSE 20

TS 4.2.6 verse 19 and VS 12.95 follow ṚV. KS, MS and KapS omit the verse. In *a*, Sāyaṇa to ṚV understands that the uprooter should not harm the herbs (*he oṣadhayaḥ* . . . *yuṣmān* . . . *mā hiṃsyāt*. . . . *bhūmeḥ khananakartā*). At TS, however, he interprets it along the lines of our rendering: "O herbs, do not let your uprooter, i.e. the performer of the digging in order to seize your root for the sake of healing, perish" (*he oṣadhayo vo yuṣmākaṃ khanitā cikitsāyai yuṣmadīyaṃ mūlaṃ grahītuṃ khananasya kartā mā riṣan mā vinaśyatu*). Mahīdhara follows this explanation almost word for word. At VS 12.100 a very similar idea is expressed (see note to verse 23, below). The herbs, being powerful beings in their own right, must be placated for the pain and insult caused to them by their uprooting. This suggests, perhaps, a development of sentiments tending towards *ahiṃsā*—the poet-healer is conscious of the harm he may cause to the herbs. Note also that the entire herb, including the root, seems to have been used.

VERSE 21

In *cd*, TS 4.2.6 verse 18 reads: *ihá saṃgátya tā́ḥ sárvā asmaí sáṃ datta bheṣajám*, "Let all those [herbs], having assembled here, bestow medicine on him (i.e. the patient)." KS 16.13 verse 17 has *ab* of ṚV only and completes the verse with *cd* of verse 16 (see verse 15 n, above). MS and KapS omit the verse; and VS 12.94 follows ṚV (note the reversal of verses 94, 95). At verse 19, Sāyaṇa to ṚV understands *asyaí* to refer to "the body of the sick man" (*rugṇatanve*); but to TS, he glosses *asmái* as "the sacrificer" (*yajamānāya*). Mahīdhara glosses *asyái* as "to the herb" (*oṣadhyai*) which is followed by Geldner (303). It is likely that *asyái* (feminine) refers to the herb (*óṣadhi*) as the contrasting use of the masculine *asmaí* at TS would confirm (cf. verse 19 n, above). Mahīdhara to VS seem to have captured the sense of *ab* in his comments: "herbs, standing near, who hear this my speech having the form of a request, and others who are fixed in the distance [and] being separated, hear only a little [of it]" (*yā oṣadhaya idaṃ madvacanaṃ prārthanārūpam upa samīpasthāḥ śṛṇvanti yāś cānyāḥ dūraṃ parāgatāḥ dūre vyavasthitā vyavahitāḥ satyaḥ īṣat śṛṇvanti* . . .).

VERSE 22

In *c*, TS 4.2.6 verse 20 has *karóti;* KS, MS and KapS omit the verse; and VS 12.96 follows ṚV. In *c*, Sāyaṇa to ṚV considers *brāhmaṇás* to be "the Brāhmaṇa-physician who knows the efficacy of the herbs [and who] practices medicine" (. . . *oṣadhisāmarthyajño brāhmaṇo vaidyaḥ* . . . *karoti cikitsāṃ* . . .); while at TS, he specifies him as the Brāhmaṇa who practices medicine with our roots, etc. (. . . *cikitsām asmadīyamūlādinā brāhmaṇaḥ karoti* . . .). Mahīdhara follows closely the commentary of TS. Rather than being only a member of the priestly class, the *brāhmaṇás* may also refer to those whose special craft is *bráhman*, supernatural utterance, spell (cf. the notion of *vípra, kaví* and *bhiṣáj* at verse 6 n above).

VERSE 23

This verse occurs unchanged at AVŚ 6.15.1; it is omitted by TS, KS, MS and KapS; while, it is found unaltered at VS 12.101. Between VS 12.96 (=ṚV 10.97.22) and 12.101, there are four additional verses, which read as follows:

12.97: *nāśayitrī balā́sasyā́rśasa upacítām asi, átho śatásya yákṣmāṇāṃ pākāról asi nā́śanī,* "You [,O herb,] are the destroyer of *balā́sa*, of hemorrhoids [and] of [those] heaped up (*upacít*). Moreover, you are the destroyer of the hundred *yákṣmas* [and] of the *pākārú*-disease." Mahīdhara glosses *upacítām* as "accumulating, i.e. they make the body swell" (. . . *upacinvanti śarīraṃ vardhayantīty upacītaḥ* . . .). Griffith renders: "tumors" (*The White Yajurveda,* 133, verse 98). Cf. the notion of *apacít* (82–86, above), of which *upacít* appears to be a variant. For the obscure *pākārór,* Mahīdhara understands: "that beginning with the inflammation of the mouth and with sores. *pāka* is inflammation of the mouth, *aru* is called sore; therefore, *pākāru* is sore by inflammation; or else, *pākā* is the digestion of food, *aru* is pain, thus, a state of weak digestion" (. . . *pākāroḥ mukhapākakṣatādeś ca* . . . *pāko mukhapākaḥ aruḥ kṣatam ucyate. pākenāruḥ pākārus tasya. yadvā pāko 'nnapākas tasyārurvyathā mandāgnitvaṃ* . . . ; so also Uvaṭa). Griffith leaves the word untranslated (ibid.), but, following Mahīdhara, suggests that it may be "dyspepsia; or some disease of the mouth, abcesses or gum-boil" (ibid. 130 n). It is difficult to know exactly to what *pākārú* refers. In the context with the other afflictions, however, a type of swelling or boil may not be out of the question. It is interesting to note the distinctive Atharvavedic quality of the verse in respect to the disease-terms.

12.98: *tvā́ṃ gandharvā́ akhanaṃs tvā́m índras tvā́ṃ bŕ̥haspátiḥ, tvā́m oṣadhe sómo rā́jā vidvā́n yákṣmād amucyata,* "The Gandharvas uprooted you; Indra [uprooted] you; Bṛhaspati [uprooted] you. Soma, the wise king, freed you, O herb, from *yákṣma*." Following the commentaries, *cd* may be rendered, "Soma, the king, knowing you (i.e. using you, Mahīdh.), O herb, was released from *yákṣma* (Mahīdh.: . . . *yakṣmād . . . mukto 'bhavat*)." Such an interpretation seems quite odd, as does the last line.

12.99: *sáhasva me árātīḥ sáhasva pṛtanāyatáḥ, sáhasva sárvaṃ pāpmā́naṃ sáhamānāsy oṣadhe,* "Vanquish my enemies; vanquish [those] who do battle [with me]; vanquish every evil. [For] you, O herb, are the vanquishing one." The vanquishing one (*sáhamānā*) suggests a herb related to the plant-goddess Arundhatī (see in particular AVŚ 8.2.6 and 8.7.5–6).

12.100: *dīrghā́yus ta oṣadhe khanitā́ yásmai ca tvā khánāmy ahám, átho tváṃ dīrghā́yur bhūtvā́ śatávalśā vírohatāt,* "O herb your uprooter [is] long-lived, and [he] for whom I uproot you [is long-lived]. Likewise, you, being long-lived, should grow up with a hundred shoots."

One of the most striking aspects exhibited by these extra verses is a use of and reference to Atharvavedic terminology. This shows that they are probably later additions.

Notes to AVŚ 8.7

Most translators consider AVŚ 8.7 to be a hymn addressed to medicinal plants.[152] At the introduction to the Sanskrit text, there is a prescription stating that it should be used "in a rite for the healing of all diseases beginning with *yakṣma*"[153] at KauśS 26.40, and that it should be used along with 5.2,3 in a Sautrāmaṇī-rite at VaitS 30.6;[154] and at KauśS 26.33, it occurs in a list of hymns entitled *gaṇakarmāgaṇa* (cf. AthPariś 34.24).

---

[152] Ludwig: "Preis der Kräuter (Praise of herbs)," *Der Rigveda,* 3: 504; Henry: "Hymne aux Plantes (curatives)," *Le livre,* VIII, 20, 58; see also *La magie,* 56; Griffith: "The hymn, which extols the excellence of medicinal herbs, is an incantation designed to restore a sick man to health," *Hymns of the Atharvaveda,* 1: 480; Bloomfield: "Hymn to all magic and medicinal plants, used as a universal remedy," *Hymns,* 41, 578; and Whitney-Lanman: "To the plants for someone's restoration to health," *Atharva-veda-saṃhitā,* Pt. 2, 498.

[153] *yakṣmādisarvavyādhibhaiṣajye karmaṇi;* cf. Keśava: *sarvavyādhibhaiṣajyaṃ. . . .*

[154] *tathā sautrāmaṇīyāge;* see also Henry, *Le livre,* VIII, 58; Bloomfield, *Hymns,* 578; and Whitney-Lanman, Pt. 2, 498.

VERSE 1

P 16.12.1 reads as Śau. On the brown herb (*babhrú*), cf. ṚV 10.97.1. Again the colors (except perhaps dark blue) seem to imply dried herbs.

VERSE 2

cd is found at AVŚ 3.23.6*ab*. At *cd* of that verse, the herbs are called divine and are requested to give a son (*tā́s tvā putravídyāya daívīḥ prā́vantv óṣadhayaḥ*). In b, P(K) 16.12.2 reads *devahitād*, 'divinely imposed,' perhaps in the sense of "inflicted by the gods," manuscript 'P' appears to follow Śau. Note that *yákṣma* is here expressly mentioned as being sent by the gods.

VERSE 3

P 16.12.3 reads as Śau. Barret, however, understands this verse as one line and adds to it the first line of 8.7.4 (AOS, 9: 14). The first line, as Whitney-Lanman notice, is fragmented (449), and therefore any rendering of it is purely conjectural. Henry renders: "Les Eaux [sont] l'origine, célestes [sont] les Plantes: . . ." (20); Griffith: "The waters are the best, and heavenly Plant . . ." (408); Bloomfield: "The waters and the heavenly plants are foremost; . . ." (41); and Whitney-Lanman: "Waters [were] the beginning, heavenly herbs: . . ." (499). The principal medicine against *yákṣma*, as we have noticed, was the plant or herb. In the beginning, however, the waters may have performed the same function that the plants did later (cf. especially ṚV 10.129, where the idea that everything began as water is found). Here the *yákṣma* is stated as being caused by sin (*enasyàm*).

VERSE 4

In *a*, P 16.12.4 has *ekaśṛṅgāḥ*, 'single-horned,' i.e. 'single-spiked' (Raghu Vira as Śau); and in *b*, K manuscript has *pradhanvatīr*, 'flowing forth'; but manuscript 'P' reads as Śau (so also Raghu Vira). Barret understands line two to be one verse (4) and breaks: *vaiśvadevīḥ/ugrāḥ* (AOS, 9: 14). In *c*, *víśākhā*, 'branched,' may, as Whitney-Lanman suggest, also mean "branchless" (499). Henry (57–58) and Bloomfield after him (579) understand the descriptions to be mere ornate epithets rather than an attempt at the classification of plants. Nevertheless, one cannot help but notice a sense of distinguishing plants by their gross anatomical structure, which shows an early phase of the Indian passion for classifying everything (cf. also verses 9, 27, and ṚV 10.97.1–3). On this basis, the herbs are as follows: *prastṛṇatī́* appears to be a small plant with spreading roots from which new plants emerge (i.e. a rhizome), contrasted with the *stambínī*, plants clumped together (i.e. like some grasses); the *ékaśuṅgā* or better P's *ekaśṛṅgā* (cf. also verse 9, below) suggest plants with a single ear or spathe of flowers and seeds, contrasted with the *pratanvatī́* (K: *pradhanvatī*), bushy plants spreading widely. The *vīrúdh* ('plants') are known to be: *aṃśumátī*, fibrous plants; *kāṇḍínī*, segmented plants and *víśākhā*, branched (branchless) plants.

VERSE 5

In *a,* K 16.12.5 omits *sáhaḥ;* in *d,* it reads: *muñcantv oṣadhīḥ* and omits *e.* The verse implies that the healer is preparing (Henry: applying, 20) a medicine which contains the herbs, while reciting this incantation.

VERSE 6

In *c,* Roth-Whitney read *puṣyā̃m. abd* are found at AVŚ 8.2.6 *abd.* For *ab,* K 16.12.6 reads: *jīvalām naghāriṣām jīvantīm uta,* which suggests that these are epithets of Arundhatī; in *c,* it has *puṣpām* (Bar: *puṣyām,* in agreement with Roth-Whitney) and omits *asmā̃ ariṣṭátātaye.* It is difficult to know exactly to what the words in the first line refer. They appear to be epithets of Arundhatī, the healing plant-goddess.

VERSE 7

K 16.12.7 reads as Śau. *ab* may also be rendered: "Let the companions, mindful of my charm, come here." This would imply that the companions, i.e. the herbs, should heed the spell of the healer (cf. verse 19). It does, however, pose some problems: in order to construe it in this manner, a violation of the normal *pāda*-break would have to occur.

VERSE 8

In *c,* K 16.12.8 has *sahasradhāmnīr* (cf. RV. 10.97.1). *pāda a* is somewhat obscure. Henry suggests that the nourishment of Agni may be the wood which burns and that the embryo could be the daughters of the waters, since the waters cause plants to grow (57 and notes). It may, however, refer to a fixed, water-dwelling plant which, when extracted from its habitat to be used as medicine, is found to grow back again (cf. verse 9 n).

VERSE 9

K 16.12.9 reads as Śáu. The *ávakā* is an aquatic plant which Bloomfield has noticed to be particularly associated with water and destructive of fire (AJPh, 11: 349–50). At AVŚ 4.37.8, the Gandharvas are said to eat it. The sharp-horned herbs (cf. verse 4, above, especially, P 16.12.4), therefore, appear to be water- or marsh-dwelling plants which are surrounded or enveloped by the aquatic *ávakā* and which have a characteristic spike at the top. Note the description of the plants both by gross morphology and by habitat.

VERSE 10

In *c,* K 16.12.10 includes *rakṣonāśanīḥ, 'rakṣas*-destroying,' between *balāsanā̃śanīḥ* and *kṛtyādū̃ṣaṇīś.* Most translators consider *vivaruṇā̃,* in *a,* to be a reference to the disease dropsy which Varuṇa is said to have sent as punishment (see Henry, 21; Griffith, 409; Bloomfield, 42; and Whitney-Lanman, 499; cf. also ṚV 10.97.16).

VERSE 11

P begins a new hymn with this verse. K 16.13.1 reads differently: *śívās te santv oṣadhīr apakrītāḥ sahīyasīr vīrudho yā abhiṣṭutāḥ; apāṃ sarasvatī jyeṣṭhā trāyantām asmākaṃ gām aśvaṃ puruṣaṃ paśum,* "Let the herbs be auspicious for you; let the very powerful plants who have been brought [and] who are extolled, save our cow, horse, man [and] draught-ox. Sarasvatī [is] the most excellent of waters." (A variant of P *a* is found at AVŚ 8.2.15*a*. The mention of Sarasvatī and the waters points to the additional use of water, perhaps from the sacred river Sarasvatī, in the healing rite.) This verse suggests that plants were fetched from a distance and were perhaps purchased or bartered. Bloomfield points out that the word *grấma*, 'clan' or 'village' in *c*, is usually the proper scene of the Atharvavedic ritualistic performances (579-80).

VERSE 12

K 16.13.2 reads *balena*(?) at the end of the first line and concludes the second line with: . . . *madhoḥ saṃbhūtā amṛtasya bhakṣo ghṛtamad duhrate gopurogavam,* ". . . [they], composed of honey, [are] the drink of immortality [and] yield [food] which possesses ghee [and] which has cow's milk as [its] principal [ingredient]." There is some controversy over the exact meaning of *gópurogavam* in the last *pāda*. Henry, considering that it refers to the food (*ánnaṃ*), renders: "la nourriture à laquelle préside la vache" (21, 59; cf. at *La magie:* "tous les dons nourriciers de vache," 57). Griffith follows Henry (409). Bloomfield understands it to be an expression similar to *gav-ādi* and translates: "and cattle chief of all" (42, 580). Whitney-Lanman construe it literally: "with milk (*gó*) as chief (*purogavấ*)" (500). The basic meaning of the word appears to be "that having the cow (*gó*) as leader (*purogava*)." In the context of other food products, however, the sense of *gó* may well be, as Whitney-Lanman suggest, "milk." The entire compound, therefore, could refer to a food (*ánna*) which has cow's milk as its chief ingredient; cf. P which seems to imply that the food had both ghee and milk as ingredients.

VERSE 13

In *c,* P 16.13.3 has *nas,* 'us' in place of *mā.* The Śáu implies that the patient is speaking, while the P keeps the speaker as the healer. In *d,* we may also render: "from the distress of death"; yet *áṃhas* usually stands alone.

VERSE 14

In *a,* P 16.13.4 reads as Śáu. The exact meaning of tigerish or 'derived from a tiger' as applied to an amulet of plants is uncertain. It could refer to an amulet by which plants are covered with a tiger skin (MWSED, s.v.) or one which possessed the power of a tiger (Griffith, 410). It may, on the other hand, refer to a tiger's claw which is today a very auspicious piece of jewelry worn by people in India. It is possible, therefore, that a tiger-claw amulet or talisman was associated with the plants and worn to ward off the attacks of the harmful demons.

VERSE 15

In *a,* P(K) 16.13.5 reads *oṣadhīnām* for *sáṃ vijante;* and *d,* based on manuscript 'P,' reads as Śau (K: *janabhyo*?). At AVŚ 8.5.9, two witchcrafts (*kṛtyā́* and *svayáṃkṛtā*) are implored to go away across ninety navigable streams; likewise at AVŚ 10.1.16, witchcraft (*kṛtyā́,* verse 15) is requested to go beyond ninety streams difficult to navigate. The implication in this verse is that both the *yákṣmas* who enter the kine and those who possess men are sent away by the plants to navigable rivers to be carried further away by those streams. The disease-demons are, therefore, sent as far away as possible.

VERSE 16

K 16.13.6 reads as Śau. In *a, mumucānā́,* may, as Henry (21) and Bloomfield (43, 480) suggest, be rendered actively. Griffith (410) and Whitney-Lanman (500) construe it passively: "The plants have become freed." Whitney-Lanman notice that the vocatives *mumucānā oṣadhayo* would be much preferred (500; cf. Henry who reads as such for *óṣadhayo,* 21, 60). The passive rendering is, however, grammatically more correct (cf. VS 12.98 to ṚV 10.97.23 n, 248, above). Bloomfield suggests, perhaps quite rightly, that Agni Vaiśvānara may represent the funeral fire (580). In this way, the first line may be understood as referring to the preservation of plants from the fire.

VERSE 17

In *c,* K 16.13.8 (Barret), 9 (Raghu Vira), begins: *vīrudho viśvabheṣajīs,* "the plants, the medicines for all [diseases]." Henry (57) and Bloomfield (580, 624) suggest that *āṅgirasī́,* in this instance, probably does not have the negative connotation of "pertaining to witchcraft" (*ābhicārika*). While it is clear that these herbs are beneficial to man, it does not mean that any plants acquired from the so-called malicious Aṅgiras are always harmful. Being experts in sorcery, it is very likely that the Aṅgiras had a rich store of herbs and the knowledge of their uses. Many of them could just as well have been used for beneficial ends. *āṅgirasī́,* therefore, in this context does not need to be considered in any way different from that by which it is normally understood. It merely refers to the source of the herbs, not to their quality (cf. verse 24, below). In *b,* the contrast between *párvateṣu* and *sanéṣu* suggests that a trade in the magico-medical herbs had already begun. Both the local flora and the material brought from afar were employed.

VERSE 18

P 16.13.7 reads as Śau (cf. verse 19 n). The healer appears to be speaking of four categories, all controlled by the relative pronouns of which the correlative is in verse 19: 1. those plants whom the healer knows; 2. those he is looking at; 3. those unknown but heard of by the healer; and 4. those from (in) whom he knows what has been compounded together, i.e. he knows the herbs who have gone into a herbal mixture. Here, the locative seems to have more of an ablative meaning.

VERSE 19

K 16.13.8*ab* (Raghu Vira) reads as Śau. Barret, however, includes *ab* as part of verse 18 (i.e. P 16.13.7), which is quite appropriate, for verses 18 and 19 logically follow one another. *cd* occurs above as verse 7*cd*.

VERSE 20

P 16.13.9 (Barret), 10 (Raghu Vira), reads as Śau (*ab* are obscure in manuscript 'P'). All the plants and plant products mentioned in this verse are quite auspicious. It is, therefore, natural for them to be included in the healing ritual and for homage to be paid to them. On the *ásvatthá*, see ṚV 10.97.5. Note the contrast in size between the great *ásvatthá* and the lowly *darbhá*-grass: the poet-healer was not influenced by their size. In *b*, Bloomfield has construed *amṛ́taṃ havíḥ* as two separate elements (43). It seems more appropriate to understand them as one, i.e. "the immortal oblation" (Whitney-Lanman, 500) or "libation d'ambroisie" (Henry, 22; also *La magie*, 57–58). It is significant that rice and barley (*vrīhí, yáva*), two important healing-plants in later Indian medicine, are here mentioned as medicines (*bheṣajá*). Likewise it is important to notice that both are mentioned as equals. In the *Ṛgveda* only *yáva*, 'barley' occurs. At AVŚ 8.2.18, we notice that rice and barley are requested to be auspicious to the patient, to be devoid of *balā́sa* and to be non-pain-causing; they are also said to have expelled *yákṣma* and to have released one from distress (*śivaú te stāṃ vrīhiyavā́v abalāsā́v adomadhaú, etaú yákṣmaṃ ví bādhete etáu muñcato áṃhasaḥ*).

VERSE 21

P 16.13.10 (Barret), 11 (Raghu Vira), reads as Śau (*cd* obscure in manuscript 'P'). *pṛ́śnimātṛ* is generally considered to be the Maruts (see ṚV 1.23.10, 38.4, 85.2, 89.7; 5.57.2, 3, 59, 6; 8.7.3, 17; 9.34.5 and AVŚ 5.21.14). It may, here, however, be taken to refer to the herbs who, in this verse are looked upon as children of the clouds, fertilized by Parjanya. On Parjanya, cf. AVŚ 1.2, 3; at ṚV 5.83.4*d*, he is said to promote [growth on] the earth with his flow of semen (*yát parjányaḥ pṛthivīṃ rétasā́vati*).

VERSE 22

P begins a new hymn with this verse. In *b*, K 16.14.1 has *phālayāmasi* "we cause . . . to burst forth with [the power of the nectar]" (?), presumably, after he has drunk it. In this verse, it appears that the patient is given a powerful substance to drink, after which the healer prepares another medicine to ensure his long life. In this way, he is given one medicine to dispel the disease and another to promote his life (cf. verse 5, above).

VERSE 23

K 16.14.2 has a slightly better reading for *cd: gandharvās sarpā yā vidus tā ihā yantv oṣadhīḥ,* "Let those herbs, whom the Gandharvas and the snakes know, come here" (*d* occurs at AVŚ 8.7.10*e* and P[K] 16.12.10*e*). At AVŚ 2.27.2*ab* and 5.14.1*ab*, it is said that the eagle discovered an auspicious plant (cf. 1.24.1) whom the swine (*sūkará*) uprooted with its snout (cf. Griffith, 411). It is also interesting to find the mongoose in a favorable relationship with the snake, for they are usually dire enemies (see AVŚ 6.139.5; cf. VS 24.26, 32, TS 5.5.12, 21). As Bloomfield suggests, however, the snakes could be considered as mythical rather than as poisonous and harmful creatures (580; cf. 540). Their association with the Gandharvas in this passage would support such an interpretation.

VERSE 24

In *b*, K 16.14.3 has the manuscript reading *vaghaṭo* (Raghu Vira as Śau) for *ragháṭo. vaghaṭo* may be related to *vághā* which, at AVŚ 6.50.3 and 9.2.22, seems to refer to sharp-toothed, noxious animals which eat grain (see also Macdonell-Keith, *Vedic Index,* 2: 237). For the obscure *ragháṭo,* the PW suggests the emendation *raghávas* which, from the root *raṅh,* 'to hasten,' may mean 'fleet' and, in the context with eagles and other birds, could refer to falcons or hawks (see Griffith, 411; Henry, 22, 60; Bloomfield, 43–44, 580–81; and Whitney-Lanman, 501). It may, however, be related to the word *rágha* which, at TĀ 1.1.3; 21.2, seems to mean 'evil,' 'malicious' (see Mayrhofer, Wb, 3: 31). It would appear that it refers, like the eagle, to some type of bird of prey. In *e*, the word *mṛgā́* may have the meaning 'bird' (cf. Avestan, *marᵉya* and ibid., 2: 669–70), for the entire verse refers to such animals, while the next verse speaks of the four-footed beasts. In this case, *mṛgā́* may be qualified by *patatríṇaḥ* in *d.* As Bloomfield notices, it appears that the poet has in mind the keen sight of certain birds of prey, which allows them to spot and identify, from great heights, certain objects (580–81; cf. also ṚV 10.97.13).

VERSE 25

For *cd,* K 16.14.4 reads as verse 26*cd.*

VERSE 26

For *cd,* K 16.14.5 reads: *tāvatīs tubhyam ābhṛtāś śarma yacchantv oṣadhīḥ,* which is almost identical with verse 25*cd.* The meaning of both this and the previous verse is altered only slightly, if at all, by the transposition of *cd* in the K; the present tense, *ā́bharāmi,* however, is preferred over the past passive tense of *ā́bhṛtāḥ.* Again, as in verse 18, the healer's knowledge of the correct medicine is expressed.

VERSE 27

K 16.14.6 reads as Śau. Cf. also ṚV 10.97.3*b,* 15*ab.* In *c,* there is some controversy surrounding the exact meaning of *saṃ mātára.* Henry accents *sáṃ* and thus makes it a verbal prefix: "toutes, qu'elles se laissent traire comme des mères . . ." (23, 60; *La magie,* 58). Bloomfield reads the text as printed, but understands the plants to be similar to calves who suck from the same mother: "as if from the same mother they shall suck sap" (44, 581). Whitney-Lanman consider that the root *duh* has rather the sense of "to yield milk" and that *saṃ mātára* refers to the plants: "like joint mothers, let them milk . . ." (501). It is likely, therefore, that it refers to the various plants mentioned in *ab,* who have, as it were, a common mother, perhaps the earth (*pṛthivī́,* cf. verse 2; see also Macdonell, *Vedic Mythology,* 88) and who yield a white sap similar to milk (cf. verse 17 where sappy plants are mentioned). In this way, the association between milking and the mother is symbolical.

VERSE 28

cd occurs at AVŚ 6.96.2*cd;* 7.112(117).2*cd* and ṚV 10.97.16*cd* with the variant *sárvasmād* for *víśvasmād* (cf. notes to ṚV 10.97.16). In *b,* K 16.14.7 has *u[t] tvā* for *átho;* and for *cd,* it reads: *u[t] tvā yamasya paḍbīśād, oṣadhībhir apīparam,* "with the herbs, I have transported you over Yama's foot-fetter." In *ab,* the word *śalá,* compounded with the cardinal numbers *páñcan* and *dáśan,* is obscure. It can mean 'a measure of distance' (MWSED, s.v.); or it may be etymologically connected with *śará* and mean 'reed,' 'arrow,' 'staff' (Mayrhofer, Wb, 3: 313–14, and 306). Ludwig (505) and Griffith (412) render it in the latter sense, while Henry (23) and Bloomfield (44, 581–82) understand it in the former sense and render: "from a depth of five fathoms, from a depth of ten fathoms." Whitney-Lanman leave the word untranslated (501). Both definitions are vague in this context; and, as Whitney-Lanman notice, the notion of distance or depth is almost senseless (ibid.). Perhaps it is some obscure reference to a disease sent by Rudra through his arrows (cf. AVŚ 6.57; 6.90) or to gigantic demons.

APPENDIX I

Sanskrit Names of Plants with Botanical Equivalents

Introduction

One of the most difficult problems facing scholars of Indian medicine is the correct identification of the flora mentioned in the medical and non-medical literature of ancient India.

The plants listed in this appendix, therefore, represent the most likely equivalents, based on an examination of numerous *nighaṇṭus*, books of Indian materia medica, and researches into ancient Indian pharmaceutics.

Given in Sanskrit alphabetical order, the appendix provides a glossary of all the plants previously mentioned in this work with their probable botanical appellations. I have, where possible, endeavored to supply significant synonyms. It is hoped that this practice may allow individual terms to be checked in other sources thereby providing further synonyms. For the botanical names, I have followed Meulenbeld, whose excellent Appendix Four in *The Mādhavanidāna and its chief commentary* (Leiden, 1974), 520–611, has spared me the laborious task of consulting the *Index Kewensis* and the *International Code* in order to obtain the currently accepted Linnaean nomenclature. I have also included the common English name of the particular plant when it was available.

akṣa (= *vibhītaka*): *Terminalia bellerica* Roxb; beleric myrobalans.

apāmārgá (= *śikharī*): *Achyranthes aspera* Linn = *A. heptapetalum* Roxb; rough-chaff tree, prickly-chaff flower.

aralu: see under *jaṅgidá*.

áriṣṭa (= *nimba*): *Melia azadirachta* Linn = *Azadirachta indica* A. Juss; nīm, margosa tree, Indian lilac.

arundhatī́ [= *sahadevī* (comm. to AVŚ 4.12.2) = *sahā* = *balā*]: *Sida cordifolia* Linn; country mallow or (= *sahadevī* = *mahāsahā* = *mahābalā*): *Sida rhombifolia* Linn; or (= *sahadevī* = *sahā* = *atibalā*): *Abutilon indicum* Linn & Sw; Indian mallow; or (= *sahadevī*): *Vernonia cinerea*, Less; fleabane.

arjuna (= *kakubha*): *Terminalia arjuna* Bedd, W & A; *arjuna*, (white) myrobalan.

alākā [= *bhṛgaka* = *bhṛṅgarājā* (comm. to KauśS 31.28)]: *Eclipta alba* (Linn) Hassk.

ávakā (= *śaivāla*): *Vallisneria spiralis* Linn = *Blyxa octandra* Rich; grassy plant growing in marshlands, moss.

aśvatthá (= *pippala* = *bodhi*): *Ficus religiosa* Linn = *Urostigma religiosum* Gasp; sacred fig, pipal tree.

ásiknī [= *nīlī* (comm. to AVŚ 1.23.1) = *nīla* = *nīlikā* = *nilinī*]: *Indigofera tinctoria* Linn; true indigo, dyer's indigo.

āmalaka (= *āmalaki* = *dhātrī*): *Phyllanthus emblica* Linn = *Emblica officinalis* Gaertn; emblic myrobalan, Indian gooseberry.

āla [= *godhūma* (comm. to KauśS 25.18) = *yavanaka* = *sumana*]: *Triticum vulgare* Linn = *T. sativum* Lam; wheat.

āsurī (= *rājikā* = *rājasarṣapa*): *Brassica juncea* Coss = *Sinapis juncea* Linn; common Indian or brown mustard.

udumbára (= *kṣīrī* = *hemadugdha* = *kṣīradru* = *kṣīravṛkṣa*): *Ficus racemosa* Wall & Linn = *F. Glomerata* Roxb; cluster-fig, gular fig, country fig.

urvārú [= *ervāru(ka)* = *karkaṭī*]: *Cucumis melo* Linn var. *momordica* Duthie et Fuller = *C. momordica* Roxb; also *C. melo* Linn var. *utilissimus* Duthie et Fuller = *C. utilissimus* Roxb. There is confusion over the exact identification: for *C. momordica,* KaiNi (101) gives *cirbhiṭa,* etc. and Nadk (1: 403) offers *ervāru,* etc.; for *C. utilissimus,* KaiNi (99) gives *ervāru* and Nadk (1: 406) offers *karkaṭi*; for *C. melo,* Nadk (1: 402–403) gives *kaliṅga,* etc.; sweet or musk melon.

uśīra (= *vīra* = *vīraṇa* = *abhaya* = *śevya*): *Vetiveria zizanioides* (Linn) Nash = *Andropogon muricatus* Retz; "khas-khas" grass.

óṣadhi [= *haridrā* (comm. to AVŚ 1.23.1)]: *Curcuma longa* Roxb; turmeric, saffron. It is generally a term for medicinal herbs or simples.

kapivallī (= *kapivallikā* = *gajapippalī*): *Scindapsus officinalis* Schott = *Pothos officinalis* Roxb.

karīra (= *karīraka* = *tīkṣṇasāra* = *gūḍhapatra*): *Capparis aphylla* Roth = *Capparis sodada* R. Br = *C. decidua* Edgew = *Sodada decidua* Forsk; caper plant, caper berry.

kúṣṭha (= *kapāla*): *Saussurea lappa* C. B. Clarke = *Aplotaxis lappa* Decne = *A. auriculata* D.C.

kṛ́ṣṇā [= *indravāruṇī* (comm. to AVŚ 1.23.1)]: *Citrullus colocynthis* Schrad = *Cucumis coloynthis* Linn; Indian wild bitter gourd, bitter apple, bitter cucumber; or (= *pippalī*: s.v.); or it is equivalent to a variety of plants, see Meulenbeld, *Mādhavanidāna,* 545–46.

khadirá (= *gāyatrī* = *kuṣṭhaghna*): *Acacia catechu* Willd = *Mimosa catechu* Linn; catechu, black catechu.

khálva [= *kṛṣṇacaṇaka* (comm. to AVŚ 2.31.1) = *caṇaka*]: *Cicer arietinum* Linn; black chick-pea; or it is equivalent to *niṣpāva: Dolichos lablab* Linn.

garī (= *kadamba*): *Andropogon caricosus* Linn = *A. serratus* Retz; a type of grass (*tṛṇa*) (comm. to KauśS 31.15); see also Caland, AZ, 101 and note.

gulgulú (= *guggulu* = *mahiṣākṣa*): *Balsamodendron mukul* Hook ex. Stocks = *Commiphora mukul* Engl; gum-gugul, Indian bedellium. It is also equated with *kapitthaparṇī*: *Boswellia glabra* Roxb = *B. serrata* Roxb ex. Coleb; Indian olibanum or frankincense. It is frequently used as a fumigant!

caṇaka (*kṛṣṇacaṇaka,* comm. to AVŚ 2.31.1), see *khálva.*

cīpúdru?: perhaps a type of tree (comm. to AVŚ 6.127.2), equal to *śīpudru* (= *sarala*): *Pinus longifolia* Roxb.

jaṅgiḍá (= *aralu* = *araṭu* = *śyonāka* = *lodhra*): *Oroxylum indicum* Vent = *Calosanthes indica* Blume = *Bignonia indica* Linn.

jayantī: *Sesbania aculeata* Pers; or (= *jayantika*): *Sesbania aegyptiaca* Pers = *Aeschynomena sesban* Roxb; or (= *balāmoṭā*): a type of *hilamocikā*: *Enhydra flutuans* Lour.

jīvantī: see under *jīvī*.

jīvalā?: it could be related to *jīvaka*, *jivantī*, etc.

jīvī [= *jīvantī* (comm. to KauśS 31.28) = *jīvā* = *maṅgalyā*]: *Leptadenia reticulata* W & A = *Dendrobium macraei* Lindl; or (= *jīvaka* = *madhura* = *maṅgalya*): *Microstylis wallichii* Lindl. There is difficulty with the correct identification of this plant: both *jīvantī* and *jīvaka* belong to the group of plants which are sweet smelling (*madhuragaṇa*) and which promote vitality (*jīvanīya*) [see TAS 31.30 (p. 458)]; cf. also *Bhāvaprakaśa*, 1: 295–96.

tíla (= *snehaphala*): *Sesamum indicum* Linn; gingili seed, sesamum, sesame.

darbhá (= *kuśa* = *uluka*): *Imperata arundinacea* Cyrill = *I. cylindrica* Beauv = *Saccharum cylindricum* Lam = *Poa cynosuroides* Retz. Meulenbeld notices that there could be a distinction between *darbhá* and *kuśa* (*Mādhavanidāna*, 562); likewise P. V. Sharma at KaiNi, 229: *kuśa*: *Desmostachya bipinnata* Stapf.

dārbhyūṣa [= *veṇudārbhūṣa* (comm. to AVŚ 7.74[78].1) = ? *vaṃśa*]: *Bambusa bambos* Druce = *B. arundinacea* Retz; bamboo, a type of reed-grass.

dūrvā (= *śiṣṭa* = *aghadviṣṭā*): *Cynodon dactylon* (Linn) Pers; bermuda grass, dog grass. Some equate it with *kuśa* (see under *darbhá*). Cf. also *nīladūrvā*: *C. dactylon* (Linn) Pers at KaiNi, 227, and TAS 31.151 (489).

dhavá (= *nanditaka* = *śakaṭākhya* = *gaura* = *dhurandhara*): *Anogeissus latifolia* Wall = *Conocarpus latifolius* Roxb; crane tree.

naḍá (= *naḷa* = *nīḷotpala*): *Nymphaea lotus* Linn = *N. rubra* Roxb ex. Salisb; water-lily.

nikaṭā?: two *Curcuma*-plants (*haridrā*, see under *óṣadhi*) growing on sides of trees (see Caland, AZ, 96 n).

nitatnī [= *kācamācī* (comm. to AVŚ 6.136.1) = *kākamācī* = *raktakākamācī*]: *Solanum nigrum* Linn.

nyagródha (= *vaṭa* = *śamī* = *vanaspati* = *yakṣavāsa*): *Ficus benghalensis* Linn = *Ficus indica* Roxb; banyan tree, Indian fig.

paraśú?: the usual meaning for this word is 'axe' or 'hatchet.' Perhaps the wooden part of the instrument is meant.

parṇá (= *palāśá*: s.v.).

palāśá (= *kiṃśuka* = *kirmī*): *Butea frondosa* Koenig ex. Roxb = *B. monosperma* (Lam) Taub; bastard teak, butea-gum.

piṅgá? (= *hiṅgu*): *Ferula foetida* Regel = *F. asafoetida* Linn; or (= *haridrā*): see under *óṣadhi*.

pippalī (= *capalā* = *kṛṣṇā* = *kaṇā*): *Piper longum* Linn; pepper-corn, long pepper.

pūtīka (= *karañja*): *Pongamia pinnata* (Linn) Merrill; Indian beech. TAS 35.27 (550) explains that it is synonymous with a variety of *karañja*; cf. also Meulenbeld, *Mādhavanidāna*, 537.

pūtúdru? (= *khadirá*: s.v.); or (*devadāru*): *Cedrus deodara* Loud = *Pinus deodara* Roxb; Himalayan cedar.

pṛśniparṇī [= *klītanī* = *dhāvanī* = *guhā* = *kalaśī* = *kumbhī* (*vṛkṣa*)]: *Uraria lagopoides* DC = *Doodia lagopodioides* Roxb = *U. picta* Desv. *Bhāvaprakāśa*, 1: 286–87 identifies two plants *pṛśniparṇī*: *Uraria picta* Desv and *U. lagopoides* DC.

pramanda [= *induka* = *aśmantaka* (Dārila to KauśS 8.17; 25.11) = *aśmanta*]: *Ficus cordifolia* Roxb; see however Caland, who does not believe it to be a plant (AZ, 15–16 n).

plakṣá (= *pippari* = *vāṭī* = *supārśa*): *Ficus infectoria* Roxb = *F. lacor* Buch.-Ham.

bajá?: a type of *sarṣapa*: *Brassica campestris* Linn var. *sarson* Prain.

mārṣā (= *mārṣaka* = *māriṣa* = *taṇḍulīya*): *Amaranthus spinosus* Linn; or [= *chaumārṣā* (Hindī)]: *A. paniculatus* Mig., See Nidk, 2: 89.

múñja (= *śara* = *sthūlagarbha* = *vipūya*): *Saccharum arundinaceum* Retz = *S. munja* Roxb = *S. sara* Roxb.

yáva (= *indrayava*): *Hordeum hexastichon* Linn = *H. sativum* Pers = *H. vulgare* Linn; barley.

rājasarṣapa (= *āsurī*: *s.v.*).

rāmā [= *bhṛṅgarājā* (comm. to AVŚ 1.23.1)]: see under *alākā*.

varaṇá (= *varuṇa* = *varāṇa* = *śamakā* = *setu* = *urumāṇa* = *kumāraka*): *Crataeva nurvala* Buch.-Ham = *C. religiosa* Hook & Forest = *C. trifoliata* Roxb; three-leaved caper.

viṣāṇaka (*viṣāṇā*)? (= *viṣāṇikā* = *karkaṭaśṛṅgī*): *Pistacia integerrima* Stew ex. Brandis; or *Rhus succendanea* Linn. TAS 51.63 (467) explains that it is a synonym for a variety of *meṣaśṛṅgī* (= *ajaśṛṅgī*): *Gymnema sylvestre* R.Br = *Asclepias geminata* Roxb; or it is equal to *sahasracakṣu* (= *indrākṣa*): *Saussurea* sp. *Dichrostachys cineria* W & A.; cf. *Bhāvaprakaśa*, 1: 98.

śamī (= *lakṣmī* = *tuṅgā* = *śivā* = *sītā* = *saktuphalā*): *Acacia sundra* DC = *A. suma* Buch.-Ham ex Wall = *Mimosa suma* Roxb; or *Prosopis spicigera* Linn. According to TAS 19.39 (308) it causes the hair to fall out.

śāla (= *sarja* = *sarjarasa* = *kānta*): *Shorea Robusta* Gaertn; śāl tree; or (= *priyāla* = *cāra*): *Buchanania latifolia* Roxb.

śalmalí (= *śālmalī* = *picchilā*): *Bombax ceiba* Linn = *B. malabaricum* (DC) S & E = *B. heptaphyllum* Roxb = *Salmalia malabarica* Schott et Endl; silk-cotton tree.

śigru (= *śo*[*au*]*bhāñjana* = *kṛṣṇagandha*): *Moringa pterygosperma* Gaertn = *M. oleifera* Lam; horse-radish. Red variety is *madhuśigru*; white variety is *haritachada* [TAS 37.26–27 (595)], or *śvetaśigru* (see Meulenbeld, *Mādhavanidāna*, 603).

śīrṣa (= *mandana*): *Randia dumetorum* Lam; bushy gardenia, emetic nut; see Caland, AZ, 96 n; or (= *śirīṣa* = *plavaga* = *kalima* = *vipra*): *Albizzia lebbeck* Benth.

APPENDIX II

Bibliographical Essay

A review of the secondary literature on traditional Indian medicine has yet to be undertaken. The purpose of this essay, therefore, is to present a critical bibliographic history of the most significant studies in western languages. Materials in modern Indian languages have been omitted as they were unavailable to me.[1] For a critical review of translated Sanskrit medical texts, I refer to my "An annotated bibliography of translations into western languages of principal Sanskrit medical treatises."[2]

A brief sketch of the early history of Indological studies in Europe and in India will help to set the stage for a survey of the research into India's medical history.

The French Jesuit missionaries working in South India in the seventeenth and eighteenth centuries have given the first indications that the Sanskrit language was being learned by people from the Occident. Unfortunately their efforts were isolated and demonstrate that they did not gain a real understanding of India's antique past.

The key figure in the development of Indology was Sir William Jones who, before taking up his post in 1783 as Supreme Court judge in Calcutta, had learned all the major European languages as well as Hebrew, Arabic, Persian and Turkish and had recognized the relationship between Persian and European languages. He studied Sanskrit under Charles Wilkins, the only member of the East India Company to have learned the language at that time, and several Sanskrit paṇḍits in Calcutta. Less than one year after his arrival he and Wilkins founded the Asiatic Society of Bengal and Jones became its first president. The Society published a journal, *Asiatic Researches*, and both Jones and Wilkins began to produce translations directly from Sanskrit, which included the *Bhagavad Gītā* and *Hitopadeśa* (Wilkins) and *Śakuntalā* and *Gīta Govinda* (Jones). In addition to his translations, Jones was the first person to affirm publicly the relationship between Sanskrit and Greek and Latin and its hypothetical connection with German, Celtic and Persian. Jones and Wilkins were followed in Calcutta by Henry Colebrooke and Horace Hayman Wilson, who continued to produce translations

---

[1] For a brief survey of the most pertinent studies, see G. J. Meulenbeld, "The surveying of Sanskrit medical literature," in G. J. Meulenbeld, ed., *Proceedings of the International Workshop on Priorities in the Study of Indian Medicine*, held at the State University of Groningen, 23–27 October 1983 (University of Groningen: Institute of Indian Studies, 1984), 33–34.

[2] *Clio Medica*, 19.3-4 (1984): 281-291.

from Sanskrit and to further Indological studies through the Asiatic Society of Bengal. In Europe, the Frenchman Anquetil-Duperron, a Persian scholar, published a Latin translation of fifty *Upaniṣads*, philosophical works of the late Vedas, which had been translated into Persian for Prince Mohammed Dārā-Shakoh, the son of Shah Jahan who is famous for commissioning the construction of the Taj Mahal as a tomb for his wife.

The early translations from Sanskrit began to create an interest in Sanskrit literature in Europe. In 1803, a founding member of the Asiatic Society of Bengal, Alexander Hamilton, detained in France at the end of the Peace of Amiens, became the first teacher of Sanskrit in Europe at the recently founded École des Langues Orientales Vivantes (1795). He taught Sanskrit to Friedrich Schlegel, the first German Sanskritist and a leader of the German Romantic School, who published, in 1808, a book on Indian language and literature containing the first German translations from Sanskrit.[3] In 1814, Leonard de Chézy was appointed to the first chair of Sanskrit founded at the Collège de France. He taught Sanskrit to Friedrich Schlegel's brother, August Wilhelm, who was in 1818 appointed the first professor of Sanskrit in Germany, at the newly founded University of Bonn. Sanskrit was first taught in England at the training college of the East India Company at Hertford. In 1832, H. H. Wilson was appointed Boden Professor of Sanskrit at Oxford, the first chair of Sanskrit in England. Chairs were then established at London, Cambridge and Edinburgh, as well as at several universities in the United States.

In 1816, the Bavarian Franz Bopp, a student of Chézy, gave birth to the new linguistic science of comparative philology with his work, *Über das Conjugations-system der Sanskrit Sprache in Vergleichung mit jenem der griechischen, lateinischen, persischen und germanischen Sprache* (Andreä: Frankfurt am Main), which, based on Jones's earlier studies, presented a very tentative reconstruction of the common ancestor of Sanskrit and the classical languages of Europe. In 1821, the French Société Asiatique was founded in Paris; and two years later the Royal Asiatic Society was established in London. The interest in editing, translating and studying Sanskrit literature grew rapidly from these beginnings.

The foundations of Vedic Studies in Europe were laid by Eugène Burnouf, who taught at the Collège de France in the early 1840s. Two of his students were Rudolf Roth who originated the study of the Vedas in Germany and Friedrich Max Müller who, while professor of Comparative Philology at Oxford, produced the excellent edition of the *Ṛgveda* with the commentary of Sāyaṇa (1849–1875) and edited and contributed to the *Sacred Books of the East*, a series of authoritative, annotated translations. Before Müller, however, Theodor Aufrecht had already published an edition of the *Ṛgveda* in romanized script (1861–1863). Perhaps the greatest achievement during

---

[3] *Über die Sprache und Weisheit der Inder. Ein Beitrag zur Begründung der Altertumskunde*, Heidelberg: Mohr und Zimmer, 1808.

the formative period of Indology in Europe was the *Sanskrit-Wörterbuch* or *St. Petersburg Lexicon,* compiled by the Germans Otto Böhtlingk and Rudolf Roth and published in seven folio volumes by the Academy of Arts and Sciences of St. Petersburg from 1852–1875. Sir Monier Monier-Williams, while professor of Sanskrit at Oxford, drew largely on this work for his *Sanskrit–English Dictionary* (Oxford, 1899). From these beginnings the study of Sanskrit and Indian history was established at the major universities in Europe and America and almost every type of Indian literature received some attention.

In India also, in the early part of the nineteenth century, Rammohan Roy, founder of the Brahmo Samāj, a religious organization which sought to unite the best of Christian and Brāhmaṇic religious ideals, translated many of the *Upaniṣads* into English. During this time the first Sanskrit editions of many treatises were published in Bengali script. Influenced and incited by the Bengal Renaissance of the latter part of the last century, Indian scholars began to take a renewed interest in their own past. Editions of Sanskrit texts were being published in many parts of India and critical scholarship was being carried out by people like Bhāū Dājī, Rājendralāl Mitra and Sir R. G. Bhāndārkar. The fervor of this Renaissance rekindled interest in all areas of the Indian arts and sciences.[4]

By the twentieth century, the four main centers of Indology were Germany, France, England and India. The United States and Holland at this time were largely a branch of the German school. From each of the four came the beginnings of the investigations into the literature of ancient Indian medicine.

Interest in the medical tradition of the ancient Indian came principally from two types of investigators: the Sanskritist who explored the literature of the Indians and the physician who was curious to know how Indian medicine compared with, and might be beneficial to, his own tradition of medicine.

The British

The first information about traditional Hindu medicine or *āyurveda* came from the pen of the British surgeon and Sanskritist stationed in Calcutta, H. H. Wilson, who, in 1823, published an article entitled "On the medical and surgical sciences of the Hindus."[5] Probably working from manuscripts, Wilson sympathetically summarized the general principles and practices

[4] This brief account of the history of Indology has been culled from Maurice Winternitz, *A history of Indian literature,* translated from the German by S. Ketkar (1927; rpt. New Delhi: Oriental Books Reprint Corporation, 1977, second edition), 1: 8–25, and A. L. Basham, *The wonder that was India* (New York: Grove Press, 1959), 4–8.

[5] Originally published in *Oriental Magazine* (Calcutta), 1: 207–12, 349–56, and reprinted in *Essays analytical, critical and philological on subjects connected with Sanskrit literature,* Vol. 1. Collected and edited by Reinhold Rost (London: Trübner & Co., 1864), 269–76, 380–91.

of *āyurveda* as outlined in the first chapters of the treatises of Suśruta, Caraka and Vāgbhaṭa.

Almost from the beginning of the British East India Company, there had been an interest in acquiring knowledge of the flora and fauna of India so that it might be used in medicine both in India and back home in England.[6] One of the first individuals to investigate the subject of Indian materia medica from the historical point of view was John Forbes Royle who was a physican of the medical staff of the Bengal army during the early part of the nineteenth century. In 1837, as professor of Materia Medica and Therapeutics at King's College, London, he published a book entitled, *An essay on the antiquity of Hindoo medicine,* including an introductory lecture to the course of materia medica and therapeutics, delivered at King's College (London: Wm. H. Allen and J. C. Churchhill), in which is presented a summary of the current knowledge of Indian medical and scientific history. Using the commerce of Indian drugs as a central theme, he appears to be the first person to posit a connection among Indian, Arabic, Greek and Chinese medicine. There is no evidence that he possessed a knowledge of Sanskrit. His information is gleaned from the existing secondary sources on the different subjects and medical traditions.[7]

Working from manuscripts with the aid of an āyurvedic paṇḍit, a physician of the Bengal Medical Service, Thomas A. Wise, undertook a study of *āyurveda.* In 1845 he published his *Commentary on the Hindu system of medicine* (Calcutta) which, he states, is "intended to describe the Hindu science of medicine" (ii). It is, therefore, not a translation, but a summary of the āyurvedic medical tradition, based principally on the texts of Caraka and Suśruta.

These British scholars and professionals attached to the East India Company in the early to the middle part of the last century were in fact the pioneers in the field of Indian medical history. After this initial burst of enthusiasm, the interest in the subject among British Indologists, physicians or historians of medicine was at best meager until the Indologist A. F. Rudolf Hoernle, principal at the Calcutta Madrasa, took up the study of Sanskrit medical treatises during the latter part of the last century and the beginning of this one. Starting with his monumental edition and translation of the *Bower Manuscript,* a large portion of which is concerned with med-

---

[6] An early essay on traditional Indian materia medica is John Fleming's "A catalogue of Indian medicinal plants and drugs, with their names in the Hindustani and Sanscrit languages," *Asiatic Researches,* 11 (1812): 153–96. The first book of the materia medica of India is Ainslie Whitelaw's *The materia medica of Hindoostan* (Madras, 1813), which was revised, enlarged and printed under the title, *Materia medica,* 2 vols. (London, 1926). See also D. V. Subba Reddy, "Dr. Whitelaw Ainslie and his contributions to materia medica and the history of medicine in India," *Bulletin of the Institute of History of Medicine,* Hyderabad, 2(1) (1972): 35–51.

[7] He also wrote *Illustrations of Botany and other branches of natural history of the Himalayan Mountains,* 2 vols. (London, 1839). See also D. V. Subba Reddy, "John Forbes Royle, botanist-medical historian; teacher and benefactor of the British Empire," *Bulletin of the Institute of History of Medicine,* Hyderabad, 3(2) (1973): 79–87.

icine, published in Calcutta from 1893 to 1912,[8] Hoernle was forced to investigate the texts of Indian medicine in order to assure the accuracy of his work. This led to studies on the authors and on the textual tradition of *āyurveda* and to investigations of the ancient Indian anatomical terminology.[9] His *Studies in the medicine of ancient India. Part I: Osteology or the bones of the human body*[10] incorporates an introduction which attempts to give a chronology of the principal āyurvedic authors and their texts, followed by a study of the historical development of the medical science of osteology in ancient India. It is a significant work on a very specialized topic. From the title of the monograph other studies focusing on different parts of Indian medical history might be expected. Unfortunately, none has appeared; and with Hoernle the investigation into ancient Indian medicine ceased to be a topic of research interest among British scholars.

Today, however, a renewed interest in the subject is taking place. The Australian born and Cambridge trained philologist Ronald Emmerick at the University of Hamburg has in the last decade published several articles pertaining to Indian medicine and āyurvedic textual studies and is completing an edition and translation of the Indian medical treatise *Siddhasāra* by Ravigupta[11] and an index of the principal Indian Sanskrit medical texts. Quite recently, Dominik Wujastyk, a young scholar trained in Sanskrit at Oxford University has been appointed to catalog a little known collection of Indian manuscripts at the Wellcome Institute for the History of Medicine in London and actively to occupy himself with Indian medical history.

The French

Around the middle of the eighteenth century, Sanskrit manuscripts were beginning to be collected and edited in India. The French abbé, J. M. F. Guérin, a parish priest at Chandernagor, collected in Bengal Sanskrit manuscripts on the Indian sciences, including medicine, with the express purpose of using them in a comparison with ancient Greek and Latin med-

---

[8] Calcutta: Office of the Superintendent of Government Printing, India [Archaeological Survey of India, New Imperial Series, Vol. 22]. Reprinted in three volumes, New Delhi, 1983.

[9] Some of Hoernle's most important articles include the following: a series under the generic title, "Studies in ancient Indian medicine," as follows: I. "The commentaries on Suśruta," JRAS (1906): 283–302, 699–700; II. "On some obscure anatomical terms," JRAS (1906): 915–41; (1907): 1–18; III. "Itsing and Vāgbhaṭa," JRAS (1907): 413–17; IV. "The composition of the Caraka Saṃhitā, and the literary methods of ancient Indian medical writers (A study in textual criticism)," JRAS (1908): 997–1028; V. "The composition of the Caraka Saṃhitā in light of the Bower Manuscript (An essay in historical and textual criticism)," JRAS (1909): 857–93. Others are: "The authorship of the Charaka Saṃhitā," *Archiv für Geschichte der Medizin,* 1 (1907): 29–40; and "The Bhela Saṃhitā in the Bower Manuscript," JRAS (1910): 830–33.

[10] Oxford: Clarendon Press, 1907; reprinted: New York: AMS Press, Inc., 1980.

[11] *The Siddhasāra of Ravigupta.* Vols. 1, 2 (Wiesbaden: Franz Steiner Verlag GMBH. 1980, 1982) [Verzeichnis der orientalischen Handschriften in Deutschland. Supplementband 23. 1, 2].

ical texts so that European doctors might derive knowledge from Indian medicine.[12]

About this same time, Indian medicine was attracting the attention of physicians in France. With the circulation of the works by Wilson and Royle, the possibility of a connection between Greek and Indian medicine began to be examined. The topic was to be one to which the French scholars of Indian medicine would constantly address themselves.

In 1843 and 1844, a certain Dr. Cerise published an article entitled, "Notice sur les doctrines pyscho-physiologiques des anciens philosophes hindous,"[13] in which the Hindu medical theory of the elements, temperaments, senses and sense faculties were examined in relation to that of the Greek philosophers. In 1853, the physician Gustave Alexandre Liétard[14] in Strasbourg defended the first thesis on Indian medicine in France, entitled, "Essai sur l'histoire de la médecine chez les Indous," printed in Strasbourg in 1858 and published under the title *Lettres historiques sur la médecine chez les Indous* (Paris: Victor Masson et Fils, 1862). It is an examination of Indian medical history from its earliest period in the Vedas to the time of the āyurvedic treatises of Caraka and Suśruta. He contributed information on the history of *āyurveda* in the *Dictionnaire encyclopédique des sciences médicales* (Paris, 1864–1889) and established himself as the current authority on Indian medicine, with numerous articles touching on Vedic and āyurvedic medicine and the possible connections with Hellenic medicine.[15] Working entirely from existing translations and secondary literature, Liétard was able to contribute significant information on Indian medicine to the general field of the history of medicine. Lacking the necessary languages, however, his work does not seem to have penetrated the circle of Sanskrit scholars, thereby keeping the study of Indian medicine on the fringes of Indology.

Liétard's work and that of Allan Webb[16] inspired the great historian of Greek medicine, Charles Daremberg, to look seriously into Hindu medicine.

---

[12] Information on French historians of medicine has been gathered from Arion Roşu's "La médecine indienne traditionnelle," *Le Courrier du CNRS*, 40 (1981): 20–25.

[13] *Annales médico-psychologiques*, T. 2: 333–42; T. 3: 1–16.

[14] See Nigel W. T. Allan's short article, "Gustave Alexandre Liétard: Orientalist and Physician," *Medical History*, 25(1) (1981): 85–88.

[15] Some of his most important essays include: "La physiologie et la cosmologie dans le Rig-Véda," *Gazette hebdomadaire de médecine et de chirurgie*, 1867, 17–23, 49–56, 65–70; "Fragments d'histoire et de bibliographie," *Gazette hebdomadaire*, 1883, 313–20, 329–34; "Notice sur les connaissances anatomiques des Indous. L'Anatomie et la physiologie dans l'Ayurvéda de Suçruta," *Revue médicale de Nancy*, T. 16 (1884): 236–40; "La littérature médicale de l'Inde," *Bulletin de l'Académie nationale de médecine* (Paris), 3rd series, T. 35 (1896): 466–84; "Le médecine Charaka. Le serment des hippocratistes et le serment des médecins hindous," *Bulletin de l'Académie nationale de médecine* (Paris), 3rd series, T. 37 (1897): 565–75; and "La doctrine humorale des Hindous et le Rig-Véda," *Janus* 3 (1898): 17–21.

[16] "The historical relation of ancient Hindu with Greek medicine, in connection with the study of modern medical science in India; being a general introductory lecture delivered June 1850," *Calcutta Review*, 14 (1850): i-vi, 541f.

Daremberg's *Recherches sur l'État de la médecine durant la Période primitive de l'Histoire des Indous* (Paris: J. B. Baillière et Fils, 1867) is an examination of the medical tradition represented in the *Ṛgveda* in relation to that typified in the Greek works of Homer. His excellent knowledge of the Greek sources allowed him to point to interesting similarities between these two medical traditions. His overall bias towards the superiority and antiquity of Greek medicine, however, led him to make unjustified statements about the influence of that medical tradition on early Indian medicine. He was, nevertheless, one of the first scholars to notice the important role which magic played in the Vedic medical tradition.

Liétard had also encouraged and guided the physician Palmyr-Uldéric-Alexis Cordier to carry on research into Indian medicine. In 1894, Cordier submitted his thesis, "Étude sur la médecine hindoue (temps védique et héroïques)," for the degree of Doctorat en Médecine at Bordeaux. Published by the medical publishers J. B. Baillière et Fils (Paris) in 1897, it encompassed a detailed examination of medically relevant passages from numerous Vedic and post-Vedic texts, culled from the existing printed texts and translations. It represents one of the pioneering efforts in the study of the earliest phases of Indian medicine. With his orientalist fervor confirmed by his residence at the French centers in India and Indo-China and by his familiarity with the relevant languages, Cordier, before his untimely death in 1914, had contributed significantly to oriental studies and Indian medical studies with his collection and study of Sanskrit and Tibetan manuscripts. He was instrumental in bringing āyurvedic studies into the purview of the Indologist.

The study of Indian medicine in France had dwindled to insignificance after Cordier, until the ophthalmologist and Indologist Jean Filliozat was called upon in 1934 to catalog the manuscripts collected by Cordier and housed in the Bibliothèque nationale in Paris. Filliozat's numerous articles and monographs on ancient Indian medicine have distinguished him as the foremost authority on the subject.[17] His *La doctrine classique de la médecine indienne; ses origines et ses parallèles grecs*, originally a thèse de lettre submitted to the Sorbonne in 1949,[18] ranks as one of the most important works on Indian medicine. Equipped with the necessary language and professional skills, he, like Cordier, was able to bring āyurvedic studies to the attention of the Indologist as well as the historian of medicine. As professor of Sanskrit at the Collège de France, he promoted the scholarly investigation of Indian medicine so that today several well qualified French scholars are engaged in the study of *āyurveda* and its history. He died in October of 1982.

---

[17] A good bibliography with reprints of some of Filliozat's articles on the history of Indian science and medicine is found in *Laghu-prabandhaḥ. Choix d'articles d'indologie par Jean Filliozat*, compiled and edited by Colette Caillat, et al. (Leiden: E. J. Brill, 1974), xi–xxv, 193–299.

[18] Paris: Imprimerie nationale, 1949; second edition: Paris: École française d' Extrême-Orient, 1975. English translation by Dev Raj Chanana, Delhi: Munshiram Manoharlal, 1964.

The Germans

Among the German scholars the focus was almost exclusively on philological and textual studies of Indian medical texts. It is perhaps not surprising that the first complete translation of a Sanskrit medical treatise was undertaken by a German. Franciscus Hessler translated the *Suśruta Saṃhitā* into Latin, under the title *Suśrutas Āyurvedas,* which was published in Erlangen in three volumes from 1844 to 1850;[19] and reading through the early Bengali editions of Caraka and Suśruta, Rudolf Roth made lexical contributions of Sanskrit medical terms to the *St. Petersburg Lexicon* in the mid-nineteenth century.

The early German interest in comparative philology, however, led to a penchant for Vedic studies. In 1864, Adalbert Kuhn published on article in which he compared Vedic and Germanic incantations, several of which were medical in content.[20] A year later appeared J. Virgil Grohmann's very important article on Vedic medicine, "Medicinisches aus dem Atharva-Veda, mit besonderem Bezug auf den Takman,"[21] in which a detailed examination of the demonic disease *takmán* and related afflictions is offered. The importance of this work lies in Grohmann's identification of *takmán* with the disease commonly known as malaria. Although subsequent advances have allowed improvements to be made on his original thesis, Grohmann's study remains a significant contribution to the understanding of Vedic medicine. It is unfortunate that he did not undertake a more comprehensive investigation of other medical topics. The need for an overview of medicine during the Vedic age was filled by Heinrich Zimmer in the chapter "Heilkunde" of his general survey of Vedic India entitled, *Altindisches Leben.*[22] Maurice Bloomfield, an American Sanskrit scholar from Johns Hopkins University, advanced the understanding of Vedic medicine with his translations and annotations of many Atharvavedic medical hymns in his *Hymns of the Atharvaveda* which appeared as volume 42 of Max Müller's *Sacred Books of the East* (Oxford, 1897).

The Sanskritist Julius Jolly was the first of the German school of Indologists to demonstrate an active interest in the later textual and doctrinal tradition of *āyurveda.* His handy *Medicin* (Strassburg: Karl J. Trübner, 1901), commissioned as Band III, Heft 10 of F. Kielhorn's and G. Bühler's *Grundriss der Indo-Arischen Philologie und Altertumskunde,* is still perhaps the best short account of Indian medicine. It offers a presentation of the principal medical authors and their texts along with an accurate and systematic outline of the basic principles of āyurvedic medicine. It has subsequently been

---

[19] Erlangae: Enke, 1844–50. The author's commentary was published under a separate title: *Commentarii et annotationes in Suśruta Āyurvedam,* Erlangae, 1852–1855.

[20] "Indische und germanische Segensspruche," *Zeitschrift für vergleichende Sprachforschung auf dem Gebiete der indogermanische Sprachen,* 3 (1864): 49–74, 113–57.

[21] *Indischen Studien,* 9 (1865): 381–423.

[22] Berlin: Weidmannsche Buchhandlung, 1879, 374–99.

updated by its English translator, C. G. Kashikar.[23] In addition to his monograph, Jolly published several important essays on the age and sources of *āyurveda*[24] and contributed articles on āyurvedic medicine in James Hasting's *Encyclopaedia of Religion and Ethics.*[25]

The first German physician and historian of medicine to take up the study of Indian medicine was A. Albert M. Esser, an ophthalmologist from Düsseldorf. Trained in Sanskrit, Esser made important contributions to āyurvedic studies with accurate translations and authoritative studies of ophthalmology in the *Suśruta Saṃhitā* and later medical treatises during the early part of this century.[26] With Esser's specialized skills, historical studies of Indian medicine were beginning to be recognized as a topic of the history of medicine and not exclusively in the domain of the Sanskrit scholar or philologist.

The most prolific writer on traditional Indian medicine was the physician from Chemnitz, Reinhold F. G. Müller, whose enthusiasm for the history of Indian medicine helped to bring the subject into focus for many historians of medicine. In 1926, Müller engaged himself full time in the study of the history of medicine and of Asian subjects when he was no longer able to keep up an active practice due to injuries he suffered during the first World War. Shortly thereafter he became friendly with Albert Grünwedel and Albert August von Le Coq, distinguished scholars of Indian and Central Asian archaeology, and began to direct his studies toward ancient Indian medicine. In 1939, he was selected to be a member of the Deutschen Akademie der Naturforscher Leopoldina zu Halle/S, through which he published a number of monographs on Indian medicine. The Akademie-Bibliothek of the Leopoldina now houses his Fachbibliothek under the title "Sammlung Reinhold Müller." In 1942, he habilitated in Leipzig and was awarded the Karl-Sudhoff-Plakette of the Deutschen Gesellschaft für Geschichte der Medizin, der Naturwissenschaft und der Technik and in 1953 he was given the title of professor. He died on 22 February 1966 at the age of eighty-three, having to his credit nearly 130 articles and monographs on all aspects of ancient Indian medicine.[27]

---

[23] Published under the title, *Indian medicine,* Poona, 1951; second edition: Delhi: Munshiram Manoharlal, 1977.

[24] Some of his important articles include four essays under the general title, "Zur Quellenkunde der indischen Medizin": 1. "Vāgbhaṭa," ZDMG, 54: 260–70; 2. "I-tsing," ZDMG, 56: 565–72; 3. "Ein alter Kommentar zu Suśruta," ZDMG, 58: 114–16; 4. "Die Cikitsākalikā des Tīsaṭācārya," ZDMG, 60: 413–68. Also significant is his "Some considerations regarding the age of the early medical literature of India," *Transactions of the International Congress of Orientalists,* 9(1) (1892): 454–61.

[25] One is on "Disease and Medicine (Hindu)" 4: 753–55; another is on "Body (Hindu)" 2: 773–74.

[26] His major study is *Die Ophthalmologie des Suśruta,* (Leipzig: Johann Ambrosius Barth, 1934). Important articles on the subject of ancient Indian ophthalmology include: "Die ophthalmologische Therapie des Bhāvaprakāśa," *Sudhoffs Archiv,* 25 (1932): 184–213, and "Die Ophthalmologie im Bower-Manuskript," *Sudhoffs Archiv,* 35 (1942): 28–42.

[27] Information for this biographical sketch derives from Rudolph Zaunick's obituary, "Rein-

A close examination of Müller's works indicates that much of his voluminous output is repetitive. He knew some Sanskrit, but it was not adequate for his task. His understanding of ancient Indian history and culture derived largely from the Indologist Johannes Hertel who was professor at Koeniglichen Real-Gymnasium, Doebel, Saxony and a friend of Müller. Relying entirely on Hertel's now untenable view that fire was the principal motivating force which dominated the lives of the Vedic Indians,[28] Müller interpreted Vedic and to some extent later Indian medicine in terms of a fire principle. Filliozat harshly criticized this over simplistic view of ancient Indian medicine,[29] and by so doing turned an already skeptical community of Sanskrit scholars and Indologists away from Müller's work.

It cannot be denied that Müller's studies of Indian medical history rest on a very weak foundation of Sanskrit philology and Indian history. His labor-of-love in marshaling an enormous quantity of data pertaining to all aspects and periods of traditional Indian medicine, nevertheless, must be applauded, for it has demonstrated the importance of the subject to historians of medicine and has provided a guide to the source materials on ancient Indian medicine. A comprehensive index of Müller's works is, however, a desideratum.

Müller had the greatest influence among the historians of medicine. The Swiss born physician and historian of medicine, Henry Sigerist, made full use of Müller's works in his rather clumsy section on "Hindu medicine" in volume 2 of his *History of medicine.*[30]

No one in Germany since Müller has taken up an intensive investigation of Indian medicine. The Indologist and historian of Indian art, Henry Zimmer, son of the aforementioned Vedic scholar Heinrich Zimmer, has been drawn into it, but only as a side interest. Consequently, his *Hindu medicine*[31] is merely an outsider's observation, wanting in substantive information. More recently the German philologist Claus Vogel began the study of Indian medicine with several articles[32] on the subject and a partial translation of the *Aṣṭāṅgahṛdaya Saṃhitā* both from the Sanskrit and the Tibetan texts.[33]

---

hold F. G. Müller, 16. April 1882–22. Februar 1966," to which is attached a useful list of Müller's publications (*Clio Medica,* 1 [1966]: 359–66).

[28] Hertel's theory of a fire principle is put forth in his *Die arischer Feuerlehre,* I. Teil, (Leipzig: H. Haessel, 1925).

[29] *La doctrine,* 40 and 72 n. See also 105, above.

[30] New York: Oxford University Press, 1961, 121–93.

[31] Baltimore: Johns Hopkins Press, 1948 [The Hideyo Noguchi Lectures, Vol.VI]. The book is a series of lectures delivered at the Johns Hopkins Institute of the History of Medicine in 1940. The final editing of the lectures was done by Ludwig Edelstein who was given the task after Zimmer's unexpected death. Edelstein's lengthy preface is particularly important for the observations made on Hellenistic similarities and differences to Indian medicine.

[32] Four articles are noteworthy: "On the humoral physiology and pathology of the hippocratics," *The Poona Orientalist,* 22 (1957): 62–73; "On the ancient Indian and Greek systems of medicine," *The Poona Orientalist,* 24 (1959): 31–34; "On the Guinea-worm disease in Indian medicine," *Adyar Library Bulletin,* 25 (1961): 55–68; and "On Bu-ston's view of the eight parts of Indian medicine," *Indo-Iranian Journal,* 6 (1962): 290–95.

[33] Wiesbaden: Franz Steiner, 1965 [Abhandlungen für die Kunde des Morgenlandes, Band 37.2].

He quickly abandoned the pursuit because it was not considered to be in the mainstream of Indological studies in Germany.

Today the Dutch psychiatrist and Indologist Garret Jan Meulenbeld is one of the leading scholars of ancient Indian medicine. His *Mādhavanidāna and its chief commentary, chapters 1–10* (Leiden: E. J. Brill, 1974) is a model study, providing an accurate translation of part of a medical treatise and its commentary as well as generally useful information on Indian medicine in appendices.

The Indians

Quite naturally the most active interest in Indian medicine has come from the Indians themselves. The early part of the nineteenth century saw the first editions of Sanskrit medical treatises printed in Bengali script. These served as the principal texts used by the Sanskritists and Indologists who wrote on topics of āyurvedic medicine. These editions are now obsolete, having been superseded to a great extent by the more recent editions of Vaidya Jādavjī Trikamjī Ācārya, published by the Nirṇaya Sāgar Press in Bombay, and those found in the Sanskrit Series of the Ānandāsrama in Poona.

Inspired by the cultural and literary renaissance in Bengal during the latter part of the last century, Indian scholars began to take an interest in their own Hindu medical tradition. The renewed focus on *āyurveda* was brought about mainly through the efforts of the āyurvedic physician Gangadhara Ray (1799–1885), who fought for the purity of āyurvedic vis-à-vis occidental medicine. Followers of Ray sought to legitimize traditional āyurvedic medical practice and to provide the basis of a professional organization which included the establishment of teaching and research, hospitals, botanical gardens, pharmacies and industries for the production of āyurvedic medicines.[34] To a great extent these aims were accomplished in more recent years by the late āyurvedic physician from Bombay, Shiv Sharma, whose wit and political prowess won him an international reputation as a leading proponent of traditional Indian medicine.

Opponents of this purist mode of thought were the advocates of a more syncretic system of *āyurveda*, who sought to combine the best of both Western and āyurvedic medicine. The leading spokesman of syncretism was C. Dwarkanath, principal of the Government and Unani College in Mysore, who outlines his approach to *āyurveda* in his three volume study entitled, *The fundamental principles of āyurveda* (Mysore: The Hindusthan Press, 1954).[35]

---

[34] Arion Roşu, "La médecine indienne traditionnelle," 23; see also Brahmanada Gupta, "Indigenous medicine in nineteenth- and twentieth-century Bengal," in *Asian medical systems, a comparative study*, ed. Charles Leslie (Berkeley: University of California Press, 1976), 371.

[35] Charles Leslie, "Interpretations of illness: syncretism in modern Āyurveda," unpublished paper, 17–19 and passim; cf. also his "The ambiguities of medical revivalism in modern India," in *Asian medical systems*, 356–67.

The renaissance was also responsible for the first English translations of the medical classics of Caraka and Suśruta by Indian scholars and practitioners of āyurveda.[36] One of the first surveys of *āyurveda* was *Aryan medical system, a short history* (Gondal, 1895), written by an Indian prince, Sir Bhagavat Sinhjee. The work was clearly an attempt to legitimize *āyurveda* and promote interest and further research in the subject by native and foreign scholars. Coming from the hand of royalty it tended to carry a special weight of authority.

A significant figure in the early studies of *āyurveda* was Girindranāth Mukhopādhyāya (Mukherjee), a physician trained at Calcutta Medical College at the end of the last and beginning of the present century. Two of his works are especially noteworthy. *The surgical instruments of the Hindus*, 2 vols. (Calcutta: Calcutta University Press, 1913–1914), is an excellent study which won him the Griffith Prize at Calcutta University in 1909. Volume 1 is a valuable study of the various surgical instruments employed by the āyurvedic physician from earliest times; volume 2 contains eighty-two plates, illustrating these instruments, most of which date from more recent centuries. The book is amply supported with citations from Sanskrit medical texts and attempts a comparative study of the surgical instruments of Indian, Greek, Roman, Arab and modern European surgeons. Unfortunately, accurate translations are wanting, and passages are merely summarized. It is a useful source for information on ancient Indian surgery and particularly the instruments of the medical profession and can serve as a point of departure for a more detailed study of comparative surgery. New translations from the Sanskrit will, however, have to be undertaken.

Mukhopādhyāya's second treatise, *History of Indian medicine*, 3 vols.,[37] was greatly influenced by P. C. Roy, the chemist at Presidency College in Calcutta, who wrote a *History of Hindu chemistry* in two volumes based mainly on āyurvedic texts.[38] Mukhopādhyāya wanted to produce a similar history for Indian medicine. Unfortunately for the modern scholar, the volumes are a disorganized jumble of names; some are physicians and some mythical healers or healing gods from antiquity. The volumes may occasionally be consulted to gain an outline and an overview of the contents of selected āyurvedic texts, but no dates may be considered as accurate.

Mukhopādhyāya's enthusiasm for *āyurveda* and penchant for studies of traditional Indian medicine gained him the appointment of editor-in-chief of the *The Journal of Āyurveda*, published in Calcutta from about 1923 and devoted to all topics of āyurvedic medicine from its ancient texts, to which

---

[36] *Carakasaṃhitā*, English translation with notes by Avinash Chandra Kaviratna and Pareshnath Sarma Kavibhusan (Calcutta, 1890–1925). The actual translator was Kisori Mohan Ganguli. *An English translation of the Sushruta Samhita based on original Sanskrit text*, 3 vols., translated and edited by Kaviraj Kunjalal Bhishagratna (Calcutta, 1907–16. Reprinted: Varanasi: The Chowkhamba Sanskrit Series Office, 1963 [The Chowkhamba Sanskrit Series, Vol. 30]).

[37] Calcutta, 1922–29. Reprint: Delhi: Orient Books Reprint Corporation, 1974.

[38] Charles Leslie, "Interpretations of illness," 20.

Mukhopādhyāya contributed numerous original essays, to modern political debates and relevant news on the status of *āyurveda* in India.[39]

The historical study of Indian medicine in India was taken over by D. V. Subba Reddy, professor of Physiology at Madras Medical College, who tirelessly wrote on every aspect of Indian medical history. He began his research in the history of medicine in 1931 by studying the works of Singer and Garrison and was greatly influenced by Henry Sigerist whom he met in 1944 when Sigerist was invited by the British Government of India to serve as adviser to the Bhore Committee for a "Health Survey." At that time, Sigerist wrote a report, recommending the creation of an Institute of History of Medicine as part of the then contemplated All Indian Medical Institute in Delhi. Problems of the war and internal strife which led to India's independence and partition in 1947 prevented the materialization of the Institute. Finally in the 1950s and 1960s, mainly through the efforts of Subba Reddy, the Central Council for Research in Indian Medicine and Homoeopathy established the Indian Institute for History of Medicine at the Osmania Medical Colleges in Hyderabad. From 1963 with Subba Reddy as editor-in-chief, it began to publish an annual *Bulletin of the Indian Institute of History of Medicine,* modeled on the *Bulletin of the History of Medicine* from The Johns Hopkins University. It includes articles on the history of both Hindu and Arabic medicine and regularly contains a bibliography of recent works on Indian medicine and news items pertaining to medical history. For the past fifty years Subba Reddy has worked to bring Indian medicine to the attention of Western scholars of the history of medicine and to bring the history of medicine to the attention of Indian scholars.[40]

A friend of Subba Reddy and leading figure in the beginnings of Indian medical history in India was Pudipeddy Kutumbiah, a devout Christian, who undertook training in medicine in India and in Europe and Britain and received his M.D. from Madras Medical College in 1931. He later became professor of medicine at Andhra Medical College in Vizag (now Vaishakapattanam), Andhra Pradesh, from 1938 to 1945 and finally was appointed professor of medicine in Madras. While in London, he became interested in the history of medicine and started to read the works of Allbutt and Osler. After taking up his post at Vizag, he began to direct his attention to the history of *āyurveda,* focusing on the works of Caraka and Suśruta, and comparative studies involving Hippocratic and Greek medicine. In 1947, he and Subba Reddy founded the Indian Society of History of Med-

---

[39] A short biographical sketch of Mukhopādhāya is given in his obituary, "Late Dr. Girindra Nath Mukherjee," *The Journal of Āyurveda,* 12(8) (1935): 82–84.

[40] Information for this biographical sketch derives from the following: D. V. Subba Reddy, "Prof. Henry E. Sigerist. Medical humanist, visionary and friend of India," *Bulletin of the Indian Institute of History of Medicine,* 5(1) (1975): 25–33; and "Report of the medico-historical functions at Kakinada," *Bulletin of the Indian Institute of History of Medicine,* 5(1–2) (1977): 63–71.

icine in Madras (in 1953 it became the Indian Association of History of Medicine) and was appointed its first president. In 1956, the society began to publish the *Indian Journal of History of Medicine* under the editorship of Subba Reddy.[41]

Kutumbiah's greatest contribution was his *Ancient Indian medicine*[42] which is a useful introduction to āyurvedic medicine. In the book, Kutumbiah demonstrates a solid knowledge of the contents of the *Caraka-* and *Suśruta-Saṃhitās*. Organizing the subject matter into nine chapters according to the general categories of modern medicine, i.e. anatomy, physiology, etc., Kutumbiah has presented a faithful survey of the medicine of these two texts to the general reader. He has provided a long introduction in which he attempts to give an historical development of Indian medicine. Relying entirely on secondary sources, however, the author merely restates earlier speculations and transmits many of the errors of his predecessors. Little new information is offered on the origins of *āyurveda.*

Perhaps the greatest value of his book is its systematic presentation of the contents of the treatises of Caraka and Suśruta. Since he did not possess a sound philological knowledge of Sanskrit, however, Kutumbiah's summaries must always be checked with the original or with standard translations. Fortunately, he has given citations to modern editions. Furnished with a glossary of important terms and an index, the book serves as a useful general introduction to ancient Indian medicine. Lacking a fundamentally critical, historical approach, the historian of medicine will find it inadequate; and wanting a philological basis, the specialist will find it of limited significance to him.

In north India, Priyavrat Sharma, an āyurvedic physician and scholar, has produced numerous important editions, translations and studies of Sanskrit medical works. Coming from a family of āyurvedic doctors, Sharma was predestined to follow the tradition. In the 1940s he received the degree of Āyurvedācārya from the Banaras Hindu University, at a time when *āyurveda* was just beginning to become part of the curriculum of the better Indian universities. He also received degrees in Sanskrit and Hindī. After graduation he gained practical experience by working with his father and running a private practice. In 1946, he joined the faculty of the newly established Ayodhya Shivakumari Āyurvedic College in Bihar. In 1963, he became lecturer in the Āyurvedic College at the Banaras Hindu University; later he was promoted to professor of Dravyaguṇa, a post from which he retired in 1980.[43] Focusing principally on the science of *dravyaguṇa* or

[41] Ibid. An interesting article on cross-cultural influences in Indian medicine is his "The historical relations between Greek, Arabic and Indian medicine," *Indian Journal of History of Medicine,* 17(2) (1972): 29–36.

[42] Bombay: Orient Longmans Ltd., 1962, 1969, 1974.

[43] Information on Sharma's life has been taken from Guruprasad Sharma's short *Life sketck* (sic) *and bibliography of works of Prof. Priyavrat Sharma* (Varanasi: Chaukhamba Orientalia, 1981 [Jaikrishnadas Āyurveda Series, no. 12]). Useful in this publication is the list of Sharma's publications both in Hindī and in English up to 1981.

āyurvedic pharmacology, Sharma has edited many of the āyurvedic *nighaṇṭus* or books on materia medica. He has also written a useful history of āyurveda in Hindī[44] and recently completed a reliable translation of the *Caraka Saṃhitā* in two volumes.[45]

On the topic of Vedic medicine, two works have appeared: one written by an āyurvedic practitioner with specific aims in mind, while the other is by an Indologist with quite a separate purpose.

The āyurvedic physician V. W. Karambelkar's *The Atharvaveda and the Āyurveda* (Nagpur, 1961) is an attempt to legitimize āyurvedic medicine by demonstrating its antiquity. He endeavors to find the basis of *āyurveda* in the *Atharvaveda*. His deep knowledge of *āyurveda* has occasionally allowed him to offer new interpretations of difficult words and concepts. Lacking an overall critical approach, however, his views and conclusions are fundamentally untenable.

Finally the Indologist G. U. Thite has written on the early aspects of Indian medicine. Covering an enormous spectrum of literature written in Sanskrit, his *Medicine in its magico-religious aspects according to the Vedic and later literature* (Poona: Continental Prakashan, 1982) is a superficial treatment of the more religious dimensions of ancient Indian medicine. He states that the work "is not meant for studying the ancient Indian medicine as a *science* but as a *religious phenomenon*" (1). Unfortunately, Thite has only made a start towards his desired ends. The book fails to treat adequately ancient Indian medicine either as a "religious phenomenon" or as a "science."

The study of ancient Indian medicine continues to grow in India. The new periodical, *Ancient Science of Life*,[46] has an international editorial board and provides good articles on aspects of Indian medical history.

Indian contributors to the study of their medical history have included a wide range of specialists: āyurvedic practitioners, Indians trained in western medicine, Indologists, scientists and Indian historians of medicine, to name the most obvious. The eclecticism which this study has generated among Indians has produced works of varying quality and continues to do so, not unlike the study of ancient medicine by individuals in the West.

Conclusions

The major traditions of Indological studies in the West and in the East have from the nineteenth century shown a varying degree of interest in the study of Indian medicine. The efforts have been fragmented, with no

---

[44] *Āyurveda kā vaijñānika itihāsa* (Varanasi: Chaukhamba Orientalia, 1975 [Jaikrishnadas Āyurveda Series, vol. 1]).

[45] *Caraka-Saṃhitā.* Agniveśa's treatise refined and annotated by Caraka and redacted by Dṛḍhabala. Text with English translation. 2 vols. (Varanasi: Chaukhamba Orientalia, 1981–1983 [Jaikrishnadas Āyurveda Series, no. 36 I, II]).

[46] Published by AVR Educational Foundation of Āyurveda as a journal of the International Institute of Āyurveda, Coimbatore, Tamilnadu, India.

sustained and intensive investigation having taken place outside of India itself. The pursuit of such research has tended to attract a few individuals with a special interest or a particular training. In India on the other hand, it has drawn a wide spectrum of individuals, perhaps, out of a nationalistic fervor. Indologists and philologists found the textual tradition of special significance, while the historian of medicine was drawn to it by a particular interest in broadening his existing knowledge.

In the West, the study of Indian medical history was thought to require a specialized knowledge which only a few possessed. Although not explicitly stated, the evidence strongly implies that Indologists shied away from Indian medicine because it was considered to be properly understood only if one had a background in medicine. Historians of medicine, on the other hand, tended to avoid the subject largely because they did not have a knowledge of the relevant languages. For these reasons, Indian medical history has been kept on the fringes of both Western Indology and history of medicine. The current trends, however, suggest that more scholars in the West are engaging in research into Indian medicine whether as a living tradition of healing, as a problem in the history of medicine, or as a topic of philological investigation.

SPECIALIZED BIBLIOGRAPHY

Primary Sources: Texts and Translations

Vedic Saṃhitās: Atharvaveda, Ṛgveda, Yajurveda.

Atharvaveda (Śaunaka) with the Pada-pāṭha and Sāyaṇācārya's commentary. 4 vols. Edited by Vishva Bandhu, et al. Hosiarpur: Vishveshvaranand Vedic Research Institute, 1960-1962.

Atharva-Veda-Saṃhitā. Herausgegeben von R. Roth und W. D. Whitney. 3rd edition. 1924; rpt. Bonn: Ferd. Dümmler, 1966.

"The Kashmirian Atharva Veda," books 1–5, 7–15, 18. Edited by LeRoy Carr Barret. *Journal of the American Oriental Society,* 26: 197–295; 30: 187–258; 32: 343–90; 35: 42–101; 37: 257–308; 40: 145–69; 41: 264–89; 42: 105–46; 43: 96–115; 44: 258–69; 46: 34–48; 48: 34–65; 47: 238–49; 50: 43–73; 58: 571–614.

"The Kashmirian Atharva Veda, book 6." Edited by Franklin Edgerton. *Journal of the American Oriental Society,* 34: 374–411.

The Kashmirian Atharva Veda, books 16 and 17. Edited by LeRoy Carr Barret. New Haven, Conn.: American Oriental Society, 1936 [AOS, 9].

The Kashmirian Atharva Veda, books 19 and 20. Edited by LeRoy Carr Barret. New Haven, Conn.: American Oriental Society, 1940 [AOS, 18].

Atharvavedīya Paippalāda Saṃhitā. First Kāṇḍa. Edited by Durgamohan Bhattarcharyya. Calcutta: Sanskrit College, 1964 [Calcutta Sanskrit College Research Series No. 26, texts, 14].

Atharvavedīya Paippalāda Saṃhitā. (Kaṇḍas 2–4). Vol. 2. Edited by Durgamohan Bhattacharyya. Calcutta: Sanskrit College, 1970 [Calcutta Sanskrit College Research Series, 62, texts, 20].

Atharvaveda of the Paippalādas. 3 vols. Edited by Raghu Vira. Lahore: The International Academy of Indian Culture, 1936-1942 [Sarasvati Vihara Series, 1, 9, 12]. Reprinted in one volume: Delhi: Arsh Sahitya Prachar Trust, 1979.

Hymns of the Atharva-Veda. Translated by Maurice Bloomfield, 1897; rpt. Delhi: Motilal Banarsidass, 1964 [SBE, 42].

Atxarvaveda. Izbrannoe, perevod, kommentarij i vstupitel'naja stat'ja [by] T. Ja. Elizarenkova. Moskva: Nauka, 1976 (in Russian).

"Das sechste Buch der Atharva-saṃhitā." Übersetzt und erklärt [von] Karl A. Florenz. *Beiträge zur Kunde der Indogermanische Sprachen,* 12: 249-314.

The Hymns of the Atharvaveda. 2 vols. Trans. by Ralph T. H. Griffith, Varanasi: The Chowkhamba Sanskrit Series Office, 1968 (reprint) [The Chowkhamba Sanskrit Studies, 66].

Les hymnes Rohitas. Livre XIII de l'Atharva-Véda. Traduit et commenté par Victor Henry. Paris: J. Maisonneuve, 1891.

Le livre VII de l'Atharva-Véda. Traduit et commenté par Victor Henry. Paris: J. Maisonneuve, 1892.

Les livres VIII et IX de l'Atharva Véda. Traduits et commentés par Victor Henry. Paris: J. Maisonneuve, 1894.

Les livres X, XI et XII de l'Atharva-Véda. Traduits et commentés par Victor Henry. Paris: J. Maisonneuve, 1896.

Hundert Lieder des Atharva-Veda. Übersetzt von Julius Grill. 2nd edition. 1888; rpt. Wiesbaden: Martin Sändig, 1971.

Atharwaweda. Übertragen von Friedrich Rückert. Aus dem ungedruckten Nachlasse des Dichters zum ersten Male herausgegeben von Herman Kreyenborg. Kleine Ausgabe. Hannover: Orient Buchhandlung Heinz Lafaire, 1923.

Himno del Atharva Veda. (Selección y traducción) [by] Fernando Tola. Buenos Aires: Editorial Sudamericana, 1968.

Atharva-veda sanka-kodai Indo no juhō. Trans. by Naoshirō Tsuji. Tokyo: Iwanami, 1979 (in Japanese).

"Erstes Buch des Atharvaveda." [Übersetzt von] Albrecht Weber. *Indische Studien,* 4: 393–430.

"Zweites Buch des Atharvaveda-Saṃhitā." [Übersetzt von] Albrecht Weber. *Indische Studien,* 13: 129–216.

"Drittes Buch der Atharva-Saṃhitā." [Übersetzt von] Albrecht Weber. *Indische Studien,* 17: 177–314.

"Viertes Buch den Atharva-Saṃhitā." [Übersetzt von] Albrecht Weber. *Indische Studien,* 18: 1–153.

"Fünftes Buch der Atharva-Saṃhitā." [Übersetzt von] Albrecht Weber. *Indische Studien,* 18: 154–288.

Atharva-veda-saṃhitā. 2 pts. Translated by William Dwight Whitney and edited by Charles Rockwell Lanman. 1905; rpt. Delhi: Motilal Banarsidass, 1971 [HOS, 7–8].

Die Hymnen des Rigveda. 2 vols. Edited by Theodor Aufrecht. 1887. rpt. Wiesbaden: Otto Harrassowitz, 1968.

The Hymns of the Rig-Veda with Sāyaṇa's commentary. 4 vols. Edited by F. Max Müller. 2nd edition. 1890–92; rpt. Varanasi: The Chowkhamba Sanskrit Series Office, 1966 [The Chowkhamba Sanskrit Series, 99].

Ṛgveda Saṃhitā with the commentary of Sāyaṇācārya. 5 vols. Edited by N. S. Sonatakke and C. G. Kashikar. Poona: Vaidika Saṃśodhana Maṇḍala, 1933–1951.

Die Apokryphen des Ṛgveda. [Herausgegeben von] Isidor Scheftelowitz. 1906; rpt. Hildesheim: Georg Olms, 1966.

Der Rig-Veda. 3 pts. Aus dem Sanskrit ins Deutsche übersetzt von Karl Friedrich Geldner. Cambridge, Mass.: Harvard University Press, 1951 [HOS, 33–35].

Rig-Veda. 2 vols. Übersetzt und mit kritischen und erlaüternden Anmerkungen versehen von H. Grassmann. Leipzig: F. A. Brockhaus, 1876–1877.

The Hymns of the Ṛgveda. 2 vols. Trans. by Ralph T. H. Griffith. Fifth edition. Varanasi: The Chowkhamba Sanskrit Series Office, 1971 (rpt.). [The Chowkhamba Sanskrit Studies, 35].

Lieder des Ṛgveda. Übersetzt von A. Hillebrandt. Göttingen: Vandenhoeck and Ruprecht, 1913.

Gedichte des Rig-veda. Auswahl und Übersetzung von H. Lommel. München-Planegg: O. W. Barth, 1955.

Der Rigveda oder die heiligen Hymnen der Brāhmana, zum ersten Male vollständig ins Deutsche übersetzt mit Commentar und Einleitung von Alfred Ludwig. 6 vols. Prag: F. Tempsky, 1876–1888.

Vedic Hymns. I. Hymns to the Maruts, Rudra, Vāyu and Vāta. Trans. by F. Max Müller. 1891; rpt. Delhi: Motilal Banarsidass, 1964. [SBE, 32].

Vedic Hymns. II. Hymns to Agni (Maṇḍalas I–V). Trans. by Hermann Oldenberg. 1897; rpt. Delhi: Motilal Banarsidass, 1964 [SBE, 46].

Hymnes spéculatifs du Véda. Tr. du sanskrit et annotés par L. Renou. Paris: Gallimard, 1956.

Kapiṣṭhala-Kaṭha-Saṃhitā. A text of the Black Yajurveda. Edited by Raghu Vira. Delhi: Meharchand Lachhmandas, 1968 (rpt.).

Kāṭhakam. Die Saṃhitā der Kaṭha-Śākhā. 3 vols. Herausgegeben von Leopold von Schroeder. 1900–1910; rpt. Wiesbaden: Franz Steiner, 1970–1972.

Maitrāyaṇī Saṃhitā. Die Saṃhitā der Maitrāyaṇīya-Śākhā. 4 vols. Herausgegeben von Leopold von Schroeder. 1881–1886; rpt. Weisbaden: Franz Steiner, 1970–1972.

Kṛṣṇayajurvedīya-Taittirīya-Saṃhitā, with the commentary of Sāyaṇācārya. 8 vols. Edited by . . . Kāśīnātha-Śāstrī Āgāśe, et al. Poona: Ānandāśrama, 1959–1966 [reprinted 1978] [Ānandāśrama Sanskrit Series, No. 42].

Die Taittirīya-Saṃhitā. 2 vols. Herausgegeben von Albrecht Weber. *Indische Studien,* 11–12 (1871–1872).

The Veda of the Black Yajus School entitled Taittirīya Sanhitā. 2 pts. Trans. by A. B. Keith. 1914; rpt. Delhi: Motilal Banarsidass, 1967 [HOS, 18, 19].

Śukla Yajurveda Saṃhitā (Vājasaneyi Mādhyandina) with the Mantra Bhāṣya of Uvaṭa, the Vedadīpa Bhāṣya of Mahīdhara, Appendices, an Alphabetical list of Mantras and a short Introduction. Edited by Pandit Jagdishlal Shastri, Delhi: Motilal Banarsidass, 1971.

The Vājasaneyi-Saṃhitā in the Mādhyandina and the Kāṇva Śākhā, with the commentary of Mahīdhara. Edited by Albrecht Weber. 1852; rpt. Vararasi: The Chowkhamba Sanskrit Series Office, 1972 [The Chowkhamba Sanskrit Series, No. 103].

The Texts of the White Yajurveda. Translated by Ralph T. H. Griffith. Third edition. Benaras: E. J. Lazarus & Co., 1957 (rpt.).

Brāhmaṇas and Upaniṣads

Aitareyabrāhmaṇam, with the commentary of Sāyaṇācārya. 2 vols. Edited by Kāśīnāth Śāstrī Āgāśe, et al. Poona: Ānandāśrama, 1931 [Ānandāśrama Sanskrit Series, No. 32].

Das Aitareya Brāhmaṇa. Mit Auszügen aus dem Commentare von Sāyaṇācārya und andere Beilagen. Herausgegeben von Theodor Aufrecht. 1897; rpt. Hildesheim: Georg Olms, 1975.

Rigveda Brāhmaṇas: The Aitareya and Kauṣītaki Brāhmaṇas of the Rigveda. Translated by A. B. Keith. 1920; rpt. Delhi: Motilal Banarsidass, 1971 [HOS, 25].

The Gopatha Brāhmaṇa of the Atharva-Veda in the original Sanskrit. Edited by Rājendralāla Mitra and H. Vidyābhūṣaṇa. 1872; rpt. Delhi: Indological Book House, 1972.

Kṛṣṇayajurvedīyaṃ Taittirīyabrāhmaṇaṃ, with Sāyaṇa's commentary. 2 vols. Edited by Nārāyana Śāstrī 'Goḍabole.' 2nd edition. Poona: Ānandāśrama, 1934-1938 [Ānandāśrama Sanskrit Series, No. 37].

The Taittirīya Brāhmaṇa of the Black Yajur Veda with the commentary of Sāyaṇācārya. 3 vols. Edited by Rājendralāla Mitra. Calcutta: Asiatic Society of Bengal, 1859–1862.

The Śatapatha-Brāhmaṇa in the Mādhyandina Śākhā with extracts from the commentaries of Sāyaṇa, Harisvāmin and Dvivedagaṅga. Edited by Albrecht Weber. 1855; rpt. Varanasi: The Chowkhamba Sanskrit Series Office,1964 [The Chowkhamba Sanskrit Series, No.96].

The Satapatha-Brāhmaṇa according to the text of the Mādhyandina school. 5 vols. Translated by Julius Eggeling. 1882–1899; rpt. Delhi: Motilal Banarsidass, 1963 [SBE, 12, 26, 41, 43, 44].

One hundred and eight Upanishads. Edited by Wasudev Laxmaṇ Shāstrī Panśikar. Fourth edition. Bombay: Pāndurang Jāwajī (Nirṇaya Sāgar Press), 1932.

Ten Principal Upanishads with Śāṅkarabhāṣya. Delhi: Motilal Banarsidass, 1964.

Sechzig Upanishad's des Veda, aus dem Sanskrit übers. und mit Einleitunger und Anmerkungen versehen [von] P. Deussen. 1921; rpt. Darmstadt: Wissenschaftliche Buchgesellschaft, 1963.

The thirteen principal Upanishads. Translated by Robert Ernest Hume. Second edition. Oxford: Oxford University Press, 1931.

The Upaniṣads. 2 vols. Translated by F. Max Müller. 1879, 1884; rpt. New York: Dover Publications, 1962 [SBE, 1, 15].

La Mahā Nārāyaṇa Upaniṣad, édition critique, avec une traduction française, une étude, des notes et, en annexe, La *Prāṇāgnihotra Upaniṣad,* par Jean Varenne. Paris: Éditions E. de Boccard, 1960 (2 vols.).

Kalpasūtras

The Śrautasūtra of Āpastamba, belonging to the Taittirīya Saṃhitā, with the commentary of Rudradatta. Edited by Richard Garbe. Calcutta: Asiatic Society, 1882–1902 [Bibliotheca Indica, No. 92].

[Āpastamba] *Śrautasūtra with the bhāṣya of Dhūrtaswāmi and the Vṛtti of Rāmāgnicit.* 3 vols. Edited by S. Narasimhacher and T. T. Srinavasagopalacharya. Mysore, 1944–1953 (1945–1954) [University of Mysore. Oriental Library Publications, Sanskrit Series, Nos. 87, 93, 104].

Das Śrautasūtra des Āpastamba. Aus dem Sanskrit übersetzt von dr. W. Caland. 1–7 Buch. Göttingen: Vandenhoeck Ruprecht; Leipzig: J. C. Hinrich, 1921.

Das Śrautasūtra des Āpastamba, 8–15 (16–24. und 31) Buch. 2 vols. Aus dem Sanskrit übersetzt von W. Caland. Amsterdam, 1924–1928.

Āpastamba-gṛhyasūtra, with the commentaries the Anākula of Haradatta Miśra and the Tātparyadarśana of Sudarśanācārya. Edited by Umesh Chandra Pandey. Banaras: Jai Krishnadas-Haridas Gupta, 1928 [Kashi Sanskrit Series, No. 59].

Āśvalāyana gṛhyasūtram. With the Sanskrit commentary of Nārāyaṇa. English translation, introduction and index by Narentra Nath Sharma. Delhi: Eastern Book Linkers, 1976.

Indische Hausregeln. 4 pts. in 1 vol. Sanskrit und Deutsch herausgegeben von Adolf Friedric Stenzler. Leipzig: F. A. Brockhaus, 1864–1878.

[Baudhāyana] *Śrauta Sūtra belonging to the Taittirīya Saṃhitā.* 3 vols. Edited by W. Caland. Calcutta: Asiatic Society, 1904–1917 [Bibliotheca Indica, New Series, No. 163].

Kātyāyana Śrautasūtra with karakavasya of Srī Karakācārya. 2 vols. Edited by Nityananda Paruta Paroatiya. Varanasi, 1928–1929.

The Kauśika Sūtra of Atharva Veda with extracts from the commentaries of Dārila and Keśāva. Edited by Maurice Bloomfield, 1889; rpt. Delhi: Motilal Banarsidass, 1972.

Kauśikasūtra-Dārilabhāṣya. Edited by H. R. Diwekar, et al. Poona: Tilak Maharashtra Vidyapitha, 1972.

Altindisches Zauberritual, Probe einer Uebersetzung der wichtigsten Theile des Kauśika Sūtra von W. Caland. 1900 (1936); rpt. Wiesbaden: Martin Sändig, 1967.

The Savayajñas (Kauśikasūtra 60–68). Translation, Introduction, Commentary by J. Gonda. Amsterdam: N. V. Noord-Hollandsche Uitgevers Maatschappij, 1965.

Zwei vedische Texte über Omina und Portenta. Von A. Weber. Berlin: F. Dümmler, 1859.

The Mānava-Śrautasūtra, belonging to the Maitrāyaṇī Saṃhitā. Edited by J. M. von Geldner. New Delhi: International Academy of Indian Culture, 1961 [Śatapiṭaka, 17].

The Mānava-Śrautasūtra, belonging to the Maitrāyaṇī Saṃhitā. Trans. by J. M. von Geldner. New Delhi: International Academy of Indian Culture, 1963 [Śatapiṭaka, 27].

Pāraskaragṛhyasūtra, with śrāddha-śauca-snāna-bhojana-kalpasūtra. Edited with introduction and index, etc., by Pandit Anantarāma Śāstrī Ḍogarā. Benares: Jaya Krishna Das Haridas Gupta, 1939 (1920) [Kashi Sanskrit Series, No. 11].

Śāṅkhāyana-Śrautasūtra, together with the commentary of Varadattasutta Ānartīya. 4 vols. Edited by A. Hillebrandt. Calcutta: Asiatic Society of Bengal, 1889–1899 [Bibliotheca Indica, New Series, 100].

Śāṅkhāyana-Śrautasūtra, being a major yājñika text of the Ṛgveda. Translated by W. Caland; edited with an introduction by Lokesh Chandra. Nagpur: International Academy of Indian Culture, 1953 [Sarasvati-Vihara Series, 32].

Vaitāna-śrauta-sūtra, with the commentary called Ākṣepānuvidhi by Somāditya. Edited by Vishva Bandhu, Bhimadeva and Pitambara Datta. Hoshiarpur: Vishveshvaranand Vedic Research Institute, 1967.

Vaitāna sūtra, the ritual of the Atharvaveda. Edited with critical notes and indices by Richard Garba. London: Trübner and Co., 1878.

Das Vaitānasūtra des Atharvaveda. Übers. von W. Caland. 1910; rpt. Wiesbaden: M. Sändig, 1968.

Vaitāna sūtra, das ritual des Atharvaveda. Aus dem Sanskrit übers. und mit Anmerkungen versehen von Richard Garbe. Strassburg: K. J. Trübner, 1878.

The Vaitānasūtra. Translation and notes by S. N. Ghosal. Calcutta, 1958–1960 (issued as a supplement to the *Indian Historical Quarterly*, 34–36, 1958–1960).

The Gṛhyasūtra, rules of Vedic domestic ceremonies. 2 vols. Translated by Hermann Oldenberg and F. Max Müller, 1886–1892; rpt. Delhi: Motilal Banarsidass, 1967 [SBE, 29, 30].

[Dharmasūtra: series] *Aṅgiraḥ prabhṛtibaudhāyanāntānām. saptaviṃsatisaṃkhyamitānāṃ smṛtīnāṃ samuccayaḥ.* Edited by V. Ganeśa Āpte. 2nd edition. Poona: Anandāśrama, 1929 [Anandāśrama Sanskrit Series, No. 48].

The sacred laws of the Āryas as taught in the schools of Āpastamba, Gautama, Vāsishtha and Baudhāyana. 2 vols. Translated by Georg Bühler. 1879–1882; rpt. Delhi: Motilal Banarsidass, 1967 [SBE, 2, 14].

Other texts and translations

The Ashṭādhyāyī of Pāṇini. 2 vols. Edited and translated into English by Śriśa Chandra Vasu. 1891; rpt. Delhi: Motilal Banarsidass, 1977.

Aṣṭāṅgahṛdayasaṃhitā of Vāgbhaṭa. Edited by Sri Taradattapanta Āyurvedācārya. Varanasi: The Chowkhamba Sanskrit Series Office, 1956 [Haridas Sanskrit Series, No. 106].

Aṣṭāṅga Hṛdaya of Vāgbhaṭa. Edited with the "Vidyotinī" Hindi Commentary of Kavirāja Atrideva Gupta, by Vaidya Śrī Yadunandana Upādhyāya. Varanasi: The Chowkhamba Sanskrit Series Office, 1970 [Kashi Sanskrit Series No. 150].

Vāgbhaṭa's Aṣṭāṅgahṛdayasaṃhitā, the first five chapters of its Tibetan version, edited and rendered into English along with the original Sanskrit by Claus Vogel. Wiesbaden: Franz Steiner, 1965 [Abhandlungen für die Kunde des Morgenlandes, 37, 2].

Vāgbhaṭa's Aṣṭāṅgahṛdayasaṃhitā. Ein altindisches lehrbuch der Heilkunde. Aus dem Sanskrit ins Deutsche übertragen mit Einleitung, Anmerkungen und Indices von Luise Hilgenberg und Willibald Kirfel. Leiden: E. J. Brill, 1941.

The Atharva-veda prātiśākhya or Śaunakīya caturādhyāyikā. Edited and translated by William Dwight Whitney. 2nd edition. 1862; rpt. The Chowkhamba Sanskrit Series Office, 1962 [The Chowkhamba Sanskrit Studies, 20].

Bhāvaprakāśa of Bhāvamiśra. Edited with the "Vidyotinī" Hindi commentary by Brahmaśaṅkara Miśra and Rūpalālajī Vaiśya. 2 vols.Varanasi: Chowkhamba Sanskrit Series Office, 1969, 1980 [Kashi Sanskrit Series, 130].

The Bhela Saṃhitā. Edited by V. S. Venkatasubramania Sastri and C. Raja Rajeswara Sarma. New Delhi: Central Council for Research in Indian Medicine and Homoeopathy, 1977.

The Narrative of Bhoja (Bhojaprabandha) by Ballāla of Benares. Trans. by Louis H. Gray. New Haven, Conn.: American Oriental Society, 1950 [American Oriental Series, 34].

The Bower Manuscript. 7 parts. Edited and translated by A. F. Rudolf Hoernle. Calcutta: Office of the Superintendent of Government Printing, India (Archaeological Survey of India), 1893–1897.

The Bṛhad-Devatā attributed to Śaunaka. 2 pts. Edited and translated by A. A. Macdonell. 1904; rpt. Delhi: Motilal Banarsidass, 1965 [HOS, 5, 6].

The Charakasaṃhitā by Agniveśa, revised by Charaka and Dṛḍhabala, with the Āyurveda-Dīpikā commentary of Chakrapāṇidatta. Edited by Vaidya Jādavajī Trikamjī Āchārya. Third edition. Bombay: Satyabhāmābai Pāṇḍurang (Nirṇaya-Sāgar Press), 1941.

The Caraka Saṃhitā of Agniveśa, revised by Caraka and Dṛḍhabala, with The Āyurveda-Dīpikā commentary, of Cakrapāṇidatta and with "Vidyotinī" Hindī commentary by Kāśīnāth Śāstrī. 2 vols. Edited by Gaṅgāsahāya Pāndeya. Varanasi: The Chowkhamba Sanskrit Series Office, 1969–70 [The Kashi Sanskrit Series, 194].

The Caraka Saṃhitā. Edited and published in six volumes with translations in Hindi, Gujarati and English by Shree Gulabkunverba Ayurvedic Society, Jamnagar, 1949.

Carakasaṃhitā. English translation with notes by Avinash Chandra Kaviratna and Pareshnath Sarma Kavibhusan. Calcutta, 1890–1925.

Agniveśa's Caraka Saṃhitā. Vols. 1, 2. Text and English translation by Ram Karan Sharma and Vaidya Bhagwan Dash. Varanasi: The Chowkhamba Sanskrit Series Office, 1976, 1977 [The Chowkhamba Sanskrit Studies, 94].

Kaiyadevanighaṇṭuḥ. Edited and translated into Hindī by Priyavrata Śarmā and Guruprasāda Śarmā. Varanasi: Chowkhamba Orientalia, 1979 [Jaikrishnadas Ayurveda Series, No. 30].

The Mādhavanidāna and its chief commentary, chapters 1–10. Introduction, translation and notes by G. J. Meulenbeld. Leiden: E. J. Brill, 1974.

The Mahābhārata. 19 vols. Critically edited by various scholars. Poona: Bhandarkar Oriental Research Institute, 1933–1959.

The Mahābhārata. 18 vols. Translated by M. N. Dutt, Calcutta: Elysium Press, 1895–1905.

The Mahābhārata. 12 vols. Translated by K. M. Ganguly and edited by P. C. Roy. Calcutta: Oriental Publishing Co., 1952 (rpt.).

The Mahābhārata. 3 vols. Translated by J. A. B. van Buitenen. Chicago: University of Chicago Press, 1973–1978.

The Mahāvagga. Edited by Bhikkhu J. Kashyap. Bihar: Pāli Publication Board, 1956 [Nālandā Devanāgarī Pali Series].

Materia Medica of Ayurveda; based on Ayurveda Saukhyaṃ of Toḍarananda. Edited and translated by Vaidya Bhagwan Dash and Vaidya Lalitesh Kashyap. New Delhi: Concept Publishing Company, 1980.

The Vinaya Piṭakaṃ, vol. 1: Mahāvagga. Edited by Hermann Oldenberg. 1879; rpt. London: Luzac and Company Ltd., 1964 [Pali Text Society].

Vinaya Texts. 3 vols. Translated from Pāli by T. W. Rhys Davids and Hermann Oldenberg. 1882–1885; rpt. Delhi: Motilal Banarsidass, 1975 [SBE, 13, 17, 20].

The Book of the Discipline (Vinaya-Piṭaka), vol. IV (*Mahāvagga*). Translated by I. B. Horner, London: Luzac & Company Ltd., 1951 [Sacred Books of the Buddhists, 14].

The Mantrapāṭha or the Prayer Book of the Āpastambins. Pt. 1. Edited and translated by M. Winternitz. Oxford: Clarendon Press, 1897.

The Manusmṛti, with the "manvartha-muktāvalī" commentary of Kullūka Bhaṭṭa and the "maṇiprabhā" Hindī commentary by Haragovinda Śāstrī. Edited by Gopāla Śāstrī Nene. Varanasi: The Chowkhamba Sanskrit Series Office, 1970 [Kashi Sanskrit Series, No. 114].

The Laws of Manu, translated, with extracts from seven commentaries by G. Bühler. 1886; rpt. Delhi: Motilal Banarsidass, 1964 [SBE, 25].

The Nighaṇṭu and The Nirukta. Text and translation by Lakshman Sarup. Delhi: Motilal Banarsidass, 1967 (2 parts in 1).

The Papyrus Ebers: The greatest Egyptian medical document. Translated by B. Ebbell. Copenhagen: Levin & Munksgaard, 1937.

The Pariśiṣṭas of the Atharvaveda. Vol. 1, pt. 1. Edited by George Melville Bolling and Julius von Negelein. Leipzig: Otto Harrassowitz, 1909.

Phāetthayasāt songkhra. Vol. 1. Bangkok: Wat Pho Traditional Medical College Association, 1961.

Ṛgvidhānaṃ. Ediditcumpraefatione Rudolf Meyeṛ Berolini: Ferḍ. Dümmler, 1878.

The Ṛgvidhāna. English translation with an introduction and notes by J. Gonda. Utrecht: N. V. A. Oosthoek's Uitgevers Mij., 1951.

Samantapāsādikā: Buddhaghosa's commentary on the Vinaya Piṭaka. Vols. 5, 6. Edited by J. Takakusa and Makoto Nagai, assisted by Kogen Mizuno, 1938; rpt. London: Luzac and Company, Ltd., 1966.

Ṛgveda-Sarvānukramaṇī of Kātyāyana and Anuvākānukramaṇī of Śaunaka. Edited by Umesh Chandra Sharma. Aligarh: Viveka Publications, 1977.

The Siddhasāra of Ravigupta. Vol. 1, 2: The Sanskrit Text. Edited by R. E. Emmerick. Wiesbaden: Franz Steiner Verlag (GMBH), 1980, 1982.

The Suśrutasaṃhitā of Suśruta with the Nibandhasaṃgraha commentary of Srī Ḍalhaṇāchārya and the Nyāyachandrikā Pañjikā of Śrī Gayadāsāchārya on Nidānasthāna. Edited by Jādavjī Trikamjī Āchārya and Nārāyana Rāma Āchārya "Kāvyatīrtha." Third edition. Bombay: Nirṇaya-Sāgar Press, 1938.

The Suśrutasaṃhitā of Suśruta. Edited by Vaidya Jādavjī Trikamjī Achārya and Nārāyan Rām Āchārya "Kāvyatīrth." Bombay: Satyabhāmābai Pāṇḍurang (Nirṇaya-Sāgar Press), 1945.

An English translation of the Sushruta Samhita. 3 vols. Translated and edited by Kaviraj Kunjalal Bhishagratna. Second edition. Varanasi: The Chowkhamba Sanskrit Series Office, 1963 [The Chowkhamba Sanskrit Studies, 30].

The Suśruta-Saṃhitā. The Hindu System of Medicine according to Suśruta. Translated by Udoy Chānd Dutt. Calcutta: Asiatic Society of Bengal, 1883–91.

The Suśruta-saṃhitā or the Hindū System of Medicine according to Suśruta. Trans. by A. F. R. Hoernle. Fasc. 1 (Sūtrasthāna 1–14). Calcutta: Asiatic Society of Bengal, 1897.

Viṣṇusmṛtiḥ: The institutes of Viṣṇu together with extracts from the Sanskrit commentary called Vaijayantī of Nanda Paṇḍita. Edited with critical notes and Anukramaṇikā and indexes of words and mantras by J. Jolly. 1881; rpt. Vanarasi: The Chowkhamba Sanskrit Series Office, 1962 [The Chowkhamba Sanskrit Series, No. 95].

Viṣṇusmṛti, with the commentary of Keśavavaijayantī of Nandapaṇḍita. 2 vols. Edited by V. Krishnamacharya. Madras: Adyar Library and Research Center, 1964 [The Adyar Library Series, 93].

The institutes of Vishnu. Translated by Julius Jolly. 1880; rpt. Delhi: Motilal Banarsidass, 1965 [SBE, 7].

Yogaśataka. Texte médical attribué à Nāgārjuna. Textes sanskrit et tibétain, traduction française, notes, indices par Jean Filliozat. Pondichéry: Institut français d'Indologie, 1979.

The Zend-Avesta. 3 vols. Translated by James Darmesteter and L. H. Mills. 1880, 1883, 1887; rpt. Delhi: Motilal Banarsidass, 1969 [SBE, 4, 23, 31].

Reference Works

Bloomfield, Maurice. *A Vedic Concordance*. 1906; rpt. Delhi: Motilal Banarsidass, 1964 [HOS, 10].

—— *Rig-Veda Repetitions*. 2 vols. Cambridge, Mass.: Harvard University Press, 1916 [HOS, 20, 24].

Bloomfield, Maurice, Franklin Edgerton and Murray B. Emeneau. *Vedic Variants*. 3 vols. Philadelphia: Linguistic Society of America, 1930–1934.

Böhtlingk, Otto und Rudolph Roth. *Sanskrit-Wörterbuch*. 7 vols. 1855–1875; rpt. Osnabrück; Otto Zeller Verlagsbuchhandlung, 1966.

Buck, Carl Darling. *A dictionary of selected synonyms in the principal Indo-European languages*. Chicago: The University of Chicago Press, 1949.

Dandekar, R. N. *Vedic bibliography*. Bombay: Karnatak Publishing House, 1946 [*New Indian Antiquary*, extra series No. 7].

—— *Vedic bibliography*. Vol. 2. Poona: University of Poona, 1961.

—— *Vedic Bibliography*. [Vol. 3]. Poona: Bhandarkar Oriental Research Institute, 1973.

Dowson, John. *A classical dictionary of Hindu mythology and religion, geography, history and literature*. 12th edition. London: Routledge & Kegan Paul Ltd., 1972 [Trübners Oriental Series].

Grassmann, Hermann. *Wörterbuch zum Rig-Veda*. Leipzig: F. A. Brockhaus, 1873.

Hoerr, Norman L. and Arthur Osol. *Blakiston's New Gould Medical Dictionary*. 2nd edition. New York: McGraw–Hill, 1956.

Jacob, Colonel G. A. *A concordance to the principal Upaniṣads and Bhagavad-Gītā*. 1891; rpt. Delhi: Motilal Banarsidass, 1971.

Macdonell, A. A. *Vedic Grammar*. 1910; rpt. Delhi: Bhartiya Publishing House, 1975.

—— *A Vedic Grammar for Students*. 1916; rpt. Bombay: Oxford University Press, 1971.

Macdonell, A. A. and A. B. Keith. *Vedic Index of Names and Subjects*. 2 vols. 1912; rpt. Delhi: Motilal Banarsidass, 1967.

Mayrhofer, Manfred. *Kurzgefasstes etymologisches Wörterbuch des Altindischen*. 3 vols. Heidelberg: Carl Winter, Universitätsverlag, 1956–1976.

Monier-Williams, Monier. *A Sanskrit–English Dictionary*. 1899; rpt. Delhi: Motilal Banarsidass, 1974.

Renou, Louis. *Bibliographie védique*. Paris: Adrien-Maisonneuve, 1931.

Rhys David, T. W. and William Stede. *The Pali Text Society's Pali-English Dictionary.* 1921–1925; rpt. London: The Pali Text Society, 1972.

Santucci, James A. *An Outline of Vedic Literature.* Montana: The American Academy of Religion, 1976 [Aids for the Study of Religion Series, No. 5].

Schmidt, Richard. *Nachträge zum Sanskrit-Wörterbuch.* Leipzig: Otto Harrassowitz, 1928.

Sharma, Aryendra. *Beiträge zur vedischen Lexikographie: neue Wörter in M. Bloomfield's Vedic concordance.* München: In Komission bei J. Kitzinger, 1959–1960.

Turner, R. L. *A comparative dictionary of the Indo-Aryan languages.* London: Oxford University Press, 1966.

Wackernagel, Jakob und Albert Debrunner. *Altindische Grammatik.* 3 vols. Göttingen: Vandenhoeck and Ruprecht, 1896–1930.

Whitney, William Dwight. *Sanskrit Grammar.* 2nd edition. 1889; rpt. Cambridge, Mass.: Harvard University Press, 1971.

Secondary Sources

Agarwal, V. S. "Roots of Indian Plants as Source for Medicine." *Indian Museum Bulletin,* Calcutta, 4(2) (1969): 81–101.

Alsdorf, L. "Gleanings from the Atharvaveda." In *Ludwig Alsdorf: Kleine Schriften.* Herausgegeben von Albrecht Wezler. Wiesbaden: Franz Steiner, 1974, 18–28 [originally published in *The Adyar Library Bulletin,* 25 (1961): 106–16].

—— "Bemerkungen zum Sūryāsūkta." In *Ludwig Alsdorf: Kleine Schriften.* Herausgegeben von Albrecht Wezler. Wiesbaden: Franz Steiner, 1974, 29–35 [originally published in *Zeitschrift der deutschen morgenländischen Gesellschaft,* 111 (1961): 492–98].

Aufrecht, Theodor. "Ein Heilspruch. Rigveda X. 137." *Zeitschrift der deutschen morgenländischen Gesellschaft,* 24 (1870): 203–204.

—— "Ueber *rápas.*" *Zeitschrift für vergleichende Sprachforschung auf dem Gebiete der indogermanischen Sprachen,* 25 (1881): 601–602.

Barret, LeRoy Carr. "Three versions of an Atharvan hymn." In *Oriental Studies in honour of Cursetji Erachji Pavry.* Edited by Jal Dastur Cursetji Pavry. London: Oxford University Press, 1933, 26–28.

Basham, A. L. *The wonder that was India. A survey of the culture of the Indian sub-continent before the coming of the Muslims.* New York: Grove Press, Inc., 1959.

—— "The practice of medicine in ancient and medieval India." In *Asian Medical Systems: A comparative study.* Edited by Charles Leslie. Berkeley: University of California Press, 1976, 18–43.

Benveniste, Emile. "La doctrine médicale des Indo-Européens," *Revue de l'histoire des religions,* 130 (1945): 5–12.

Bergaigne, Abel Henri Joseph. *La religion védique d'après les hymnes du Rig-Veda.* 4 vols. 1878–1883; rpt. Paris: Libraire Honoré Champion, 1963. English translation by V. G. Paranjpe, Poona: Aryasaṃskṛti-Prakāsana, 1969–1973 again, bound in 1 vol., Delhi: Motilal Banarsidass, 1978.

Bergaigne, A. and V. Henry. *Manuel pour étudier le sanscrit védique.* Paris: Émile Bouillon, 1890.

Bernhard Wolfram. "Human skeletal remains from the cemetery of Timargarha." *Ancient Pakistan,* 3 (1967): 291–407.

Biswas, T. K. and P. K. Debnath. "Aśvattha (*Ficus Religiosa,* Linn): a cultural and medicinal observation." *Vishveshvaranand Indological Journal,* 12 (1–2) (1974): 39–47 [Archarya Dr. Vishva Bandhu Commemoration Volume].

Bloomfield, Maurice. "Seven hymns of the Atharva-Veda." *American Journal of Philology,* 7 (1886): 466–88.

—— "Contributions to the interpretations of the Veda. Second series. "*American Journal of Philology,* 11 (1890): 319–56.

—— "Contributions to the interpretation of the Veda. [Third series]." *Journal of the American Oriental Society,* 15 (1891): 143–88.

—— "Contributions to the interpretation of the Veda. Fourth series." *American Journal of Philology,* 12 (1891): 414–43.

—— "Contributions to the interpretation of the Veda. [Fifth series]." *Journal of the American Oriental Society,* 16: 1–42.

—— "Contributions to the interpretation of the Veda. Sixth series." *Zeitschrift der deutschen morgenländischen Gesellschaft,* 48: 541–79.

—— "Contributions to the interpretation of the Veda. Seventh series." *American Journal of Philology,* 17: 399–437.

—— *The Atharvaveda.* Strassburg: Karl J. Trübner, 1899. [Grundriss der Indo-Arischen Philologie und Altertumskunde, Bd. II, Heft 1].

Bolling, G. M. "Charms and Amulets (Vedic)." In *Encyclopaedia of Religion and Ethics.* Vol. 3. Edited by James Hastings. Edinburgh: T & T Clark, 1910, 468–72.

—— "Disease and Medicine (Vedic)." In *Encyclopaedia of Religion and Ethics.* Vol. 4. Edited by James Hastings. 1912; rpt. New York: Charles Scribner's Sons, 1955, 762–72.

Borradaile, L. A. *The Invertebrata.* 3rd edition. Cambridge: Cambridge University Press, 1958.

Brandenburg, Dietrich. "Avesta und Medizin. Ein literaturgeschichtlicher Beitrag zur Heilkunde im alten Persien." *Janus,* 59 (1972): 269–307.

Burrow, T. "Sanskrit *jálāṣa.*" In *W. B. Henning Memorial Volume.* Edited by Mary Boyce and Ilya Gershevitch. London: Lund Humphries, 1970, 89–97.

Bussagli, Mario. "Recent Research on Ancient Indian Medicine." *East and West,* 2(3) (1951): 147–50.

Carnoy, A. "The Iranian Gods of Healing." *Journal of the American Oriental Society,* 38: 294–307.

Castiglioni, Arturo. *A history of medicine.* Translated from the Italian by E. B. Krumbhaar. 2nd rev. ed. New York: Alfred A. Knopf, 1958.

Chakraborty, Chhanda. *Common life in the Ṛgveda and Atharvaveda—an account of the folklore in the Vedic Period.* Calcutta: Punthi Pustak, 1977.

Chowdhury, Tarapada. "On the Interpretation of some Doubtful Words in the Atharva-Veda." *Journal of the Bihar and Orissa Research Society,* 17 (1930–31): 25–100.

Clements, Forrest E. *Primitive Concepts of Disease.* Berkeley, Calif.: University of California Press, 1932.

Coomaraswamy, Ananda K. *History of Indian and Indonesian Art,* 1927; rpt. New York: Dover Publications, 1975.

Contenau, Georges. *La médecine en assyrie et en babylonie.* Paris: Librairie Maloine, 1938.

Cordier, Palmyr-Uldéric-Alexis. "L'enseignement médical dans l'Inde ancienne. Temps védico-brahmaniques." *Bulletin de la société française d'histoire de la médecine,* 1 (1902): 177–91.

Dani, Ahmad Hasan, ed. "Timargarha and the Gandhara Grave Culture." *Ancient Pakistan,* 3 (1967): 1–407.

Das, Abinas Chandra. *Ṛg Vedic Culture.* Calcutta: R. Cambrary & Co., 1925.

Das, Rahul Peter. Review of G. U. Thite's *Medicine. Its magico-religious aspects according to the Veda and later literature* in *Indo-Iranian Journal,* 27(3) (1984): 232–44.

Dasgupta, Surendra Nath. *A history of Indian philosophy.* 5 vols. Cambridge: Cambridge University Press, 1932–1955.

Dey, Karry Loll and William Mair. *The indigenous drugs of India: short descriptive notices of the principal medicinal products met with in British India.* 2nd edition. Calcutta: Thacker, Spink and Co., 1896.

Dumézil, Georges. "A propos de latin 'jūs.' " *Revue de l'histoire des religions,* 134 (1947/1948): 95–112.

Dumont, Paul-Emile. "The Iṣṭis to the Nakṣatras (or Oblations to the Lunar Mansions) in the Taittirīya-Brāhmaṇa." *Proceedings of the American Philosophical Society,* 98(3) (1954): 204–223.

Dutt, Uday Chand and George King, et al. *The Materia Medica of the Hindus.* Revised edition. Calcutta: Madan Gopal Dass, 1922.

Edelstein, Emma J. and Ludwig Edelstein. *Asclepius: A collection and interpretation of the testimonies.* 2 vols. New York: Arno Press, 1975.

Eliade, Mircea. *Shamanism. Archaic techniques of ecstasy.* Translated from French by Willard R. Trask. Princeton: Princeton University Press, 1972 [Bollingen Series, 76].

Emmerick, R. E. "Indo-Iranian concepts of disease and cure." Unpublished paper delivered at the International Conference on Traditional Asian Medicine, Canberra, Sept. 1979.

Fairservis, Walter A., Jr. *The Roots of Ancient India.* 2nd revised edition, Chicago: The University of Chicago Press, 1975.

Filliozat, Jean. *Magie et médecine.* Paris: Presses Universitaires de France, 1943.

—— *La doctrine classique de la médecine indienne; ses origines et ses parallèles grecs.* Paris: Imprimerie nationale, 1949. Second edition, Paris: École française d'Extrême Orient, 1975. English translation by Dev Raj Chanana, Delhi: Munshiram Manoharlal, 1964.

Fleming, John. "A Catalogue of Indian Medicinal Plants and Drugs, with Their Names in the Hindustāni and Sanscrit Languages." *Asiatic Researches,* 11 (1812): 153–96.

Frazer, James George. *The Golden Bough: A study in magic and religion.* 12 vols. 3rd edition. London: Macmillan & Co., Ltd., 1911–1915.

—— *The Golden Bough.* Abridged Edition. New York: The Macmillan Company, 1963.

Geldner, K. F. *Der Rigveda in Auswahl.* 2 vols. Stuttgart: W. Kohlhammer, 1907–1909.

Gonda, Jan. "The so-called secular, humorous and satirical hymns of the Ṛgveda." In *Selected Studies.* Vol. 3, *Sanskrit: Grammatical and Philological Studies.* Leiden: E. J. Brill, 1975, 361–97 [originally published in *Orientalia Neerlandica.* Leiden, 1948, 312–48].

—— "The Indian mantra." In *Selected Studies,* 4: 248–301.

—— *The meaning of the Sanskrit term dhāman.* Amsterdam: N. V. Noord-Hollandsche Uitgevers Maatschappij, 1967 [Verhandelingen der koninklijke Nederlandse Akademie van Wetenschappen, AFD Letterkunde 173, no. 2].

—— *Eye and Gaze in the Veda.* Amsterdam, Holland: North-Holland Publishing Company 1969 [Verhandelingen der koninklijke Nederlandse Akademie van Wetenschappen, AFD Letterkunde, Nieuwe reeks-Deel LXXV, no. 1].

—— *Vedic literature: (Saṃhitās and Brāhmaṇas).* Wiesbaden: Harrassowitz, 1975.

—— *The ritual sūtras.* Wiesbaden: Harrassowitz, 1977.

Grapow, Hermann, et al. *Grundriss der Medizin der alten Ägypter.* Vols. 1–4. Berlin: Akademie-Verlag, 1954–1958.

Grégoire, Henri, avec la collaboration de R. Goossen et de M. Mathieu. *Asklèpios, Apollon Smintheus et Rudra: études sur le dieu à la taupe et le dieu au rat dans la Grèce et dans l'Inde.* Bruxelles: Bureau de la Société, 1950.

Grimm, Jacob. *Teutonic Mythology.* 4 vols. Translated by James Steven Stallybrass. 1883 (vols. 1–3), 1883 (vol. 4); rpt. Gloucester, Mass.: Peter Smith, 1976.

Grohmann, J. Virgil. "Medicinisches aus dem Atharva-Veda, mit besonderem Bezug auf den Takman." *Indische Studien,* 9 (1865): 381–423.

Gupta, P., P. C. Dutta, A. Basu. *Human Skeletal Remains from Harappā.* Calcutta: Anthropological Survey of India, Government of India, 1962 [Memoirs of the Anthropological Survey of India, no. 9].

Hammett, Frederick S. "The Anatomical Knowledge of the Ancient Hindus." *Annals of Medical History* (New Series) 1 (1929): 325–33.

Harrison, T. R. et al., eds. *Principles of Internal Medicine.* 5th edition. New York: McGraw-Hill, 1966.

Hazra, R. C. "The word 'Sthapati, —its derivation and meanings." *Our Heritage,* 1974 (special number), 397–423 [Calcutta Sanskrit College Research Series, no. CXIX].

Henry, Victor. "Vedica: second series." *Mémoires de la société de linguistique de Paris,* 9 (1896): 233–52.

—— "Un mot sémitique dans le Véda, *hrū̆ḍu.*" *Journal Asiatique,* 10 (1897): 511–16.

—— *La magie dans l'Inde antique.* 2nd edition, Paris: Émile Nourry, 1909.

Hertel, Johannes. "Nachtrag zu Ṛgveda X, 163 Vendidad VIII, 35–72." *Asia Major,* 6 (1930): 377–87.

Hillebrandt, Alfred. *Vedachrestomathie.* Berlin: Weidmannsche Buchhandlung, 1885.

—— *Vedische Mythologie.* 2 vols. 1927; rpt. Hildesheim: Georg Olms, 1965.

Hoffmann, Karl. "Altpers. afuvāya." In *Corolla Linguistica: Festschrift Ferdinand Sommer.* Ed. Hans Krahe. Wiesbaden: Otto Harrassowitz, 1955, 80–85.

—— "Notizen zu Wackernagel-Debrunner, Altindische Grammatik II.2." *Münchener Studien zur Sprachwissenschaft,* Heft 8 (1956): 5–24.

—— "Remarks on the new edition of the *Paippalāda-Saṃhitā.*" *Indo-Iranian Journal,* 11 (1968): 1–10.

Hora, S. L. "Lac and the lac-insect in the Atharva-Veda." *Journal of the Asiatic Society of Bengal, Letters,* 18 (1952): 13–14.

Huizinga, J. "Over eenige Euphemismen in het Oud-Indisch." *Album-Kern.* Leiden: Brill, 1903, 153–56.

Jog, K. P. "On *amṛ́tasya cákṣaṇam* in *Ṛgveda* 1.13.5." *Vishveshvaranand Indological Journal,* 8 (1970): 38–47.

Jolly, Julius. *Medicin.* Strassburg: Karl J. Trübner, 1901 [Grundriss der Indo-Arischen Philologie und Altertumskunde, Bd. III, Heft 10]. English translation by C. G. Kashikar, Poona, 1951; second edition, Delhi: Munshiram Manoharlal, 1977.

Karambelkar, V. W. *The Atharva-Veda and The Āyur-Veda.* Nagpur, 1961.

Kashyap, Rulia Ram. "Parasitology in the Atharva Veda." *Indian Culture,* 2 (1935–1936): 93–113.

Keith, Arthur Berriedale. *The Religion and Philosophy of the Veda and Upanishads.* 2 pts. 1925; rpt. Delhi: Motilal Banarsidass, 1970 [HOS, vols. 31 and 32].

Kirtikar, K. R. and B. D. Basu. *Indian Medicinal Plants.* 4 vols. + 4 vols. of plates. 2nd edition. 1918, 1935 (2nd ed.); rpt. Delhi: M/S. Bishen Singh Mahendra Pal Singh, 1975.

Kohlbrugge, Dina Johanna. *Atharvaveda-Pariśiṣṭa über Omina.* Wageningen: H. Veenman, 1938.

Kuhn, Adalbert. "Indische und germanische Segenssprüche." *Zeitschrift für vergleichende Sprachforschung auf dem Gebiete der indogermanischen Sprachen,* 13 (1864): 49–74, 113–57.

Kuiper, F. B. J. "Two Rigvedic loanwords." In *Sprachgeschichte und Wortbedeutung. Festschrift Albert Debrunner.* Edited by G. Redard. Bern: A. Francke, A. G. Vulag, 1954, 241–50.

—— "*nyañcanī*—'refuge' Ath.S. V. 5.2d." *Indo-Iranian Journal,* 2 (1958): 158.

—— "Remarks on *The Avestan Hymn to Mithra.*" *Indo-Iranian Journal,* 5 (1961): 36–60.

Kutumbiah, P. *Ancient Indian medicine.* 1969; rpt. Bombay: Orient Longman Ltd., 1974.

Kurup, P. N. V., et al. *Handbook of medicinal plants.* New Delhi: Central Council for Research in Ayurveda and Siddha, 1979.

Lanman, Charles Rockwell. *A Sanskrit Reader.* Cambridge, Mass.: Harvard University Press, 1971.

Law, Bimala Churn. *Historical Geography of Ancient India.* Paris: Société Asiatique, n.d.

Leake, Chauncey D. *The Old Egyptian Medical Papyri.* Lawrence, Kansas: University of Kansas Press, 1952.

Lommel, Hermann. "Eine arische Form magischer Gotteranrufung." *Acta Orientalia,* 10 (1932): 372–79.

Lüders, Heinrich. *Varuṇa.* 2 vols. Aus dem Nachlass hrsg. von L. Alsdorf. Göttingen: Vandenhoeck & Ruprecht, 1951–1959.

Macdonell, A. A. *Vedic Mythology.* 1898; rpt. Delhi: Motilal Banarsidass, 1974.

—— *A History of Sanskrit Literature.* 1899; rpt. Delhi: Motilal Banarsidass, 1971.

—— "Magic (Vedic)." In *Encyclopaedia of Religion and Ethics.* Vol. VIII. Edited by James Hastings. Edinburgh: T. & T. Clark, 1915, 311–21.

Mackay, Ernest J. H. *Further Excavations at Mohenjo-Daro, being an official account of archaeological excavations at Mohenjo-Daro carried out by the Government of India between the years 1927 and 1931.* 2 vols. Delhi: Manager of Publications, Government of India Press, 1938.

—— *Chanhu-Daro Excavations, 1935–36.* New Haven, Conn.: American Oriental Society, 1943 [AOS, vol. 20].

Mackie, Colonel Thomas T., et al. *A Manual of Tropical Medicine.* Prepared under the auspices of The Division of Medical Science of The National Research Council. Philadelphia: W.B. Saunders Company, 1945.

Majumdar, Girijaprasanna. "Vedic Plants." In *B.C. Law Volume, Part 1.* Edited by D. R. Bhandarkar, et al. Calcutta: The Indian Research Institute, 1945, 644–68.

Malaviya, Maya. "Magic in the Vedas." *The Journal of the Ganganatha Jha Kendriya Sanskrit Vidyapeetha,* 27 (3–4) (1971): 319–22.

Mallin, Robert and Ted A. Rathbun. "A Trephined Skull from Iran." *Bulletin of the New York Academy of Medicine,* 32 (1976); 782–87.

Marshall, Sir John, ed. *Mohenjo-Daro and The Indus Civilization, being an official account of archaeological excavations at Mohenjo-Daro carried out by the Government of India between the years 1922 and 1927.* 3 vols. London: Arthur Probsthain, 1931.

Meyer, J. J. "Über den anatomisch-physiologischen Abschnitt in der Yājñavalkya- und in der Vishṇusmṛiti." *Wiener Zeitschrift für die Kunde des Morgenland,* 35 (1928): 51–58.

Mitra, Sarat Chandra. "On a Few Ancient Indian Amulets and Charms." *Journal of the Royal Asiatic Society of Bengal* (New Series) 29 (1933): 81–88.

Modak, B. R. "Employment of the Atharvaveda Mantras." *Journal of the Karnatak University* (Humanities) 10 (1966): 11–19.

—— "Magic in Atharvavedic Literature." *Journal of the Karnatak University* (Humanities) (1969): 8–30.

Muir, John. *Original Sanskrit texts on the origin and progress of the religion and institutions of India.* London, William and Norgate, 1858–1874 (rpt. Amsterdam: Oriental Press, 1967).

Müller, Reinhold F. G. "Die Medizin im Ṛg-Veda." *Asia Major,* 6 (1930): 315–76; 386–87.

—— "Die Gelbsucht der Alt-Inder." *Janus,* 34 (1930): 177–95; 226–39.

—— "Zur anatomischen Systematik im *Yajus.*" *Sudhoffs Archiv für Geschichte der Medizin und der Naturwissenschaften,* 27 (1934): 20–31.

—— "Über *Pitta* oder Galle, unter Bezug zur *Tridoṣa*-Lehre der altindischen Medizin." *Janus,* 38 (1934): 77–106.

—— "Zu altindischen Anschauungen von den Einigeweiden des Leibes." *Sudhoffs Archiv für Geschichte der Medizin und der Naturwissenschaften,* 28 (1935): 229–63.

—— "Vom *manas* (Geist) und seinen Krankheiten in der altindischen Medizin." *Janus,* 39 (1935): 74–93.

—— "Der *Takman* des *Atharvaveda* (Eine medizingeschichtliche Skizze)." *Artibus Asiae* (Leipzig) 6 (1937): 230–42.

—— "Über die *dṛṣṭi* oder das Sehen nach altindischen Vorstellungen." *Janus,* 43 (1939): 177–88.

—— "Zu Vorstellungen altindischer Ärzte über Fortpflanzungs-Stoffe." *Quellen und Studien zur Geschichte der Naturwissenschaften und der Medizin,* 8 (1942): 154–76.

—— *Grundlagen altindischer Medizin.* Halle, 1942 [Nova Acta Leopoldina, NF, Nr. 74, Bd.11].

—— "Altindische Lehren von den Knochenbrüchen." *Ergebnisse der Chirurgie und Orthopadie* 35 (1949): 230–45 [In memoriam Friedrich Pels Leusden].

—— *Grundsätze altindischer Medizin.* København: Ejnar Munksgaard, 1951.

—— "Soma in der altindischen Heilkunde." *Asiatic* (Festschrift Friedrich Weller). Edited by Johannes Schubert and Ulrich Schneider. Leipzig: Otto Harrassowitz, 1954, 428–41.

—— "Über Krankheiten, Behandlungen und Fürsorge bei Kindern im alten Indien." *Kinderärztliche Praxis,* 23 (1955): 365–72.

—— "Kannten die altindischen Ärzte die Lunge? (Zur Bedeutung von *kloman* und *phupphusa*)." *Sudhoffs Archiv für Geschichte der Medizin und der Naturwissenschaften,* 39 (1955): 134–44.

—— *Altindische Embryologie.* Leipzig: Johann Ambrosius Barth, 1955 [Nova Acta Leopoldina, NF 115, Bd. 17].

—— "Yakṣma. Medizingeschichtliche Untersuchungen zur Entwicklungswertung der indischen Krankheitslehre." *Mitteilungen des Instituts für Orientforschung,* 4 (1956): 278–313.

—— "Über begriffliche Bewertungen altindischer Ärzte." *Mitteilungen des Instituts für Orientforschung,* 4 (1956): 368–410.

—— "Wundarzt und Priester im alten Indien." *Mitteilungen des Instituts für Orientforschung,* 5 (1957): 225–34.

—— "Semasiologisches indischer Medizin." *Mitteilungen des Instituts für Orientforschung,* 6 (1958): 266–83.

—— *Eigenwertungen in altindischer Medizin.* Leipzig: Johann Ambrosius Barth, 1958 [Nova Acta Leopoldina, NF, Nr. 138, Bd. 20].

—— "Die Sagen vom Katheterisieren der Inder bei Harnverhaltung." *Sudhoffs Archiv für Geschichte der Medizin und der Naturwissenschaften,* 42 (1958): 377–87.

—— "Bemerkungen zu einigen Erkenntnisgrundsätzen indischer Ärzte." *Wiener Zeitschrift für die Kunde Sud-und Ostasiens und Archiv für indische Philosophie,* 3 (1959): 12–33.

—— "Schädeleröffnungen nach indischen Sagen." *Centaurus,* 6 (1959): 68–81.

—— "Die beiden indischen Götterärzte." *Archiv Orientalni,* 28 (1960): 399–413.

—— "Wörterheft zu einigen Ausdrücken indisches Medizin." *Mitteilungen des Institut für Orientforschung,* 7 (1961): 64–159.

—— "Vedisch: *pataya* = fliegen lassen?" *Die Sprache,* 7 (1961): 64–69.

—— "Der vedisch-arisch Arzt und seine Auswirkungen." *Rivista Degli Studi Orientali,* 36 (1961): 95–107.

—— "Wörter und Sachen." *Die Sprache,* 8 (1962): 264–72.

—— "Über einige Denkarten indischer Ärzte und ihre eigenen Auswertungen." *Rivista Degli Studi Orientali,* 37 (1962): 265–78.

—— "Über indische Vorstellungen von der Verdauung." *Mitteilungen des Instituts für Orientforschung,* 7 (1959): 198–223.

—— "Über indische Farben." *Sudhoffs Archiv für Geschichte der Medizin und der Naturwissenschaften,* 47 (1963): 325–33.

—— "Zusammenfassungen einiger derzeitiger Beurteilungen indischer Medizin." *Centaurus,* 9 (1963): 194–211.

—— "Über einige indische, zumal ärztliche Denkarten." *Wiener Zeitschrift für Kunde Süd-und Ostasiens und Archiv für indische Philosophie,* 8 (1964): 32–42.

—— "Indische Würmerkrankheiten." *Gesnerus,* 21 (1964): 14–22.

—— "Einige Beurteilungen alter Denkweisen der Inder und ihrer Ärzte." *Zeitschrift für philosophische Forschung,* 18 (1964): 681–89.

—— "Über indische Bewertungen der Sinne." *Wiener Zeitschrift für Kunde Süd-und Ostasiens und Archiv für indische Philosophie,* 9 (1965): 39–47.

—— "Medizin der Inder in kritischer Übersicht." *Indo-Asian Studies.* Pt. 2. Edited by Lokesh Chandra. New Delhi: International Academy of Indian Culture, 1965, 3–127.

—— "Indische Blut-Bewertungen." *Centaurus,* 11 (1965): 57–62.

—— "Einige Bemerkungen über Salz in Bewertung der Inder und ihrer Ärzte." *Clio Medica* 1 (1965): 60–64.

—— "Zum dem Fremdling im Ṛgveda." *Wiener Zeitschrift für die Kunde Süd-und Ostasiens und Archiv für indische Philosophie,* 10 (1966): 1–5.

—— "*Indisch: Dravya* (medizingeschichtlich)." *Centaurus,* 11 (1966): 259–69.

—— "Über Abort oder Fehlgeburt nach indischen Bewertungen." *Gesnerus,* 24 (1967): 78–80.

—— "Über verschiedene Ergebnisse indischer Textuntersuchungen durch Sprachwissenschaftler oder einen Medizingeschichtler." *Rocznik Orientalistyczny,* 30 (1967): 95–113.

Murthy, R. S. Shivaganesha. "The *Brāhmaṇas* on Medicine and Biological Sciences." *Indian Journal of History of Science,* 5(1) (1970): 80–85.

Nadkarni, A. K. *Dr K. M. Nadkarni's Indian Materia Medica.* 2 vols. 3rd edition, Bombay, 1954.

Narten, Johanna, ed. *Karl Hoffmann: Aufsätze zur Indoiranistik.* 2 vols. Wiesbaden: Dr Ludwig Reichert Verlag, 1975–1976.

—— "Ved. *āmáyati* und *āmayāvín.*" *Studien zur Indologie und Iranistik,* Heft 5/6 (1980): 153–66.

Oertel, Hanns. "Contributions from the *Jaiminīya Brāhmaṇa* to the history of the *Brāhmaṇa* Literature." Series 1. *Journal of the American Oriental Society,* 18 (1897): 15–48.

Oldenberg, Hermann. *Die Hymnen des Rigveda. Band 1: Metrische und textgeschichtliche Prolegomena.* Berlin: Wilhelm Hertz, 1888.

—— *Ṛgveda, Textkritische und exegetische Noten, erstes bis sechstes Buch.* Berlin: Weidmann, 1909, [In Akademie der Wissenschaften Göttingen. *Philologisch-Historische Klasse. Abhandlungen,* n.F., Bd. 11].

—— *Ṛgveda, textkritische und exegetische Noten, siebentes bis zehntes Buch.* Berlin: Weidmann, 1912. [In Akademie der Wissenschaften, Göttingen. *Philologisch-Historische Klasse. Abhandlungen,* n.F., Bd. 13.T.2].

—— *Die Religion des Veda.* Stuttgart: J. G. Cotta, 1923.

Patyal, Hukam Chand. "Significance of *Varaṇa-(Crataeva Roxburghii)* in the Veda." *Oriens,* 21–22 (1968–1969): 300–306.

—— "Critical examination of some readings in the Paippalāda Saṃhitā (Kāṇḍa II). [With special reference to D. Bhattacharyya's edition]." *Journal of the Oriental Institute,* Baroda 21 (1972): 275–82.

—— "Ātharvaṇic Practices with Roots of Plants (*Mūlakarmans* or *Mūlakriyās*)." *Vishveshvaranand Indological Journal,* 15(1) (1977): 13–19.

Pisani, Vittore. "Review of Manfred Mayrhofer: *Kurzgefasstes etymologisches Wörterbuch des Altindischen.*" *Paideia: revista letterana di informazione bibliografica,* 20 (1965): 327–29.

—— "Avest. *hizuma-, staman-*und verwandtes." In *Monumentum H. S. Nyberg.* Vol. 2. Téhéran: Bibliothèque Pahlavi, 1975, 163–64.

Pischel, Richard and K. F. Geldner. *Vedische Studien.* Band I. Stuttgart: W. Kohlhammer, 1888–1889.

Possehl, Gregory L., ed. *Ancient cities of the Indus.* Durham, North Carolina: Carolina Academic Press, 1979.

Puhvel, Jaan. "Mythological Reflections of Indo-European Medicine." In *Indo-European and Indo-Europeans: Papers presented at the Third Indo-European Conference at the University of Pennsylvania.* Ed. by George Cardona, Henry M. Hoenigswald and Alfred Senn, Philadelphia: University of Pennsylvania Press, 1970, 369–82.

Rao, K. Bhasker. "Medicine in the Rig Vedic Period." *Indian Journal of History of Medicine* (Madras) 3 (1958): 33–36.

Rao, S. R. "Excavations at Rangpur and other Explorations in Gujarat." *Ancient India,* 18 and 19 (1962 and 1963): 5–207.

—— *Lothal and The Indus Civilization.* New York: Asia Publishing House, 1973.

Rau, Wilhelm. *Staat und Gesellschaft in alten Indien: nach den Brāhmaṇa-Texten dargestellt.* Wiesbaden: Otto Harrassowitz, 1957.

Renou, Louis. *Les écoles védiques et la formation du Veda.* Paris: Imprimerie nationale, 1947.

—— "Études védiques: 4. Les passages communs au Ṛg- et à l'Atharva- Véda; 5. Atharva-Véda et rituel." *Journal Asiatique,* 243 (1955): 405–17; 417–35.

—— "Védique *nirṛti.*" *Indian Linguistics,* 16 (1955): 11–15 [Suniti Kumar Chatterji Jubilee Volume].

—— *Études védiques et pāṇinéennes.* 17 vols. Paris: É. de Boccard, 1955–1969.

—— *Vedic India.* Translated from the French by Philip Spratt. Calcutta: Susil Gupta (India) Private Ltd., 1957.

—— "Notes sur la version 'Paippalāda' de l'Atharva-Veda. (Première série)." *Journal Asiatique,* 252 (1964): 421–50.

—— "Notes sur la version 'Paippalāda' de l'Atharva-Veda (Deuxième série)." *Journal Asiatique,* 253 (1965): 15–42.

Rolland, Pierre. "Un fragment médical 'védique': Le premier khaṇḍa du Vārahapariśiṣṭa Bhūtotpatti." *Münchener Studien zur Sprachwissenschaft,* 30 (1972): 129–38.

Roth, Rudolf. *Zur Litteratur und Geschichte des Weda: drei Abhandlungen.* Stuttgart: A. Liesching, 1846.

—— "Das Lied des Arztes, Rigveda 10, 97." *Zeitschrift der deutsche morgenländische Gesellschaft,* 25: 645–48.

Roy, Mira. "Methods of Sterilization and Sex-Determination in the *Atharvaveda* and in the *Bṛhadāraṇyakopaniṣad.*" *Indian Journal of History of Science,* 1(2) (1966): 91–97.

—— "Anatomy in the Vedic Literature." *Indian Journal of History of Science,* 2(1) (1967): 35–46.

—— "Family Relations in Some Plants in the *Atharvaveda.*" *Indian Journal of History of Science,* 5(1) (1970): 162–77.

Roy Chowdhury, Amiya Kumar. "Trepanation in ancient India." *Asiatic Society of Calcutta,* Communications, 25 (1973): 203–206.

—— *Bharatavarsha—An Evolutionary Synthesis of India, Vol. 1: Dandakaranya and Makakantara—Central Highlands.* Calcutta: Rupa & Co., 1975.

Sarma, P. J. "The art of healing in Rigveda." *Annals of Medical History* (Series 3) 1 (1939): 538–41.

Schlerath, Bernfried. "Zu den Merseburger Zaubersprüchen." *Innsbrucker Beiträge zur Kulturwissenschaft,* Sonderheft 15 (1962): 139–43.

Schmidt, Hanns-Peter. "The origin of Ahiṃsā." In *Mélanges d'Indianisme:* à la mémoire de Louis Renou. Paris: Éditions E. De Boccard, 1968, 626–55.

—— "Ṛgvedic *madhyāyú* and *madhyamaśī́.*" *Annals of the Bhandarkar Oriental Research Institute,* 1977–1978, 309–17.

—— *Some women's rites and rights in the Veda.* Poona: Bhandarkar Oriental Research Institute, 1985.

Schroeder, Leopold von. *Mysterium and Mimus in Rigveda.* 1908; rpt. Amsterdam: Philo Press, 1974.

Sharma, A. K. "Neolithic human burials from Burzahom, Kashmir." *Journal of the Oriental Institute,* Baroda 16(3) (1967): 239–42.

—— "Kalibangan human skeletal remains—an osteo-archaeological approach." *Journal of the Oriental Institute,* Baroda 19 (1969): 109–14.

Sharma, Jagan Nath, Jagadish Narain Sharma and Ram Behari Arora. "Arthritis in Ancient Indian Literature." *Indian Journal of History of Science,* 8(1–2) (1973): 37–42.

Sharma, P. V. *Dravyaguṇa-vijñāna.* 6 vols. Varanasi: Chowkhamba Bharati Academy, 1977–1983 [The V. Ayurveda Series, no. 3].

Shende, N. J. *The Religion and Philosophy of the Atharvaveda.* Poona: Bhandarkar Oriental Research Institute, 1952 [Bhandarkar Oriental Series, no. 8].

Sigerist, Henry E. *A History of Medicine.* 2 vols. New York: Oxford University Press, 1951–1961.

Simon, Richard. *Index Verborum zu Leopold Von Schroeder's Kāṭhakam-Ausgabe.* Leipzig: F. A. Brockhaus, 1912.

Singer, Charles and E. Ashworth Underwood. *A Short History of Medicine.* 2nd edition. Oxford: Clarendon Press, 1962.

Specht, Franz. "Zu dem Wechsel von *p* und *m* und ein idg. Wort für die 'Bohne.' " *Zeitschrift für vergleichende Sprachforschung auf dem Gebiete der indogermanischen Sprachen,* 69: 133–38.

Thieme, Paul. "Mitra and Aryaman." *Transactions of the Connecticut Academy of Arts and Sciences,* 41 (1957): 1–96.

Thompson, R. Campbell. *The Devils and Evil Spirits of Babylonia.* 2 vols. 1903, rpt. New York: AMS Press, 1976.

Vats, Madho Sarup. *Excavations at Harappā: Being an account of archaeological excavations at Harappā carried out between the years 1920–21 and 1933–34.* 2 vols. Delhi: Manager of Publication, Government of India Press, 1940.

Velankar, H. D. "Similes in the Atharvaveda." *Journal of the Asiatic Society of Bombay* (New Series) 38 (1963): 19–43.

Vishva Bandhu. "Vedic textuo-linguistic studies. 8. An Atharvan Hymn to lac (*lākṣā*)—AV. V. 5." *Vishveshvaranand Indological Journal* 9 (1971): 1–20; 281–89.

—— "An Atharvan Hymn to lac (*lākṣā*)." In *Siddha-Bhāratī or The Rosary of Indology*. Edited by Vishwa Bandhu. Hoshiarpur: V.V.R. Institute, 1950, 201-13.

von Negelein, Julius. "Das Pferd in der Volksmedizin." *Globus*, 80 (1901): 201–204.

Wasson, Gordon R., *Soma: divine mushroom of immortality*. Harcourt Brace Jovanovich, Inc. 1970

Webster, Hutton. *Magic: a sociological study*. California: Stanford University Press, 1948.

Winternitz, M. "Folk-Medicine in Ancient India." *Nature*, 58 (7 July 1898): 233–35.

—— "Witchcraft in ancient India." *The Indian Antiquary*, 28 (1899): 71–83.

Wise, T. A. *Commentary on the Hindu System of Medicine*. Calcutta, 1845.

Witzel, Michael. "On the reconstruction of the authentic *Paippalāda Saṃhitā*." *Journal of the Ganganath Jha Kendriya Sanskrit Vidyapeetha*, 29 (1973): 463–88.

Zimmer, Heinrich. *Altindisches Leben. Die cultur der vedischen Arier nach den saṃhitā dargestellt*. Berlin: Weidmannsche Buchhandlung, 1879.

Zysk, Kenneth G. "A note on ancient Indian medicine." *Bulletin of the Indian Institute of History of Medicine*, 8 (1978): 14–23.

—— "Studies in traditional Indian medicine in the Pāli Canon: Jīvaka and Āyurveda." *Journal of the International Association of Buddhist Studies*, 5 (1982): 70–86.

—— "The evolution of anatomical knowledge in ancient India, with special reference to cross-cultural influences." *Journal of the American Oriental Society*, 106.4: (1986): 687-705.

—— "An annotated bibliography of translations into Western languages of principal Sanskrit medical treatises." *Clio Medica*, 19.3-4 (1984), 281-91.

—— "Mantra in *āyurveda*: a study of the use of magico-religious speech in ancient Indian medicine." in Harvey Alper, ed., *Understanding Mantra*. Albany: SUNY Press, 1985, 1989, 123-43.

appear.

—— "Fever in Vedic India." *Journal of the American Oriental Society*, 103.3 (1983): 617–21.

—— "Towards the notion of health in the Vedic phase of Indian medicine." *Zeitschrift der deutsche morgenländische Gesellschaft*, 135(2) (1985): 312–18.

—— *Aceticism and healing in ancient India. Medicine in the Buddhist monastery*. New York and Oxford: Oxford University Press, 1991.

—— "Reflections on an Indo-European system of medicine," in *Perspectives on, Indo-European Language, Culture and Religion. Studies in Honor of Edgar Polomé*. Vol. 2. McLean, Virginia: Institute for the Study of Man, 1992, 321-36.

INDEX OF SANSKRIT TEXT-PLACES
(N.B. Index follows English alphabet)

Atharvaveda Saṃhitā (Paippalāda)

INDEX OF SANSKRIT WORDS

AVESTAN WORDS

GENERAL INDEX